Tracheostomies:

The Complete Guide, 2nd Edition

Linda L. Morris, PhD, APN, CCNS, FCCM
M. Sherif Afifi, MD, FCCM, FCCP
Editors

Benchmark Health Publishing Company
Wilmette, Illinois

For permission to use content or illustrations, contact:
Benchmark Health Publishing Company
BenchmarkHealthPublishing.com
P.O. Box 354, Wilmette, Illinois 60091
Wilmette, IL
benchmarkhealthpublishing@gmail.com

Editors: Linda L. Morris and M. Sherif Afifi
Cover Design: Michael Garzel
Copy Editor: Karen Rought
Book Designers: Goran Tovilovic and Dragan Tovilovic

Print ISBN: 978-1-7366998-0-5
E-book ISBN: 978-1-7366998-1-2

Library of Congress Control Number 2021907525
Morris, Linda L, 1954-
Afifi, M.Sherif, 1959-
Tracheostomies: The Complete Guide, 2nd ed. / Linda L. Morris, M. Sherif Afifi

I dedicate this book to my mother, Louise Hostert Morris, who has taught me strength and courage. At 96 years young, she is still in charge and learning new things. I also admire the thousands of tracheostomy patients who have taught me so much and provided the opportunity to hone my skills and the passion to advance care for tracheostomy patients everywhere.

LLM

In today's healthcare settings, clinicians often embellish on daily successes; but, at the end of the day, it is truly their patients' progress that shapes their psyche.

Writing with a purpose to deliver a crisp concept is a life-long practice. And, so, I dedicate this book to my very supportive family and wish them success to push through boundaries of comfort zones and achieve highest potential.

MSA

Table of Contents

Chapter Contributors

M. Sherif Afifi, MD, FCCM, FCCP
Professor of Anesthesiology, Critical Care, & Surgery
Northwestern Medicine
Chicago, IL

Michiel J. Bové, MD
Assistant Professor of Otolaryngology
Northwestern University
Feinberg School of Medicine
Chicago, IL

Itzhak Brook, MD, MSc
Professor of Pediatrics
Georgetown University
Washington, DC

Linda L. Morris, PhD, APN, CCNS, FCCM
Director, Nursing Research
Advanced Practice Nurse, Pulmonary Services
Shirley Ryan AbilityLab
Associate Professor, Physical Medicine and Rehabilitation & Anesthesiology
Northwestern University
Feinberg School of Medicine
Chicago, IL

John Parson, BA, RRT
Registered Respiratory Therapist
Past Department Manager, Rehabilitation Institute of Chicago
(Retired)

Samuel Racette, MD
Otolaryngology Resident Physician
Northwestern Memorial Hospital
Chicago, IL

Heather M. Starmer, MA CCC-SLP, BCS-S
Clinical Associate Professor
Department of Otolaryngology,
Head and Neck Surgery
Director, Head and Neck Cancer Speech and Swallowing Rehabilitation
Stanford Cancer Center
Stanford, CA

Karen Watters, MB BCh BAO, MPH
Attending in Pediatric Otolaryngology
Boston Children's Hospital
Assistant Professor, Department of Otolaryngology and Head and Neck Surgery
Harvard Medical School
Boston, MA

Lisa Wolfe, MD
Professor of Medicine, Pulmonology and Neurology
Northwestern University
Feinberg School of Medicine
Chicago, IL

Preface to the Second Edition

The first edition of Tracheostomies: The Complete Guide documented nuances of care required for the patient with a tracheostomy. The goal of first edition was to focus on a niche practice and provide an overview of the continuum of care of the patient with a tracheostomy tube in different phases and settings. We hoped the manual would decompartmentalize silos of expertise of clinicians caring for these patients.

This second edition takes our goal to a new level. Contributing authors, each with very specialized expertise, provide a thorough, up-to-date, and detailed resource. The second edition highlights several substantive changes from the first edition. The format is changed to include review questions at the end of each chapter. The questions should be used not only as a review, but also to ensure complete understanding of key concepts discussed in the text.

The chapter on care of the patient with a laryngectomy was completely transformed by two experts: a speech language pathologist and a physician who has very personal experience with a laryngectomy. The unique collaboration of these two expert clinicians makes this chapter especially meaningful.

The chapter on care of the pediatric patient is completely revised and provides a different perspective from a pediatric otolaryngologist. The chapter on rehabilitation and recovery has an added perspective from a pulmonologist who specializes in long-term care of pulmonary patients. An additional section on care of the patient in the office and in the community is especially valuable.

Similar to the first edition, significant effort was made to get updated product information from as many international manufacturers as possible, including the US. We did our best to bridge language and legal barriers to include new manufacturers' products and their description. Additional manufacturers provide much diversity in design and function of their products. The list of manufacturers, however, though exhaustive, is not complete, as a few did not officially agree to be included.

As we go to press, we are in the midst of the COVID-19 pandemic, with guidelines and recommendations changing frequently as we continue to learn more. For current guidelines and recommendations for tracheostomy care during the COVID-19 crisis, refer to the following associations' websites: American Society of Anesthesiologists (https://www.asahq.org/in-the-spotlight/coronavirus-covid-19-information), Society of Critical Care Medicine (https://www.sccm.org/disaster), National Tracheostomy Safety Project (http://www.tracheostomy.org.uk/healthcare-staff/improving-tracheostomy-care/covid-19), the American Association of Otolaryngology- Head and Neck Surgery (https://www.entnet.org/content/coronavirus-disease-2019-resources), and the American Association of Critical Care Nurses (https://www.aacn.org/clinical-resources/covid-19), the American Thoracic Society, (http://www.thoracic.org), the American College of Surgeons, (https://www.facs.org), the American College of Chest Physicians (https://www.chestnet.org), and the Ammerican Association of Critical Care Nurses.

Finally, in keeping up with readerships' preferences and trends, emphasis was placed on an electronic version of this edition, while still maintaining paperback availability of the manual. Publishing platforms were chosen that encompassed both PC- and OS-based devices for ease of mobile access to our book. In conclusion, this unique topic is indeed a niche practice, and we hope the second edition provides good value to those who care for complex patients. Consequently, we continue to encourage and welcome feedback and reviews from our readership via all sales and social media venues (Apple, Google, Amazon, Facebook, Twitter), specialty medical journals, as well as our website, https://www.TrachResource.com.

Preface to the First Edition

The first edition of the clinical resource is written for health care professionals of all disciplines who care for patients with tracheostomies. The nature of compartmentalized care in medicine today does not allow for a clear overview of the continuum of care for a patient with a tracheostomy. Surgeons are skilled in the procedure of placing a tracheostomy but are often unaware of the myriad of tubes available and the advantages and disadvantages of each. Intensivists make decisions every day regarding the optimal time to place a tracheostomy but may not have the opportunity to follow the complete process of downsizing and decannulation. Nurses routinely do tracheostomy care but may not realize its significance in preventing complications. Respiratory therapists are experts in managing the ventilator but may not be comfortable with other aspects of care such vocalization. In this book, we provide the fine details of the daily care of patients with tracheostomies to help health care practitioners make appropriate decisions and educate their patients.

Some medical centers have the benefit of a tracheostomy specialist to manage these patients, but it frequently falls to junior residents or others who are often unaware of the available options and necessary precautions. We hope the reader will come to appreciate the importance of this work as we describe in detail the art and science of caring for the patient with a tracheostomy. The book spans the entire spectrum of care—from surgical placement to choices and fitting of tubes, to restoration of voice, and finally, to rehabilitation and recovery. Because care of the tracheostomy patient involves many disciplines, chapter authors have been chosen to share their unique perspectives and expertise.

We are certain the reader will find this book a useful clinical reference and refer to it again and again. We invite comments, questions, and alternative approaches and techniques to trachs@yahoo.com or visit our Web site at www.TrachResource.com. Perhaps a future edition can include any omissions.

Biographies

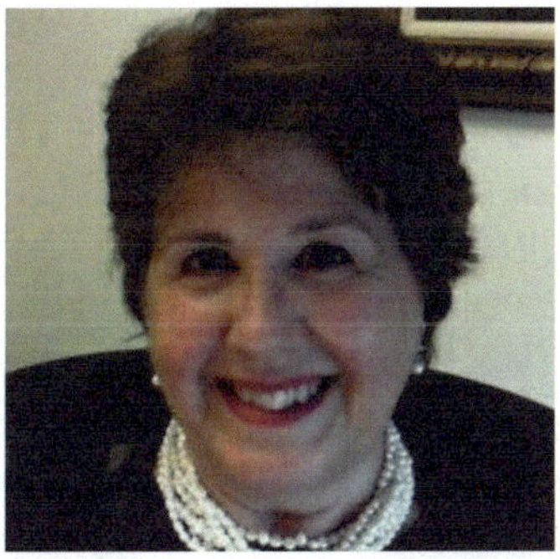

Linda L. Morris, PhD, APN, CCNS, FCCM has unique experience in critical care, education, research, and rehabilitation nursing. She has over 17 years' experience as a tracheostomy specialist and is currently director of nursing research and advanced practice nurse for pulmonary services at the Shirley Ryan AbilityLab (formerly the Rehabilitation Institute of Chicago). She also holds a faculty appointment as Associate Professor of Physical Medicine & Rehabilitation and Anesthesiology for the Northwestern University Feinberg School of Medicine in Chicago, Illinois. She has published extensively in the field of critical care and tracheostomies. Current research interests include tracheostomy outcomes, including quality of life, body image perception, and decannulation of tracheostomy patients.

Board certified as a critical care advanced practice nurse (clinical nurse specialist) and registered nurse in Illinois, Dr. Morris holds a baccalaureate degree from Southern Illinois University at Edwardsville, Illinois, a Master of Science in Nursing from Loyola University, and a PhD in Nursing Research from the University of Illinois at Chicago. She is an elected Fellow of Critical Care Medicine from the American College of Critical Care Medicine. As one of its original members, Dr. Morris continues to be very active with the Global Tracheostomy Collaborative (www.globaltrach.org), an international group of specialists dedicated to research and quality outcomes of patients with tracheostomies.

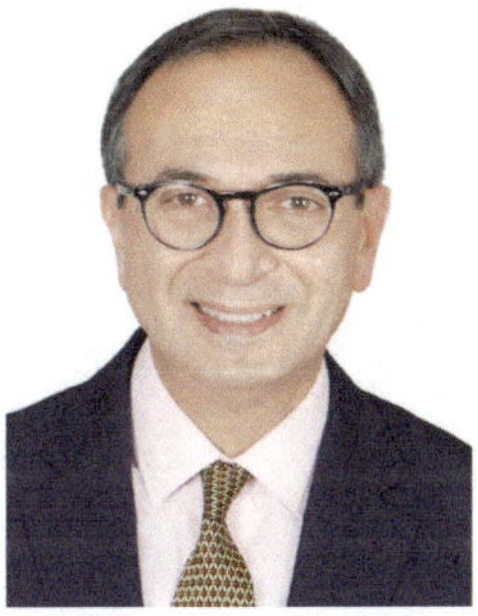

M. Sherif Afifi is Professor of Anesthesiology, Surgery, and Critical Care Medicine at Northwestern Medicine, Chicago, Illinois, and a past member of the Board of Directors for the Commission on Accreditation of Respiratory Care (CoARC).

His career spans multiple roles in post-graduate medical education including program directorships and curriculum design. He fulfills editorial functions for multiple journals, and publishes articles and manuals addressing topics in Perioperative Care and Tracheostomies.

Following medical school education, Dr. Afifi completed clinical and research training in respiratory physiology, then clinical training in general and cardiothoracic anesthesiology as well as critical care medicine. He has served on the medical staff of the Cleveland Clinic Foundation, Yale School of Medicine, Advocate Healthcare, and Northwestern Medicine. He is consulted widely on needs assessments of clinical services, resource utilization, and compliance with healthcare regulatory requirements.

Acknowledgments

The editors wish to thank the numerous people involved in the creation and the production of this work. First, we thank the chapter authors who who shared their unique expertise and extensive experience to carefully sketch their niche practices. We thank Michael Garzel, graphic designer, for adding fresh live colors to our recognizable book cover. We thank Karen Rought, our copy editor and our book designers, Goran Tovilovic and Dragan Tovilovic who answered our many questions quickly and completely.

We would like to acknowledge other groups with the same mission as ours: Improving tracheostomy care around the globe. Specifically, we salute the Global Tracheostomy Collaborative (GTC, globaltrach.org), the National Tracheostomy Safety Project (NTSP, tracheostomy.org.uk), and the Tracheostomy Resource and Management Service (TRAMS, tracheostomyteam.org).

Finally, we are indebted to our patients who entrust us with their care; and to our students, we are grateful to you for allowing us to share our passion.

1

Normal Functional Anatomy of the Airway and Selected Disorders

by M. Sherif Afifi

Objectives

- Review the functional anatomy of the upper airway
- Introduce alterations of the upper airway that cause obstruction
- Illustrate functions of the larynx encompassing phonation and coordination of breathing with swallowing
- Provide selected alterations in laryngeal function and their associated clinical disorders
- Describe the process of swallowing and its impediment in specific disorders
- Contrast anatomical differences between adult and pediatric upper airways

Introduction

Normal air passages start from the nose and end at the bronchioles of the lung. They are vital to the delivery and modification of respiratory gas to and from the alveoli, which are the center of gas exchange. For descriptive purposes, the airway is divided into the upper airway, which includes the nose, mouth, pharynx, and larynx, and the lower airway, which includes the trachea, bronchi, and the subdivisions of the bronchi. Each structure has its own independent constitution, vascular supply, and nerve supply, all of which facilitate different and coordinated functions. The functions of the airway include olfaction, deglutition (swallowing), phonation, and, of course, gas exchange.

Any interruption to the normal anatomy of the constituents of the airway results in altered function of its various organs. This chapter will review the anatomical landmarks of the upper and lower airways, identify the airway's vascular and nerve supplies, and review the function of its various parts. A comparison of changes in the anatomy from infancy to adulthood will also be provided.

THE UPPER AIRWAY

The upper airway is composed of the nose, mouth, pharynx, and larynx. Besides providing a natural conduit for gas exchange, the structures of the upper airway have additional functions in humidification of gases, protection of the lower airway, deglutition, and phonation.

The Nose

The external nose consists of a bony vault and a cartilaginous vault. The bony vault comprises the nasal bones, the frontal processes of the maxillae, and the nasal portion of the frontal bone. The cartilaginous vault is formed by the upper lateral cartilages, which meet the cartilaginous portion of the septum in the midline. The cavities of each nostril are continuous with the nasopharynx posteriorly. The nasal cavities are bounded posteriorly by the nasopharynx. The adenoids are located posteriorly in the nasopharynx just above the nasal surface of the soft palate. The soft palate rests on the base of the tongue during quiet nasal respiration, sealing the oral cavity.

Functional Anatomic Relevance

- The nose provides moisture to approximately 10,000 liters of ambient air that passes through the nasal airway every day.[1] The moisture is constituted from transudated fluid through the mucosal epithelium as well as secretions from glands and goblet cells. These secretions have bactericidal properties.
- The floor of the nose is tilted slightly downward at approximately 10 to 15 degrees. Thus, when a nasal tube or fiberscope is inserted through the nose, it should be directed slightly inferiorly to follow this major channel.
- The nasal mucosa is exquisitely sensitive to topically applied vasoconstricting medications such as phenylephrine, epinephrine, or cocaine. Cocaine has the added advantage of providing profound topical anesthesia and is the only local anesthetic agent that produces vasoconstriction; the others cause vasodilation.
- The contiguity of the paranasal sinuses with the nasal cavity leads to infections of the paranasal sinuses with prolonged nasotracheal intubation. Consequently, surveillance for infected paranasal sinuses is important with long-term placement of airways or nasogastric tubes in the nasal passages.

The Mouth

The mouth, or oral cavity, is divided into two parts: the vestibule and the oral cavity proper. The vestibule is the space between the lips and the cheeks externally and the gums and the teeth internally. The oral cavity proper is bounded anterolaterally by the alveolar arch, teeth, and gums; superiorly by the hard and soft palates; and inferiorly by the tongue. Posteriorly, the oral cavity communicates with the palatal arches and pharynx.

The Tongue

The tongue is a noncompressible muscular structure. The tongue is attached to the symphysis of the mandible anteriorly and anterolaterally and the stylohyoid process and hyoid bone posterolaterally and posteriorly, respectively. The posterior limit of the tongue corresponds to the position of the hyoid bone. The sensory and motor innervations of the tongue include different sources. Sensory fibers for the anterior two-thirds are provided by the lingual nerve. Taste fibers are furnished by the chorda tympani branch of the nervus intermedius. Sensory fibers for the posterior third come from the glossopharyngeal nerve (IX). Some sensory innervation is provided by the superior laryngeal nerve. The major motor supply is from the hypoglossal nerve (XII).

Functional Anatomic Relevance

- During laryngoscopy, the tongue is ordinarily displaced into the mandibular space; thus, the larynx is exposed for intubation under direct vision. Also, encroachment of the mandibular space by a large tongue, a small mandible, infection (e.g., Ludwig's angina), or masses limit displacement of the tongue into this space, and thus makes orotracheal intubation difficult or impossible.
- A forward jaw-thrust maneuver pulls the mandible and tongue forward to open the upper airway and alleviate upper airway obstruction. Normally, the mandibular condyles articulate within the temporomandibular joint for the first 30 degrees of mouth opening. Beyond 30 degrees, the condyles translate out of the temporomandibular joint anteriorly into the zygomatic arches. The jaw-thrust maneuver can prove life-saving for many patients with upper airway obstruction, and it facilitates ventilation with a face mask as well as the insertion of orogastric tubes.

The Pharynx

The pharynx is a U-shaped musculo-membranous tube that extends from the base of the skull to the inferior border of the cricoid cartilage anteriorly, and the lower border of the sixth cervical vertebra (C6) posteriorly. It is approximately 15 cm long and, in the adult, has its widest point at the level of the hyoid bone and its narrowest at the lower end, where it joins the esophagus. Anteriorly, it opens into the nasopharynx, oropharynx, and laryngopharynx (**Figure 1.1**). The pharynx is the common pathway for food and respiratory gases.

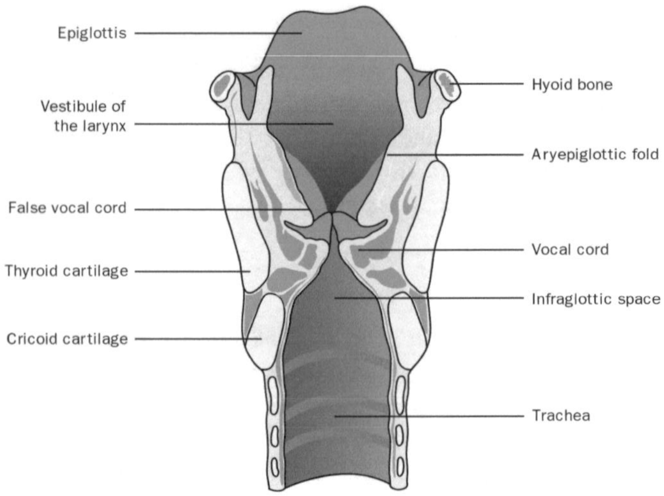

Figure 1.1. Anatomy of the pharynx and larynx

Functional Anatomic Relevance

- Oropharyngeal muscle tone keeps the upper airway open during quiet breathing. Respiratory distress is associated with pharyngeal muscular activity attempting to open the airway further. Sedative hypotic and opiate agents may attenuate some of this tone and precipitate partial or total airway obstruction.
- The pharynx defends against pathogens through the presence of lymphoid tissue at its base. Inhaled micro-particles are removed by impaction as they pass in the posterior pharynx. An inhaled airstream changes direction sharply by 90 degrees at the nasopharynx, thus causing some loss of momentum of the suspended particles. The particles are then trapped by a circular array of lymphoid tissue located at the entrance of the respiratory and gastrointestinal tracts. The ring includes the tonsils, which, if infected or enlarged, often impede the passage of endotracheal tubes. Abscess formation, hemorrhage, or tumor growth may cause airway obstruction.
- Patency of the pharynx is a critical component for proper gas exchange. Upper airway obstruction in patients who are sedated or anesthetized (with or without an endotracheal tube) or who have altered levels of consciousness is caused by a tongue with loss of muscle tone falling back against the posterior pharyngeal wall. Shorten, Opie, Graziotti, Morris, and Khangure[2] used magnetic resonance imaging (MRI) to demonstrate a different mechanism for upper airway obstruction in patients sedated with midazolam. A decrease in the anterior-posterior dimension at the level of the soft palate and epiglottis occurred while sparing the tongue. Thus, the soft palate and epiglottis may have a more important role than muscle tone in the development of upper airway obstruction.
- Obstructive sleep apnea (OSA) results from a reduction in the size of the pharynx, among other causes. Normally, the longer axis of the pharyngeal airway is transverse; however, in OSA patients, the anterior-posterior axis is predominant. It is believed this orientation is less efficient for airway muscle function. Imaging studies using MRI, computed tomography (CT), nasopharyngoscopy, fluoroscopy, and acoustic reflections divulged differences in anatomical structure between awake and asleep males.[3] In awake males with OSA, CT demonstrated a reduced airway caliber at all levels of the pharynx when

compared with normal patients, with the narrowest point posterior to the soft palate.[4] The application of continuous positive airway pressure (CPAP) increases the cross-sectional area, and thus, volume of the oropharynx, especially in the lateral axis.[5]

The Larynx

The larynx is the organ of phonation and is located in the anterior portion of the neck. It extends from its oblique entrance formed by the aryepiglottic folds, the tip of the epiglottis, and the posterior commissure between the arytenoid cartilages (interarytenoid folds) through the vocal cords to the cricoid ring (**Figure 1.2**). It is a boxlike structure, 4 to 5 ml in volume, and is made up of cartilages, ligaments, muscles, and mucous membrane. In adults, it is situated in the anterior portion of the neck at the level of C3 through C6. The larynx is shorter in women and children and is situated at a slightly higher level. The larynx consists of three single cartilages—the epiglottis, the thyroid, and the cricoid—and three paired cartilages—the arytenoids, the corniculates, and the cuneiforms. The laryngeal cavity is a space between the true vocal cords (VC) and the arytenoid cartilages and is known as the rima glottidis. It divides the larynx into two parts: The upper compartment extends from the laryngeal outlet to the VC and contains the vestibular folds and the sinus of the larynx; the lower compartment extends from the VC to the upper portion of the trachea. The piriform sinus is the space between the epiglottis and the aryepiglottic folds medially and the hyoid bone, thyrohyoid ligament, and thyroid cartilage laterally (known as the piriform fossa).

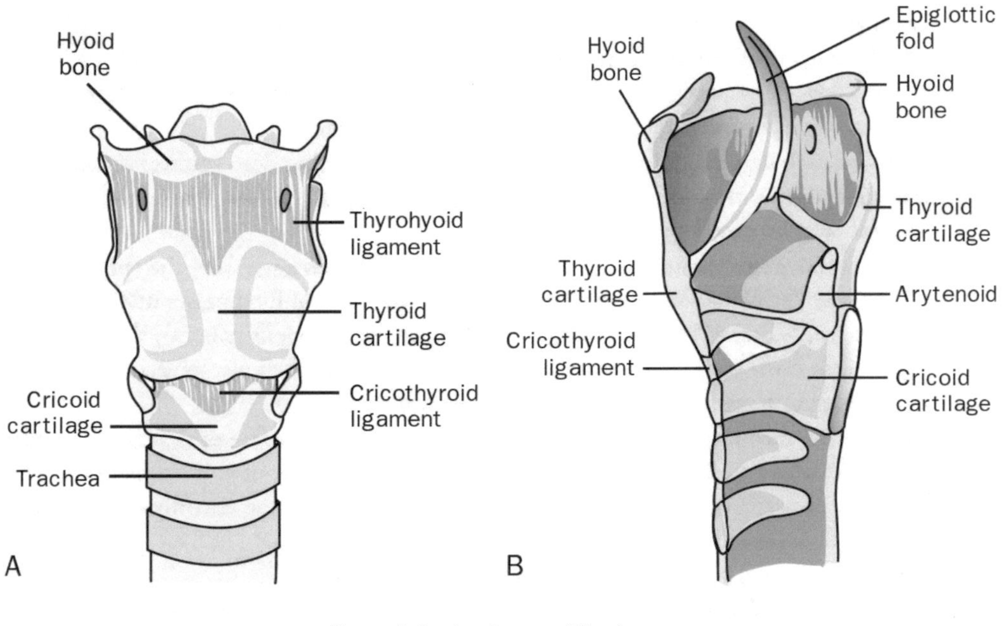

Figure 1.2. Anatomy of the larynx:
A) Anterior view, B) Sagittal view

The larynx is innervated by two branches of the vagus: the superior laryngeal and the recurrent laryngeal nerves. The superior laryngeal nerve reaches the internal side of the larynx. It divides into an external (motor) branch, which descends to supply the cricothyroid membrane, and upper and lower branches, which supply the mucous membrane of the base of the tongue, pharynx, epiglottis, and larynx. The superior laryngeal branch of the vagus nerve supplies sensation to the undersurface of the epiglottis, all of the larynx to the level of the false VC, and the pyriform recesses posterolaterally to either side of the larynx.

The recurrent laryngeal nerve (RLN) arises from the vagus nerve and loops around the subclavian artery on the right and the aortic arch on the left. After ascending between the trachea and the esophagus, it passes behind the thyroid gland and innervates all the intrinsic muscles of the larynx except the cricothyroid. In addition, it supplies sensory branches to the mucous membranes or the larynx below the VC.

Functional Anatomic Relevance

- The larynx is the most heavily innervated sensory structure in the body, followed closely by the carina. Stimulation of the unanesthetized larynx during intubation causes tremendous reflex sympathetic activation, with significant elevation in heart rate, blood pressure, and intracranial pressure (particularly in patients with loss of autoregulation). This elevation of heart rate and blood pressure may precipitate a marked increase in myocardial oxygen demand and significant afterload that could potentially lead to large vessel dissection or rupture (e.g., injured or dissected carotid artery, thoracic artery, or abdominal aorta).
- The pyramidal arytenoid cartilages sit on the posterior aspect of the larynx. The intrinsic laryngeal muscles cause them to swivel, opening and closing the VC. An endotracheal tube that is too large may, over time, compress these structures, causing mucosal and cartilaginous ischemia and resulting in permanent laryngeal damage. A traumatic intubation may dislocate these cartilages posteriorly (most commonly from a MAC, or curved blade) or anteriorly (most commonly from a Miller, or straight blade). Early diagnosis and intervention may avoid permanent hoarseness.
- The larynx bulges posteriorly into the hypopharynx, leaving deep recesses on either side called pyriform recesses or sinuses. Foreign bodies (e.g., plastic, glass, or fish bones) occasionally become lodged there.
- During active swallowing, the larynx is elevated and moves anteriorly, the epiglottis folds down over the glottis to prevent aspiration, and the bolus of food passes midline into the esophagus. When not actively swallowing (e.g., the unconscious patient), the larynx rests against the posterior hypopharynx such that a nasogastric tube must traverse the pyriform recess to gain access to the esophagus and stomach.
- The cricoid membrane extends between the upper anterior surface of the cricoid cartilage to the inferior anterior border of the thyroid cartilage. Its height approximates the tip of the index finger in adults. Locating the cricoid cartilage and the cricothyroid membrane quickly in an airway emergency is crucial. It is usually easily done in men because of their obvious laryngeal prominence (Adam's apple).
- Upper airway edema characteristically affects the upper portion of the larynx down to the level of the VC. Edema usually occurs between the mucosal layer and underlying connective tissue and gravitates down the larynx. The epithelium forming the superficial surface of the mucosa covering the vocal folds is tightly bound to the connective tissue covering the vocalis muscle and prevents flow of fluid below that point.
- Clinical examination of the VC with laryngoscopy and fiberoptic bronchoscopy determines their position, mobility, and structure as well as their pathology and dysfunction during inspiration, expiration, and phonation. Under normal conditions, the

VC meet in the middle in the production of phonation. On inspiration, they part from each other and then return to midline during expiration, leaving a small opening between them (**Figure 1.3**). A reflexive, forceful contraction of all laryngeal muscles, as commonly occurs when a foreign body lodges in the larynx, is referred to as a laryngospasm. When laryngospasm occurs, both true and false VC lie tightly in the midline.

- VC palsies result from interrupted innervations of the larynx. The RLN may be traumatized during surgery (commonly thyroid or parathyroid or aortic arch repair procedures), damaged from a tumor growth or trauma in the neck, or stretched due to pressure from an endotracheal tube (ETT).[6] The left RLN is more likely to be paralyzed than the right because of its close proximity to many intrathoracic structures, making it liable to injury from neoplasms, organ enlargement (aortic aneurysm or left atrial dilation), ice-cold solutions, or erroneous surgical ligation.
- The RLN carries both abductor and adductor fibers to the vocal cords. The abductor fibers are more vulnerable, and moderate trauma causes a pure abductor paralysis, whereas severe trauma causes both abductor and adductor fiber injury.
- In pure unilateral abductor palsy, both VC meet at the midline during phonation because adduction can still occur on the affected side. However, only one cord abducts during inspiration: the unaffected one. By contrast, in complete unilateral RLN palsy, both abductors and adductors are affected, and the affected VC lies in a paralyzed position midway between complete abduction and complete adduction. During phonation, the unaffected VC crosses the midline to meet the paralyzed cord (**Figure 1.4**). On inspiration, the unaffected VC adducts normally, while the affected VC does not move.
- Bilateral RLN palsy produces a different result. In incomplete bilateral abductor damage to the RLN, the adductor fibers draw the VC toward each other, and the glottis opening is reduced to a thin slit, which leads to significant respiratory distress. By contrast, in complete bilateral palsy of the RLN, each VC lies midway between adduction and abduction, producing a moderate glottis opening. Therefore, bilateral incomplete RLN palsy is more life-threatening than complete bilateral palsy.[7]

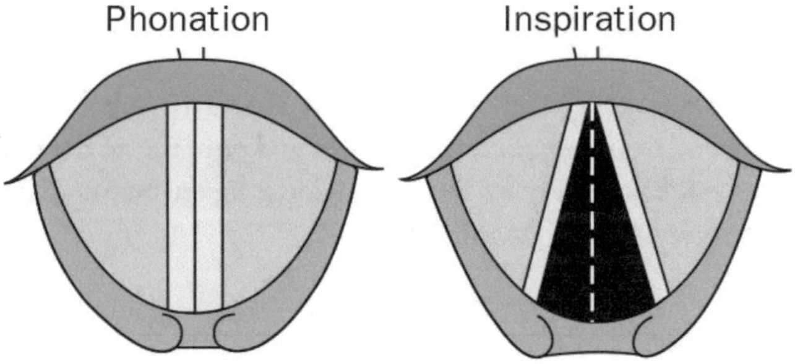

Figure 1.3. Vocal cord position during phonation and inspiration

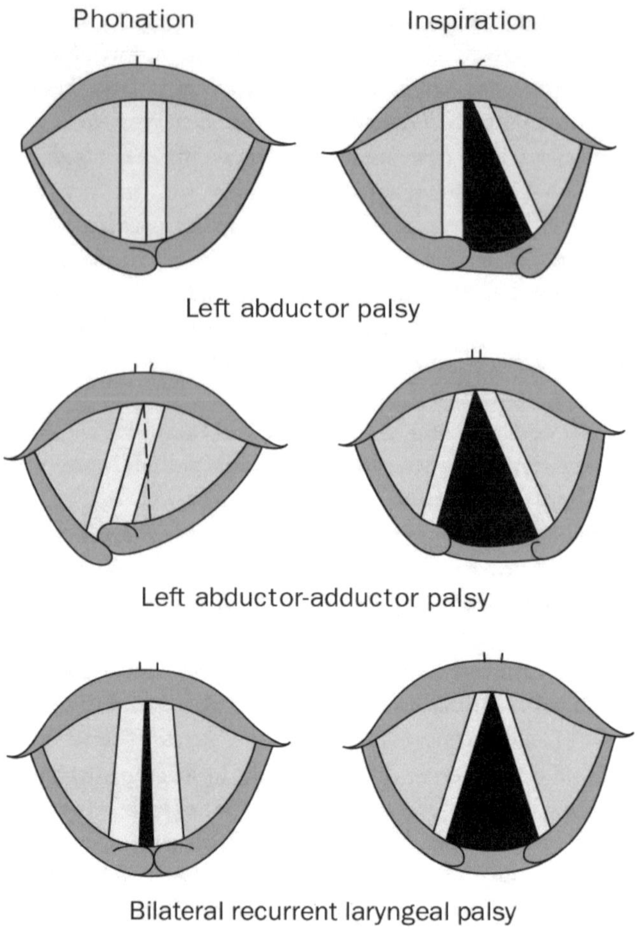

Figure 1.4. Vocal cord position during inspiration and expiration in the presence of nerve palsies. Top: Left abductor palsy. Middle: Left abductor-adductor palsy. Bottom: Bilateral recurrent laryngeal palsy.

The Epiglottis

The epiglottis is shaped like a leaf, with its lower end attached to the thyroid cartilage by the thyroepiglottic ligament and its upper, rounded part free and posterior to the tongue. The epiglottis is attached to the hyoid bone anteriorly by the hyoepiglottic ligament. Small depressions on either side of this ligament are referred to as the valleculae.

Functional Anatomic Relevance

- During swallowing, as the laryngeal muscles contract, the downward movement of the epiglottis and the closure and upward movement of the glottis prevent food from entering the larynx.
- When the epiglottis becomes acutely inflamed and swollen (acute epiglottitis), a life-threatening airway obstruction may occur.

PHYSIOLOGY OF SWALLOWING

Normal swallowing consists of three phases: oral preparatory and transport, pharyngeal, and esophageal. The oral preparatory phase consists of the opening and closing of the mouth, moistening food, masticating, and preparing an appropriate size bolus with the movement of the tongue and cheek muscles. The oral transport (or "buccal") phase lasts one second and begins with the compression of the food bolus against the hard palate. Next, the tongue retracts in a posterior direction to force the bolus into the oropharynx. Then, the posterior tongue is lifted by the styloglossus and palatoglossus muscles, which also elevate the uvula and seal the nasopharynx to prevent nasal aspiration. This phase is voluntary and involves important cranial nerves: V (trigeminal), VII (facial), and XII (hypoglossal). In the pharyngeal phase (one second), the bolus is advanced from the pharynx to the esophagus through the sequential contraction of the constrictor muscles. The soft palate is elevated to the posterior nasopharyngeal wall through the action of the levator veli palatini. The palatopharyngeal folds on each side of the pharynx are brought close together through the superior constrictor muscles so only a small bolus can pass. Then the larynx and hyoid are elevated and pulled forward to the epiglottis to relax the cricopharyngeus muscle. This passively shuts off the pharyngeal entrance and pulls the VC close together, narrowing the passageway between them. This phase is passively controlled reflexively and involves cranial nerves V, X (vagus), XI (accessory), and XII (hypoglossal). The respiratory center of the medulla is directly inhibited by the swallowing center for the very brief time it takes to swallow. This means it is briefly impossible to breathe during this phase of swallowing, and the moment where breathing is prevented is known as deglutition apnea. The bolus moves through the pharynx at a speed of 25 feet per second (8 m/s). During the esophageal phase (8-20 seconds), the upper esophageal sphincter relaxes to let food pass. The various striated constrictor muscles of the pharynx, in addition to peristalsis and relaxation of the lower esophageal sphincter, sequentially push the bolus of food through the esophagus into the stomach. Difficulty in moving food from the mouth to the stomach is called dysphagia.

Neural Regulation of Swallowing

- Swallowing is initiated by sensory impulses transmitted as a result of the stimulation of receptors on the fauces, tonsils, soft palate, base of tongue, and posterior pharyngeal wall.
- Sensory impulses reach the brainstem primarily through the 7th, 9th, and 10th cranial nerves, while the efferent (motor) function is mediated through the 9th, 10th, and 12th cranial nerves. The cricopharyngeal sphincter opening is reflexive; relaxation occurs when the bolus reaches the posterior pharyngeal wall prior to reaching the sphincter.
- Strokes can affect the normal swallowing reflex and result in dysphagia. A right-hemisphere stroke affects the left side of the patient's body and results in dysphagia characterized by lengthened time for food to move through the pharynx. By contrast, patients with left-hemispheric strokes show weakness on the right side of their body and are more likely to exhibit oral-stage swallowing problems.

Cranial Nerves

- CN V—The trigeminal nerve contains both sensory and motor fibers that innervate the face and is important in chewing.

- CN VII—The facial nerve contains both sensory and motor fibers and is important for the sensation of the oropharynx and taste to the anterior two-thirds of the tongue.
- CN IX—The glossopharyngeal nerve contains both sensory and motor fibers and is important for taste to the posterior tongue and the sensory and motor functions of the pharynx.
- CN X—The vagus nerve contains both sensory and motor fibers, provides taste to the oropharynx, as well as sensation and motor function to the larynx and laryngopharynx, and is important for airway protection.
- CN XII—The hypoglossal nerve contains motor fibers that primarily innervate the tongue.

Thyroid Cartilage

The thyroid cartilage is a shield-like structure composed of two plates that meet to form a notch. The thyroid notch is more prominent in men than in women. The prominence of the Adam's apple in males is due to the more acute angle at which the thyroid laminae meet, with a greater anteroposterior diameter. At the posterior aspect of each lamina, there are horns on the superior and inferior aspects. The inferior horn has a circular facet that allows it to articulate with the cricoid cartilage.

Thyroid Cartilage

The cricoid cartilage is shaped like a signet ring. It has articular facets that attach to the thyroid cartilage and the arytenoids. It is separated from the thyroid cartilage by the cricothyroid ligament, or membrane.

- It is important to identify the cricoid cartilage because the cricothyroid membrane is contiguous with it inferiorly. In acute airway obstruction, the cricothyroid membrane may be penetrated with a needle, knife, or tube and connected to an oxygen source via a standard 15-mm connector. Cricothyrotomy is the first procedure performed to relieve asphyxiation in situations where intubation and mask ventilation are impossible. The hyoid bone, which is not part of the larynx proper, is attached to the thyroid cartilage by the thyrohyoid ligament. The inferior horn of the thyroid cartilage, joined by the cricothyroid ligaments, articulates with the cricoid cartilage bilaterally. Cricothyrotomy is performed by penetrating this ligament.

Paired Cartilage

The arytenoids are triangular structures located on the posterosuperior aspect of the cricoid cartilage.

THE LOWER AIRWAY

The lower airway is composed of the trachea, two mainstem bronchi, and terminal and respiratory bronchioles. The scope of this section will be limited to the trachea and bronchi in relation to the patient with a tracheostomy.

Trachea

The trachea is a tubular structure, about 15 cm long in adults, extending from the cricoid cartilage to the bronchial bifurcation. It has an outer diameter of 2.5 cm. It consists of 16 to 20 C-shaped cartilages joined by fibroelastic tissue and closed posteriorly by the trachealis muscle. At the level of the fifth thoracic vertebra, the trachea bifurcate into right and left mainstem bronchi. The right (more than the left) mainstem bronchus appears to be a vertical continuation of the trachea; furthermore, the right upper lobe bronchus has its origin about 2 cm from the carina, compared to the left, which arises about 5 cm from the carina. For these reasons, aspiration of food, liquid, or foreign bodies is far more likely to occur on the right side, and right mainstem intubations are more common than the left.

The trachea begins at the inferior border of the cricoid ring. The sensory supply to the tracheal mucosa is derived from the recurrent laryngeal branch of the vagus nerve. The trachea is between 9 and 15 mm in diameter in the adult and is 12 to 15 cm long. It may be somewhat larger in the elderly. The adult male trachea will generally easily accept an 8.5-mm inner diameter (ID) ETT; a 7.5-mm ID ETT may be preferable in women. If the patient being intubated might require bronchoscopic pulmonary toilette (e.g., due to COPD or airway burns), consider increasing to a 9.0-mm ID tube for men or an 8-mm ID tube for women.

- It is physiologically important to note that the upper part of the trachea is extrathoracic, whereas the lower half is intrathoracic. This relationship creates different behaviors during inspiration and expiration. The extrathoracic trachea, which is subject to the effects of ambient atmospheric pressure, decreases slightly in caliber during inspiration and increases during expiration. By contrast, the intrathoracic trachea undergoes expansion during inspiration as a result of negative intrathoracic pressure from the pleural cavity. During expiration, however, surrounding pleural pressure diminishes the tracheal caliber, which may be exaggerated in the setting of marked increased expiratory effort in airway obstruction.
- Forces affecting airflow through the airways can be categorized as those that facilitate airflow and those that oppose it. In general, differences in pressure drive airflow in and out of the respiratory system from areas of higher to lower pressure. The lung contains two different pressure systems, whereas the chest wall exerts a separate one. The force driving airflow is the difference between the airway opening, or mouth (P_m), and the pressure in the alveoli (P_{alv}) and the pleural space (P_{pl}). The difference between these two pressures is called the transpulmonary pressure (P_L, the pressure across the lung). The pressure across the chest wall (P_{cw}) is the difference between the pleural pressure (P_{pl}) and the atmospheric pressure (P_B) (**Table 1.1**).
- Forces opposing airflow in the airways result from elastic, flow resistive, or inertial properties of the respiratory system. Inertance deals with the mass of the lung and the acceleration of these tissues and the linear acceleration of gas in the lung. Thus, pressure losses due to inertial forces increases progressively as respiratory frequency increases but are generally negligible during quiet breathing. Elastance, and its reciprocal compliance, reflect the relationship between pressure and volume when there is no airflow. Hence, these measures are static. By contrast, resistance is dependent on the rate of changes of lung volume (i.e., flow) during active breathing and are, thus, dynamic pressures.

Table 1. Respiratory System Difference Across the Pleura and Atmosphere	
Airway (P_{aw})	$P_{alv} - P_m$
Lung (P_L)	$P_{alv} - P_{pl}$
Chest wall (P_{cw})	$P_{pl} - P_B$
Total respiratory system (P_{RS})	$P_{alv} - P_B$

P_{aw}: airway pressure; P_{alv}: pressure in alveolar spaces; P_B: atmospheric pressure; P_{cw}: pressure of the chest wall; P_L: lung pressure; P_{pl}: intrapleural pressure (estimated at esophageal pressure); P_m: mouth pressure (or airway opening); P_{RS}: total pressure within the respiratory system

Comparative Anatomy of the Adult and Infant Airways

The anatomical differences between the adult and infant airways include the position and shape of the larynx, tongue, epiglottis, and bronchi (**Figure 1.5**). In proportion to the rest of the body, the infant's head is much larger than the adult's, so its weight forces the cervical spine to assume a more flexed position, which easily produces airway obstruction. The infant's tongue is proportionately larger than that of the adult's and, with lack of muscle tone, may "fall back," obstructing the flow of air during inspiration and expiration. Furthermore, the epiglottis is omega-shaped, longer, and stiffer.

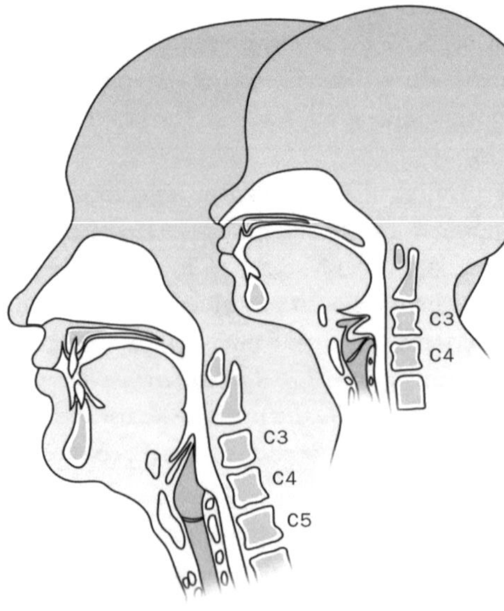

Figure 1.5. Comparative anatomy of adult and infant airways

The larynx is situated at a higher level in relation to the cervical spine in infants. At birth, the rima glottidis lies at the level of the interspace between the third and fourth cervical vertebrae. Upon reaching adulthood, it lies one vertebra lower. The narrowest part of the infant's laryngeal airway is at the level of the cricoid cartilage, whereas that of the adult is at the rima glottidis. At age eight, the larynx of the child closely resembles that of the adult except in size. The infant's vocal cords are concave and lie more horizontally. The biggest difference between the adult and infant larynx is that the overall diameter of the adult's airway is 10 to 12 mm wider than that of the newborn. If the internal diameter of a neonate's larynx is 4 mm at the level of the cricoid cartilage, a 1-mm circumferential reduction in this diameter (caused by either trauma or infection) would reduce the overall cross-sectional area of the airway by approximately 75%. A similar reduction in the diameter of the adult airway would reduce the cross-sectional area by about 44%.

The major conducting airways are both narrower and shorter in infants, leaving less room for error in positioning endotracheal tubes. The trachea of a premature infant may be as short as 2 cm. In infants, the bifurcation of the trachea (into right and left mainstem bronchi) projects at an angle of about 30 degrees from tracheal axis, whereas the angle of the left mainstem bronchus and tracheal axis is more acute. Thus, in infants, the right mainstem bronchus is less vertical than in adults.[8]

Summary

Functional anatomy is important to understand when treating the patient with a tracheostomy tube. Paying attention to the nuances of anatomy in relation to technique will often mean the difference between success and failure in tracheostomy tube placement and eventual removal, along with the day-to-day functions (respiratory, swallowing, and vocalization) in between. A clear understanding of the relevant anatomical structures, their blood supply, and their innervation will enhance understanding of their interdependent relationship. This understanding will guide approaches for instrumentation and intervention, as well as provide a basis for understanding how complications are best avoided or detected.

Key Points

- The upper airway provides a natural conduit for gas exchange; it humidifies and protects the lower airway and participates in the functions of deglutition and phonation.
- Alteration of pharyngeal anatomy may lead to the development of upper airway obstruction.
- The larynx is the organ of phonation. Disruption of its highly innervated structure immediately interferes with upper airway patency and, thus, impedes respiration.
- Deglutition and phonation are highly coordinated processes between several structures of the upper airway and gastrointestinal tracts and are dependent on intact sensory and motor innervation.
- Pediatric airway anatomy varies from that of adult anatomy in the size of the head, the position of the larynx, the shape of the epiglottis, the angle of the mainstem bronchi, and, most importantly, the diameter of the upper airway.

REVIEW QUESTIONS

1. When an emergency opening into the airway is required, the cricothyroid membrane should be pierced immediately:
   a. Superior to the thyroid cartilage
   b. Inferior to the thyroid cartilage
   c. Inferior to the cricoid cartilage
   d. Superior to the thyroid isthmus

   ANSWER: B. The cricothyroid membrane is in the anterior midline of the neck between the inferior border of the thyroid cartilage and the cricoid cartilage. It is palpable between the two cartilages, especially if the neck is extended.

2. A patient presents to you with a very hoarse voice. There is most likely damage to:
   a. Both sides of internal laryngeal nerve
   b. One side of internal laryngeal nerve
   c. Both sides of recurrent laryngeal nerve
   d. One side of the recurrent laryngeal nerve

   ANSWER: D. If one side of the recurrent laryngeal nerve is damaged, fixed VC and hoarseness can result. If both sides are damaged, then asphyxiation is possible. The internal laryngeal nerve only supplies parasympathetic and sensory fibers to the larynx at the vocal fold and above.

3. Compared to the adult larynx, a child's larynx is characterized by:
   a. The major conducting airways are both wider and longer
   b. The rima glottidis lies at a lower cervical vertebral interspace
   c. The overall diameter of the adult's larynx is 10 to 12 mm wider than that of the newborn
   d. In infants the right mainstem bronchus is more vertical than in adults

   ANSWER: C. The biggest difference between the adult and infant larynx is that the overall diameter of the adult's airway is 10 to 12 mm wider than that of the newborn. If the internal diameter of a neonate's larynx is 4 mm at the level of the cricoid cartilage, a 1-mm circumferential reduction in this diameter (caused by either trauma or infection) would reduce the overall cross-sectional area of the airway by 75%.

4. A three-year-old girl aspirates a small peanut and begins coughing and choking. In which area of the tracheobronchial tree is the peanut most likely lodged?
   a. Left main bronchus
   b. Left tertiary bronchus
   c. Proximal trachea
   d. Right main bronchus

   ANSWER: D. The right main bronchus is more vertical, shorter, and wider than the left main bronchus, so most aspirated objects pass into this bronchus. The tertiary bronchus is usually too small for an object as large as a peanut to be aspirated into it.

5. The critical role of the epiglottis during swallowing can be described as follows:
    a. The epiglottis is innervated by the recurrent laryngeal nerve, which initiates swallowing
    b. The epiglottis is controlled by the swallowing center of the brain
    c. The larynx and hyoid are elevated forward to the epiglottis to relax the cricopharyngeus muscle, which passively closes the pharyngeal entrance
    d. The epiglottis has no role during swallowing

ANSWER: C. The larynx and hyoid are elevated and pulled forward to the epiglottis to relax the cricopharyngeus muscle. This passively shuts off the pharyngeal entrance and pulls the vocal cords close together, narrowing the passageway between them. This phase is passively controlled reflexively and involves cranial nerves V, X (vagus), XI (accessory), and XII (hypoglossal).

References

1. Grande CM, Ramanathan S, Turndorf H. The structural correlates of airway function. *Prob Anesth.* 1988;2:175-182.
2. Shorten GD, Opie NJ, Graziotti P, Morris I, Khangure M. Assessment of upper airway anatomy in awake, sedated, and anaesthetized patients using magnetic resonance imaging. *Anaesth Intensive Care.* 1994;22:165.
3. Ayappa I, Rapoport DM. The upper airway in sleep: Physiology of the pharynx. *Sleep Med Rev.* 2003;7:9.
4. Haponik EF, Smith PL, Bohlman ME, Allen RP, Goldman SM, Bleeker ER. Computerized tomography in obstructive sleep apnea: Correlation of airway size with physiology during sleep and wakefulness. *Am Rev Respir Dis.* 1983;127:221.
5. Schwab RJ, Gefner WB, Pack AL, Hoffman EA. Dynamic imaging of the upper airway in normal subjects. J Appl Physiol. 1993;74(4):1504.
6. Ellis H, Feldman S. Anatomy for anaesthetists. 6th ed. Oxford, England: Blackwell Scientific; 1993.
7. Redden RJ. Anatomic considerations in anesthesia. In Hagburg CA. ed. *Handbook of Difficult Airway Management.* Philadelphia, PA: Churchill Livingstone, 2002:1-13.
8. Morris IR. Functional anatomy of the airway. *Emerg Med Clin N Am.* 1988;6:639-669.

2

The Tracheotomy Procedure

by Samuel Racette, Michiel J. Bové, M. Sherif Afifi

Clinical Scenario

A 55-year-old male with known squamous cell carcinoma of the base of the tongue presents to the emergency room with progressive difficulty breathing. On exam, he is leaning forward, is in moderate distress with inspiratory stridor and increased work of breathing. The decision is made to proceed to the operating room (OR) for intubation and possible tracheotomy. During awake fiber-optic intubation, the presence of a large ulcerative base of tongue mass extending to the supraglottis is noted, and following successful intubation, the decision is made to proceed with tracheotomy.

Objectives

- Present the history of tracheotomy
- Describe the indications for tracheotomy and the appropriate preoperative management
- Provide a rationale for the optimal timing of tracheotomy
- Outline the techniques of open as well as percutaneous dilatational tracheotomy
- Highlight important differences in pediatric tracheotomy
- Review the post-operative management after tracheotomy

Introduction

The tracheotomy procedure is one of the most commonly performed surgical procedures throughout the world. Nonetheless, the patients who require this procedure present significant challenges owing to their medical comorbidities, anatomy, and the emergent need for a definitive surgical airway. These difficulties as well as the procedure itself will be discussed throughout this chapter.

The first successful account of a tracheotomy is attributed to Antonio Musa Brasavola, who published his account of the procedure in 1546 AD, although it should be noted there were multiple accounts of surgical airways in animals prior to this account. In fact, the procedure was initially described nearly 3,500 years ago, making it one of the earliest recorded surgical procedures. Alexander the Great was alleged to have performed the procedure in the fourth century BC.[1]

The initial indications for the procedure were limited to life-threatening airway obstruction, and associated rates of mortality were therefore extremely high.

The indications for the procedure eventually expanded due to the work of Chevalier Jackson, who described modifications to the procedure, published in 1909, which improved the overall efficiency and safety as well as decreased mortality from 25% to 2%. The modifications also decreased the overall incidence of tracheal stenosis as a sequalae of the procedure. These modifications included the recognition of multiple factors, such as avoiding too high an incision, dividing the cricoid cartilage, using an appropriate cannula, and providing appropriate postoperative care.

Indications for Tracheotomy

The indications for tracheotomy placement in the adult population can be grouped into four broad categories: the relief of a mechanical obstruction, management of aspiration, need for long-term ventilation (while avoiding the long-term complications of translaryngeal intubation), and promotion of weaning from mechanical ventilator support. The expanded indications for tracheotomy were recently published by the American Academy of Otolaryngology—Head and Neck Surgery in the Clinical Indicators Compendium[2] as seen in **Table 2.1**.

Table 2.1. Indications for Tracheotomy as Defined by the American Academy of Otolaryngology—Head and Neck Surgery (Clinical Indicators 2.1 Compendium)
Prolonged or expected prolonged intubation
Inability of patient to manage secretions
Facilitation of ventilation support
Inability to intubate
Adjunct to manage head and neck surgery
Adjunct to manage significant head and neck trauma

The decision to perform a tracheotomy and in which manner to perform the procedure remains complex. However, the consideration of multiple factors is necessary to ensure optimal patient outcome. Factors include the relative risk of tracheotomy versus an alternative means of providing an artificial airway, characteristics of the patient's respiratory anatomy and physiology, the patient's specific pathological process and prognosis, available institutional facilities, and skilled personnel.

Whenever possible, acute upper airway obstruction should be managed with endotracheal intubation while other prioritized supportive care is provided. This is especially true if the need for mechanical ventilation is anticipated to be a short and defined period of time. As in the clinical case, the patient was found to have an obstructive mass for which a surgical airway was necessary to allow for safe respiration. Angioneurotic edema, temporary bilateral vocal cord paralysis, and epiglottitis are examples of acute airway obstruction in which temporary orotracheal intubation usually obviates the need for a surgical airway. Alternatively, if planned interventions such as radiation therapy or surgery predict airway obstruction, a tracheotomy can be performed prior to treatment to protect the airway. An example of this is the use of tracheotomy in head and neck surgical procedures involving free tissue transfer reconstruction in the oral cavity, oropharynx, hypopharynx, or larynx. In these cases, postsurgical edema may be deleterious to the viability of the newly placed flap and may lead to obstruction and re-intubation because of altered anatomy. This would be detrimental to both patient survival as well as surgical success; therefore, a surgical airway is frequently used to secure the airway.

Tracheotomy may be necessary in cases of laryngotracheal trauma, facial trauma, obstructing upper aero-digestive tract neoplasm as in the clinical case, or even severe angioneurotic edema, in which intubation may not be technically feasible. Tracheotomy is even described in severe cases of obstructive sleep apnea in which all medical treatments have failed and other surgical procedures are not appropriate.

TIMING OF TRACHEOTOMY

As with the timing and pre-operative decision-making related to any surgical procedure, the success of tracheotomy is dependent on appropriate patient selection and timing. The most appropriate time to perform a tracheotomy should balance the likelihood of laryngeal injury due to the continued use of an endotracheal tube versus the likelihood of surgical or stoma-related complications following tracheotomy (see **Table 2.2**).[3]

Table 2.2. Issues with Tracheotomy vs. Endotracheal Intubation

Tracheotomy	**Endotracheal Intubation**
Reduced need for sedation Reduced damage to glottis Reduced work of breathing (by reducing dead space) Reduced patient discomfort More invasive and complicated compared with endotracheal tube placement Scar formation Tracheostomy site can bleed or become infected Requires skill to perform the procedure May be associated with long-term complications (e.g., swallowing difficulties)	Easier and quicker to perform compared with tracheotomy Tolerated well for short periods Weaning more difficult after long-term placement Requires sedation Lessens risk of aspiration of secretions Can be used to give certain medications (e.g., adrenalin) Need to warm and filter gases as the nose, which would normally provide this function, is bypassed Improper placement can occur (e.g., esophageal placement)

There is no convincing evidence that endotracheal intubation should be limited to a specific time frame to prevent laryngeal dysfunction. However, many clinicians believe only patients who are unstable or unlikely to benefit from tracheotomy should be ventilated via an endotracheal tube for more than 21 days.[4,5,6] Part of the rationale is that tracheotomy improves patient comfort and communication, and facilitates nursing care.[7] These studies have influenced clinical practice, as evidenced by a multicenter international study of 1,638 patients which found that tracheotomy is performed after a median of 11 days.[8]

There is widespread evidence that early tracheotomy is advantageous to patients in reducing morbidity, mortality, length of stay in an ICU setting, as well as improved communication and comfort. In a randomized trial, Rumbak and co-investigators[9] compared early tracheotomy (within 48 hours) to late tracheotomy (14 to 16 days) in 122 medical patients with respiratory failure who were expected to require mechanical ventilation for more than 14 days.[6] They found the early group had significantly decreased mortality (31.7% versus 61.7%), incidence of hospital-acquired pneumonia (5% versus 25%), length of intensive care unit (ICU) stay (4.8 versus 16.2 days), and duration of mechanical ventilation (7.6 versus 17.4 days). A recent study by Patel and others[10] found a 40% increase in mortality among patients undergoing late tracheotomy (defined as after 14 days) compared to patients undergoing early tracheotomy.[7]

Furthermore, patients undergoing late tracheotomy were 1.72 times more likely to remain ventilator dependent. Early tracheotomy (within 7 days) has also been associated with a shorter length of an ICU stay by Griffiths and colleagues[11] in a meta-analysis of five studies. In a retrospective cohort study of more than 10,000 tracheotomy patients, Scales and investigators[12] compared those who underwent early tracheotomy (within 10 days) with those who underwent late tracheotomy (after 10 days). The early tracheotomy group had more ventilator-free days and a significant reduction in 90-day mortality (34.8% versus 36.9%), 1-year mortality (46.5% versus 49.8%), and study mortality (63.9% versus 67.2%). Better outcomes were associated with early tracheotomy in all of the diagnostic subgroups except for patients with a history of cardiac disease, in whom early tracheotomy was associated with an increased risk of death at 90 days (relative risk 0.135, 95% CI 0.003–0.285).

It is important to note that there may be drawbacks to early tracheotomy. One observational study of 54 male veterans found that laryngeal pathology, namely edema and ulcerative lesions, were significantly worse among patients who had undergone a tracheotomy 24 hours previously compared to patients who were extubated without a tracheotomy.[13] This study and others have demonstrated no association between severe laryngeal complications and duration of endotracheal intubation.[14] Additionally, a random multi-center trial of early (prior to 4 days) versus late tracheotomy by Young and colleagues[15] showed no significant difference in overall mortality, tracheotomy complications, and ICU length of stay. They also reported that clinicians were unable to accurately predict which patients would require long term ventilation. This result is similar to the randomized study by Blot and coauthors,[16] where 123 patients requiring prolonged intubation were randomized to early tracheotomy (within 4 days) versus prolonged intubation. There were no significant differences in any clinical outcome, including mortality, incidence of pneumonia acquired in the ICU, number of ventilator-free days, time in the ICU, number of septic episodes, sedation requirements, and laryngeal or tracheal complications. The trial was underpowered, however, since it was terminated early due to poor recruitment.

Based on this data, a recommendation for early tracheotomy (i.e., within 7 to 10 days of mechanical ventilation) would be appropriate for stable patients for whom liberation from mechanical ventilation is not likely before day 14. Regarding those patients for whom early tracheotomy is not chosen, a daily evaluation of the probability that mechanical ventilator support will be needed beyond 21 days should determine the timing of tracheotomy as long as the patient is able to safely undergo the procedure and benefits are anticipated. In fact, the recommendation from several sources is that the expected length of mechanical ventilation should be considered the most important factor in the pre-operative decision to proceed with tracheotomy.[17,18,19]

Preoperative Management

The patient with an unstable airway represents the most acute of medical emergencies. The patient with an obstructive base of tongue tumor requires immediate intervention in order to decrease the risk of mortality. In this acute setting, proper management requires the coordinated mobilization of a well trained team of physicians, nurses, and respiratory care practitioners. Initial intervention, if feasible, should be via oro-tracheal intubation or rigid bronchoscopy. If these modalities are contraindicated or not possible, tracheotomy should be performed in the OR where resources are readily available. In elective situations, bedside tracheotomy can be performed via the open or percutaneous dilation method. Bedside tracheotomy has the advantages of decreased transport-related risks, OR cost, and schedule burden. Regardless of the setting, adequate lighting (especially headlights), suction, and assistance should be available. If possible, it may be beneficial to have an anesthesia team present during tracheotomy for intensive cardiovascular and respiratory monitoring, to assist with mechanical ventilation, or in any necessary cardiopulmonary resuscitation. Frequently, patients with chronic respiratory obstruction are likely to have elevated carbon dioxide levels, which warrants close monitoring of respiratory drive after the establishment of a surgical airway. Preoperative laboratory profiles, including coagulation, hemoglobin, and electrolytes, should be reviewed. Any abnormalities should be corrected and remain stable prior to elective tracheotomy.

The patient should be optimally positioned, namely the neck should be extended (unless otherwise contraindicated) with a shoulder roll. The patient's face, neck, chest, and shoulders should be sterilized with prep solution. The face should not be draped in order to allow easy access to the endotracheal tube as well as to avoid the collection of flammable, oxygen-enriched vapors beneath the drapes. A further fire-safety precaution includes strict adherence to the proper use of alcohol-based antiseptics, including observing the required drying time. It is also recommended that whenever electrocautery or diathermy is used on the skin, an aqueous-based antiseptic is to be used. If an alcohol-based antiseptic is used, it should be cleaned off with a dry swab before applying diathermy.

Anesthetic Management

It is common for patients who require tracheotomy to have difficult airways; therefore, the anesthesiologist must be appropriately prepared in the peri-operative setting. Preparation for a difficult airway includes ensuring availability of adjunctive intubation equipment including a GlideScope or a fiber-optic bronchoscope. Features of the history and physical exam that may be associated with a difficult airway are listed in **Table 2.3**.[20] Fortunately, the airway of most patients who present for tracheotomy have previously been secured with orotracheal intubation.

Table 2.3. Factors Predicting Difficult Airway
Anatomic characteristics (e.g., bull neck, large tongue, receding jaw, limited mouth opening, difficulty visualizing posterior pharynx, diminished cervical spine range of motion, and morbid obesity)
Either inspiratory stridor (signifying obstruction at or above the level of the larynx) or expiratory stridor (signifying subglottic or intrathoracic obstruction
Hoarseness (vocal cord lesion or dysfunction)
Tachypnea and marked respiratory effort, dyspnea
Previous history of thyroid gland or neck surgery, trauma, or radiation therapy
History of previous difficult intubation or vocal cord paralysis
Infections such as epiglottitis or Ludwig's angina

Pre-anesthetic Evaluation

Regarding pulmonary status, patients with respiratory insufficiency may require mechanical ventilation with positive end-expiratory pressure (PEEP) to maintain adequate oxygenation. The continued application of PEEP is important during transport from the ICU to the OR. Based on the assessment, the decision must be made whether to choose direct laryngoscopy, awake fiberoptic intubation, or awake tracheotomy under local anesthesia to secure the airway. Often, these patients have a long history of smoking, with consequent chronic obstructive pulmonary disease (COPD). If symptoms of worsening pulmonary function are present, helpful preoperative testing includes pulmonary function tests (PFT) and arterial blood gases.

The most valuable cardiovascular history is exercise tolerance and the presence of any symptoms with exertion. Often, the tracheotomy is brief and urgent enough to preclude the need for any further cardiac screening. Hematologic profiles are essential to exclude anemia or abnormal coagulation, especially in cases of malignancy or chronic disorders. Preoperative laboratory data should survey a complete blood count (CBC), prothrombin time (PT), activated thromboplastin time (aPTT), and platelet count. Any existing preoperative neurologic deficits should be documented clearly. Finally, as with any elective procedure, the patient should have nothing by mouth or feeding tube for at least six hours prior to the procedure.[21]

In elective cases, the standard premedication is an anxiolytic such as a benzodiazepine; however, sedation is best avoided in patients whose airway is compromised or in emergency procedures. If the case is performed electively, the procedure is most commonly conducted under general anesthesia and orotracheal intubation. It may also be performed under local anesthesia while the patient is awake, particularly in situations where passage of an endotracheal tube is not possible.

The ASA (American Society of Anesthesiologists) standard monitoring is used and includes continuous pulse oximetry, capnography, and electrocardiography (ECG), along with frequent blood pressure measurements (every 3–5 minutes). For patients with critical end-organ dysfunction (neurologic or cardiovascular), arterial blood pressure should be used for closer monitoring. Peripheral intravenous access must be ensured with the placement of, at minimum, a 20-gauge intravenous catheter that infuses well. Additional equipment should be set up at the patient's bedside if the tracheotomy is scheduled to take place in the ICU (see **Figure 2.1**).

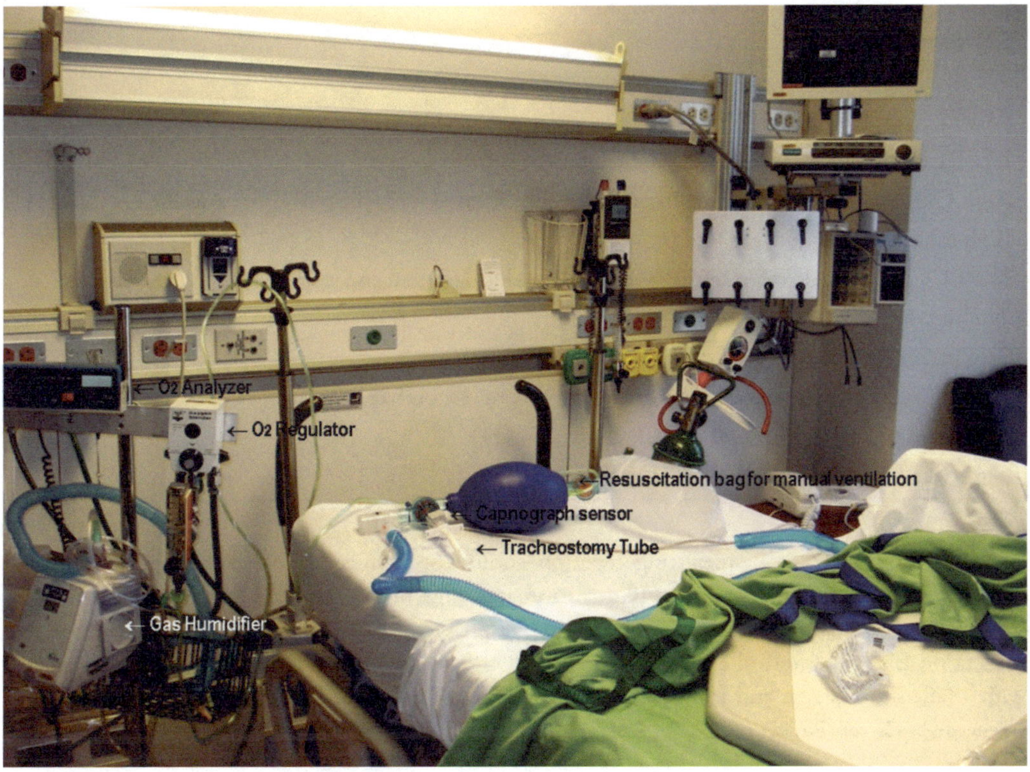

Figure 2.1 Oxygen Regulator Set-up

The FiO_2 (%) can be dialed up or down on the O_2 regulator depending on use of electrocautery and patient O_2 saturation. An oxygen analyzer calibrates the concentration of oxygen from the O_2 regulator. An air/O_2 gas mixture is delivered through a humidifier to a resuscitation ventilation bag, which the anesthesiologist uses to deliver manual breaths in concert with surgical maneuvering. A capnograph is a standard monitor in tracheotomy procedures to confirm adequate ventilation and access to the upper airway.

A pre-procedure patient safety checklist for bedside tracheotomies in the ICU is provided in **Table 2.4** for reference. Low FiO2 avoids airway fires when electrocautery is needed during surgery. A regulator for mixing oxygen and air should target FiO2 at around 30% oxygen concentration, ensuring the patient's blood oxygen saturation stays > 94%.

Table 2.4. Bedside Pre-Procedure Checklist

Members Present

Surgeon: ______________________________

Anesthesiologist: ________________________

Nurse: ________________________________

Key Elements

Patient is stable to undergo procedure.

Bipolar vs. monopolar cautery has been considered.

Both CO_2 and ABC fire extinguishers have been located with their triggers, and the responsible person has been appointed.

Main O_2 gas shut-off valve in the ICU has been located, and the responsible person has been appointed.

Skin asepsis: product is confirmed alcohol-free.

Drape does not cover mouth, endotracheal tube, or Ambu bag.

FiO_2 level has been coordinated with electrocautery.

Time Out has been performed and documented.

If already intubated, preexisting sedation should be converted to general anesthesia using carefully titrated induction agents. If not intubated and no airway problems are anticipated, a standard induction may be appropriate. If airway problems are anticipated, an awake fiberoptic intubation is the method of choice. In any event, the anesthesiologist should be prepared to deal with a failed intubation and must have a surgeon immediately available to perform an emergency tracheotomy if ventilation proves impossible.

A popular anesthetic regimen is propofol for hypnosis, fentanyl for analgesia, and a muscle relaxant to keep the patient immobile during the surgical procedure, particularly at the point of airway incision and device insertion. If a difficult intubation is anticipated, propofol dosage for induction is 1-1.5 mg/kg and a short-acting muscle relaxant such as succinylcholine at 1.5–2 mg/kg is generally recommended (half-life for succinylcholine is 5 min). By contrast, if a difficult intubation is not anticipated, a nondepolarizing muscle relaxant such as rocuronium can be administered at a dosage of 0.6 mg/kg (half-life is 20–30 min).

The O_2 regulator can be adjusted to dial the FiO_2 up or down depending on the use of electrocautery and patient requirements. An oxygen analyzer is used to calibrate the concentration of oxygen from the O_2 regulator. An air/O_2 gas mixture is delivered through a humidifier to a resuscitation ventilation bag, which the anesthesiologist uses to deliver manual breaths in concert with surgical maneuvering. A capnograph must be used as a standard monitor for tracheotomy procedures to confirm adequate ventilation and access to the upper airway. It is crucial for clear and open communication between surgical and anesthesia teams during the procedure to ensure patient safety.

Total intravenous anesthesia can be delivered using a propofol infusion (40-100 mcg/kg/min) and a fentanyl infusion (3 mcg/kg/hr total dosage approximately 250 mcg for the entire procedure). It is helpful to administer fentanyl a few minutes before the surgeon enters the trachea, as it is the time of highest stimulation. A fentanyl dose of 150–200 mcg IV can ablate a significant increase in intracranial pressure in patients with intracranial hypertension and presumed loss of autoregulation of cerebral blood flow. Fluid requirements average 1–2 ml/kg/hr for the entire procedure, and blood loss is minimal, particularly when tracheotomy is done as an isolated procedure.

A rigid bronchoscope should be available to re-establish the airway in case of a failed re-intubation after a lost airway. Alternatively, in patients at high risk for failed reintubation, a small-bore airway exchange catheter can be advanced through a flexible bronchoscope fitted into the existing ETT prior to tracheotomy tube insertion. Frequently, when tracheotomy is a prelude to a major procedure, an anode tube is inserted through the tracheotomy and sutured in place. It is replaced at the end of surgery by a cuffed tracheotomy tube.

Emergence

Besides analgesia, surgical site hemostasis, and adequate gas exchange, there are no special considerations for emergence following tracheotomy. Opioid sedation and analgesia will blunt any reactions to suctioning in the early postoperative period.

Complications

Immediately, postoperative surveillance for complications should be directed toward detection of pneumothorax, hemorrhage in the form of an obstructing hematoma, aspiration of blood, loss of airway requiring re-intubation, and pneumo-mediastinum. Pneumothorax may also occur with low neck dissection. The use of a postoperative chest radiograph will define the position of the tracheotomy tube and may act as a survey for the presence of pneumothorax or pneumomediastinum.

SURGICAL TECHNIQUE

The intimate knowledge of relevant anatomy is crucial in performing this procedure safely. The sternal notch and thyroid and cricoid cartilages are usually easily palpable through the skin. A key surface landmark, the cricoids, is usually found by using the thyroid cartilage above, and the sternal notch below, as reference points. The cricothyroid membrane spans the anterior aspect of the thyroid and cricoid cartilages. It is identified by palpating a slight indentation in the skin inferior to the thyroid notch. The paired cricothyroid arteries traverse horizontally along the superior aspect of this membrane and anastomose in the midline.

The cricothyroid muscles arise from the anterior surface of the cricoid and extend superiorly and posteriorly to attach to the lateral surfaces of the thyroid alae. The innominate, or brachiocephalic, artery crosses from left to right, just anterior to the trachea at the superior thoracic inlet and deep to the sternal notch. Its pulsations are often felt during dissection of the anterior tracheal wall. The trachea comprises 18 to 22 semicircular cartilaginous rings and is posteriorly separated from the esophagus by a membranous portion. The average width of the adult tracheal lumen is 2.3 cm in the coronal dimension and 1.8 cm in the sagittal dimension. The average length of the adult trachea is 11 cm, with a range of 12 to 15 cm.

The thyroid gland lies anteriorly to the trachea with each thyroid lobe lying laterally, with the isthmus crossing it anteriorly at the level of the second to fourth tracheal rings. The endocrine tissue is highly vascular and must be identified and handled carefully to prevent bleeding. The recurrent laryngeal nerves and inferior thyroid veins travel in the tracheoesophageal grooves laterally and are out of the surgical field unless dissection strays significantly. The great vessels are lateral to the intended dissection and proper surgical technique will avoid them.

The surgical technique for tracheotomy has evolved throughout history. The division of the thyroid isthmus was first described by Degarengot in 1720.[22] Tracheotomies continued to be performed high until the 20th century because of the relative speed and ease of this approach. This practice was not altered until 1909, when Jackson described the increased rates of subglottic stenosis associated with high tracheotomy placement. Today, many variations in technique are still commonplace. Current technique can nonetheless be divided into two broad categories: the open surgical approach and percutaneous dilatational tracheotomy.

Open Tracheotomy

The open surgical tracheotomy can be performed in the operating room or at the bedside in a monitored setting such as the ICU. The procedure is most commonly performed under general anesthesia in a previously intubated patient. Occasionally, when the patient presents in acute distress, the procedure is performed as an "awake tracheotomy" in the non-intubated patient under local anesthesia, while the patient breathes spontaneously.

Prior to the procedure, the patient is placed with a roll underneath the shoulders to extend the neck and expose surgical landmarks (**Figure 2.2A**). This maneuver is contraindicated in patients with cervical spine injuries or atlanto-axial instability, as seen in Trisomy 21 syndrome, where neck extension can result in spinal cord compression. Certain patients with tenuous airways may not be able to tolerate either neck extension or even the supine position, requiring tracheotomy to be performed with the patient in a sitting position without neck extension. Patients with significant kyphoscoliosis, cervical osteoarthritis, or other conditions in which the neck cannot be hyperextended can present a significant technical challenge.

The procedure begins with the palpation of the landmarks of the neck, including the thyroid cartilage, cricoid cartilage, and sternal notch. A marking pen may be used to indicate the relative position of each of these crucial landmarks on the skin of the extended neck prior to sterile cleansing (**Figure 2.2B**). Lidocaine with epinephrine is injected into the skin and subcutaneous tissues where the incision will be placed. The neck and upper chest are prepared in a povidone-iodine (Betadine) solution, and the surgical site is draped to allow easy access to the oral cavity so the endotracheal tube can be easily mobilized and manipulated by the anesthesiologist during the procedure. A critical precaution involves avoiding the use of Bovie cautery in the presence of alcohol-based surgical prep solution (DuraPrep). The risk of surgical fire associated with the incomplete drying of this agent in the context of electrocautery has been described previously.[23,24] This risk is further increased in awake tracheotomy during the use of oxygen-rich gas delivery from nasal cannulas or ventilation masks. The use of electrocautery in these circumstances constitutes a significant hazard.

Figure 2.2 Position & landmarks

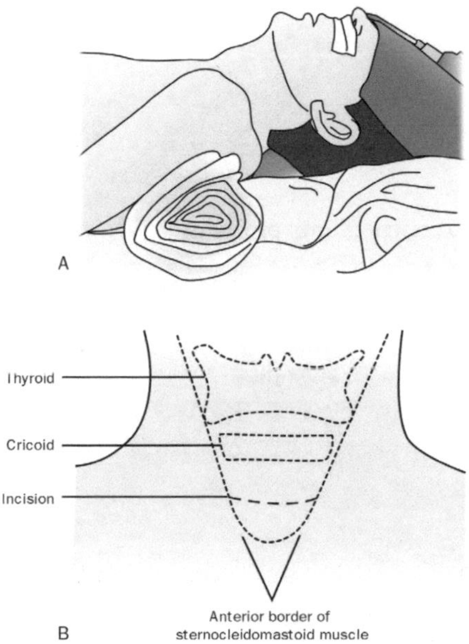

Surgical tracheotomy preparation.

A) Patient positioning with roll under shoulders.

B) Surface landmarks showing the thyroid, cricoid, intended location of the skin incision, and anterior border of the sternocleidomastoid muscle.

A 2–3 cm incision is carried out in a vertical or horizontal fashion (**Figure 2.3**). The horizontal incision provides a more cosmetically pleasing postoperative scar, as it follows the relaxed skin tension lines. However, this benefit decreases the longer the tracheostomy remains in place. Vertical incision avoids the anterior jugular venous system, therefore minimizing cumbersome bleeding in cases of emergency tracheotomies. Vertical incisions start just below the cricoid cartilage, whereas horizontal incisions are made either two fingerbreadths below the cricoid cartilage or halfway between the cricoid cartilage and the sternal notch, typically over the interspace between the second and third tracheal rings. The subcutaneous tissues are then divided with either a 15 blade or Bovie electrocautery to the level of the strap muscles. Care should be exercised at this stage to avoid damage to the anterior jugular vein, which, when identified, should be lateralized or ligated in order to avoid unnecessary bleeding. Once identified, the strap muscles should be divided vertically along their midline raphe until the thyroid isthmus is exposed (**Figure 2.4**).

Figure 2.3. Incision & spreaders

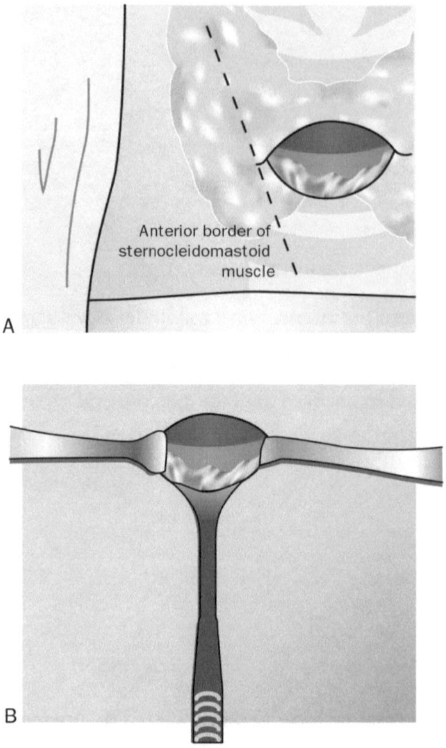

Surgical tracheotomy procedure.

A) Initial incision. Note the anterior border of the sternocleidomastoid muscle.

B) Incision with spreaders

Figure 2.4. Exposure, cross clamping thryoid isthmus

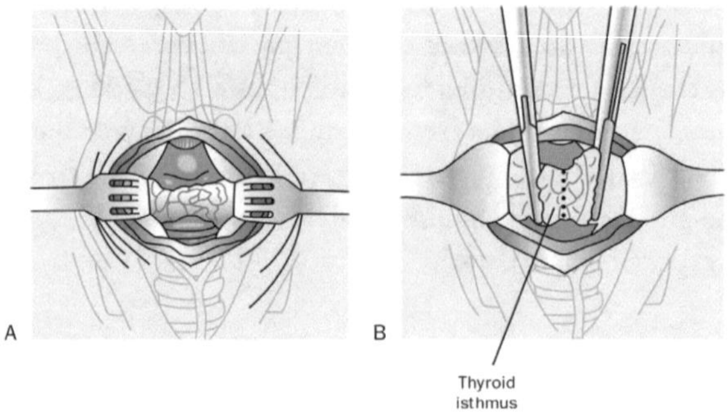

Surgical tracheotomy procedure.

A) Exposure of the thyroid isthmus. Note the thyroid isthmus is exposed over the proximal trachea.

B) The thyroid isthmus is cross-clamped and divided.

The thyroid gland can be handled in a number of ways. Depending on the location of the isthmus within the surgical wound, the isthmus can be retracted superiorly, inferiorly, or divided and ligated to expose the second and third tracheal rings where the tracheal window will be performed (**Figure 2.5**). The cricoid cartilage serves as an important landmark during this portion of the dissection. Often, traction placed on the cricoid cartilage using a cricoid hook mobilizes the laryngotracheal complex into a more favorable, superior, and superficial position to allow easier access into the trachea.

The pretracheal fascia is dissected off the proximal trachea using a Kitner sponge. With patients having tracheotomy under local anesthesia, it is important to inject local anesthetic into the pretracheal tissues prior to opening the trachea in order to provide proper analgesia. In addition, a 2% lidocaine solution can be applied trans-tracheally to provide topical endoluminal anesthesia. There are multiple incision types for entrance into the trachea. Some surgeons prefer a single horizontal inter-cartilaginous incision, while others perform an H-type incision, or make a tracheal window by removing a centimeter-wide portion of the anterior aspect of the second or third tracheal ring. The type of incision does not seem to affect the development of postoperative tracheal stenosis in either animal models[25,26] or humans. An inferiorly based trap door flap (Bjork flap) can be created by incising the interspace between the second and third tracheal rings as well as the third tracheal ring laterally on both sides, extending inferiorly from the interspace incision. The superior aspect of the flap is then sutured to the inferior aspect of the skin incision with a non-absorbable suture. This flap facilitates reinsertion of the tracheostomy tube in cases of accidental decannulation, which is especially important in obese patients or those with difficult anatomy. Despite commonly expressed concerns, one study[27] suggests there is no increased rate of either tracheostenosis or tracheocutaneous fistula with use of the Bjork flap. Another option for managing the anterior tracheal wall is the removal of an anterior section of the second or third tracheal rings using a scalpel, Metzenbaum scissors, or tracheal punch. This technique, although debated, has been associated with greater tracheal stenosis in comparison to the Bjork flap.[28] It is important to note that most causes of tracheal stenosis are related to high tracheostomy, infection at the stoma site, trauma, and urgency of the performed tracheotomy.[29]

Figure 2.5 Removing tracheal ring

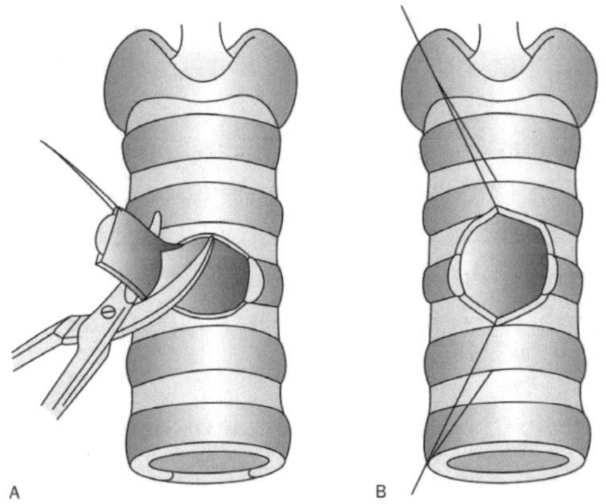

Surgical tracheotomy procedure.

A) Removing tracheal ring to form window.

B) Stay sutures are placed superiorly and inferiorly to the stoma.

Once the trachea is entered, a tracheotomy dilator is used to optimize exposure to the tracheal lumen, taking care to prevent excess trauma to the cartilaginous framework of the trachea. Upon visualization of the endotracheal tube within the lumen, the anesthesiologist is asked to withdraw the ETT until the posterior tracheal wall is visualized. The tracheostomy tube is then introduced into the lumen of the trachea under direct vision. In cases of patients with a history of difficult intubation, the endotracheal tube can be withdrawn over a tube exchanger to facilitate reintubation in case tracheostomy tube placement proves difficult. After introduction of the tracheostomy tube, proper placement should be confirmed before the endotracheal tube is removed. Proper placement is confirmed by detecting carbon dioxide return from the tracheostomy tube, and, if needed, confirming placement within the trachea by flexible bronchoscopy. If proper placement of the tracheostomy tube cannot be confirmed via these steps, the endotracheal tube should be reintroduced by the anesthesiologist. Once successfully placed, the tracheostomy tube should be secured into place with non-absorbable sutures placed through the flanges of the tube (**Figure 2.6**) as well as tracheostomy ties placed around the patient's neck.

Figure 2.6 Suturing neck flange

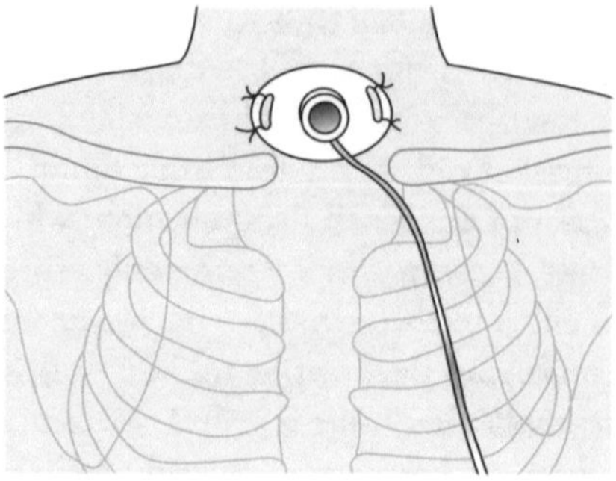

Neck flange sutured in place.

Percutaneous Dilatational Tracheotomy (PDT)

In 1953, Seldinger introduced the technique of percutaneous guidewire needle placement in arterial catheterization.[30] Soon thereafter, the guidewire technique, now known as the Seldinger technique, was adapted to various procedures, including percutaneous tracheotomy. The first modern percutaneous dilatational tracheotomy (PDT) was reported by Shelden, Pudenz, Freshwater, and Crue in 1955, but the complication rate was high due to the laceration of adjacent structures by the trocar.[31] In 1969, Toy and Weinstein developed a tapered straight dilator with a recessed cutting blade for performing percutaneous tracheotomy over a guiding catheter.[32] The technique of PDT using serial dilators over a guidewire was first described in 1985 by Ciaglia, Firshing, and Synlec. In 1989, Schachner and colleagues developed a dilating tracheotomy forceps over a guidewire.[33] In 1990, Griggs, Worthley, Gilligan, Thomas, and Myburg developed another guidewire dilating forceps specifically for percutaneous tracheotomy. Shortly thereafter, convenient kits to create a full-sized percutaneous tracheotomy became readily available.[34]

PDT involves the placement of a tracheostomy tube without direct visualization of the tracheal lumen through a surgical wound. The general consensus is that PDT should only be performed on intubated patients, although it has been performed on awake patients under local anesthesia. It is considered a minimally invasive procedure that can be performed at the bedside in monitored settings.

Bronchoscopic guidance is considered the standard of care, and a single surgeon or intensivist aided by a bronchoscopist can easily accomplish the procedure. The main benefit derived from direct bronchoscopic visualization during PDT is close, real-time surveillance for any potential immediate complications, as well as confirmation of proper positioning of the tracheostomy tube.

The criteria for PDT are similar, albeit more stringent, than for surgical tracheotomy (see **Table 2.5**).[35] The relative contra-indications include obesity, coagulopathy, un-extended neck, repeat tracheostomy, marginal oxygenation and/or ventilation on mechanical ventilator settings, extensive tumor of the upper airway, and hypotension. Patients with a BMI over 30 have been shown to be at increased risk of complications compared to patients with a BMI below 30 (15% vs 8%).[36] Although, this increased complication rate is also seen in morbidly obese patients (BMI>40) undergoing open surgical tracheotomy.[37]

Table 2.5. Contraindications to Percutaneous Dilatational Tracheotomy
Relative Contraindications
Children under 12 years of age
Anatomic abnormalities of the trachea, including tracheomalacia
Palpable pulses over tracheotomy site
Active infection over tracheotomy site
Thyroid mass or goiter over tracheotomy site
Obese neck or nonpalpable laryngotracheal landmarks
PEEP greater than 15 cm H_2O
Platelet count less than 40,000/mm3
Bleeding time greater than 10 minutes
Absolute Contraindications
Prothrombin time or partial thromboplastin time greater than 1.5 times control
Limited ability to extend the neck, especially in the unstable spine
History of difficult intubation
Need for urgent surgical airway

Abnormal coagulopathies should be corrected and anti-coagulants should be stopped prior to undergoing the procedure. Abouzgheib and colleagues[38] demonstrated the safety of PDT in patients actively taking anti-platelet therapy. Their findings agreed with previous retrospective reviews of ICU patients showing increased bleeding complications with INR greater than 1.7 or a platelet count less than 50,000.[39] The un-extended neck presents challenges, but has not been shown to increase complication rates.[40] Moreover, PDT has been shown to be safe in patients requiring a repeat tracheotomy,[41] whereas patients with hypotension on significant pressor infusions may not be suitable for PDT, and clinical judgement is required for patient safety. Clinicians performing PDT should be well-trained in the technique, prepared to convert to an open surgical tracheotomy if needed, and be ready to manage any immediate complications.

For this procedure, the patient is positioned and draped as for standard, open tracheotomy. A skin incision is made and the pretracheal tissue cleared with minimal blunt dissection. The endotracheal tube is withdrawn until the cuff is just at the level of the glottis. The endoscopist can place the tip of the bronchoscope such that the light from its tip is visible through the surgical wound, thus highlighting the target area. The operator then enters the tracheal lumen below the second tracheal ring with a needle introducer (**Figure 2.7A–B**).

Figure 2.7A Perc needle insertion

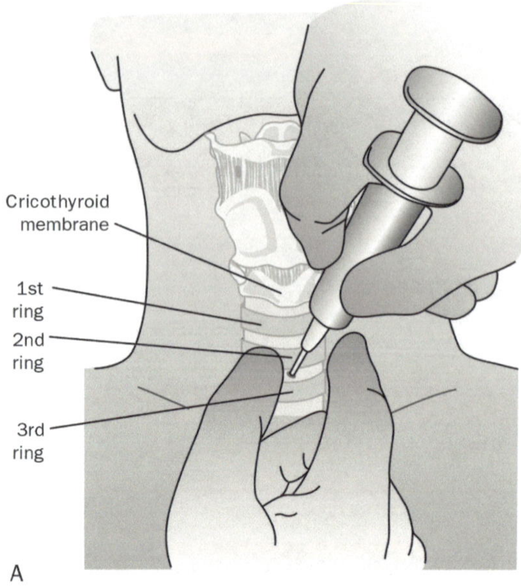

Percutaneous tracheotomy procedure.

A) Insertion of needle between second and third tracheal rings.

B) Bronchoscopic view of needle insertion into trachea. (Bronchoscopic image courtesy of Alberto de Hoyos, MD)

Figure 2.7B Bronchoscopic View: Needle entry

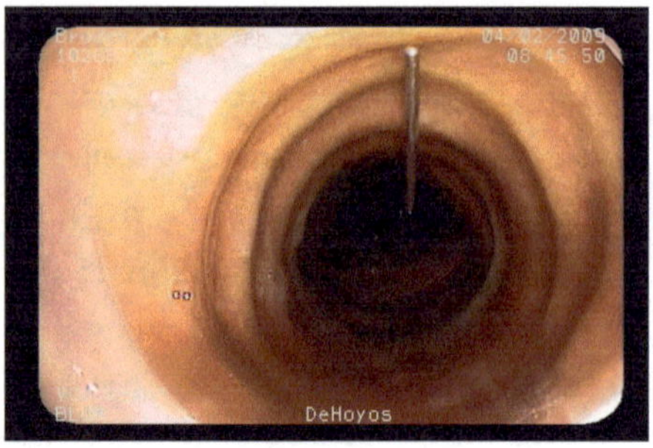

A guidewire is then inserted through the needle (**Figure 2.8A–B**).

Figure 2.8A Guidewire through needle

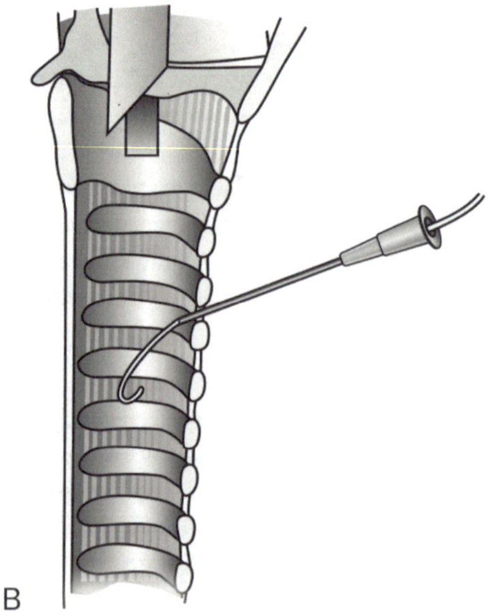

A) Guidewire is placed through needle introducer.

B) Bronchoscopic view of guidewire through needle. (Bronchoscopic image courtesy of Alberto de Hoyos, MD)

Figure 2.8B Bronchoscopic View: Guidewire through needle

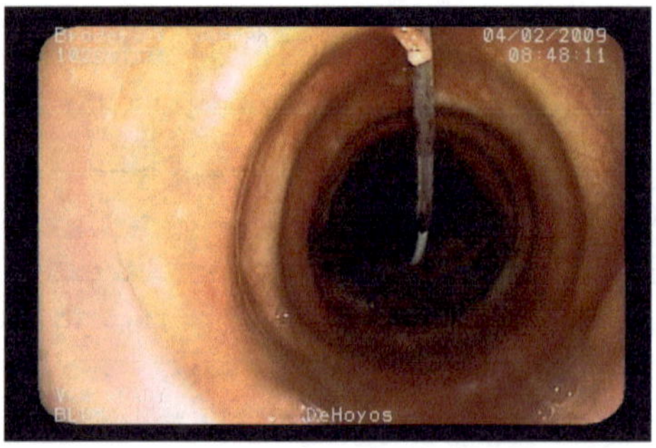

The track extending from the skin to the tracheal lumen is then serially dilated over a guidewire (**Figure 2.9A–B**).

Figure 2.9A Dilator over guidewire

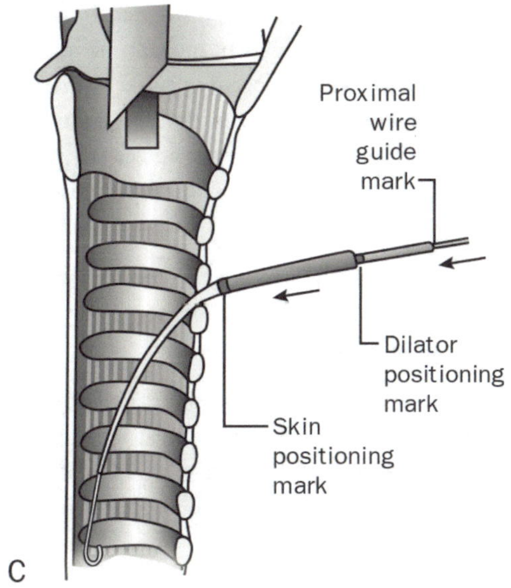

A) Insertion of tracheostomy tube over dilator. B) Bronchoscopic view of tracheostomy tube placed over dilator. (Bronchoscopic image courtesy of Alberto de Hoyos, MD)

Figure 2.9B Bronchoscopic View: Dilator insertion

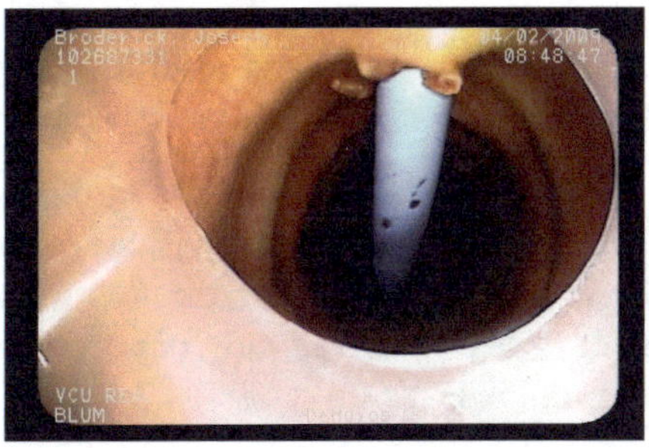

A tracheostomy tube is then introduced under direct bronchoscopic view over the dilator (**Figure 2.10A–B**).

Figure 2.10A Tracheostomy tube over dilator

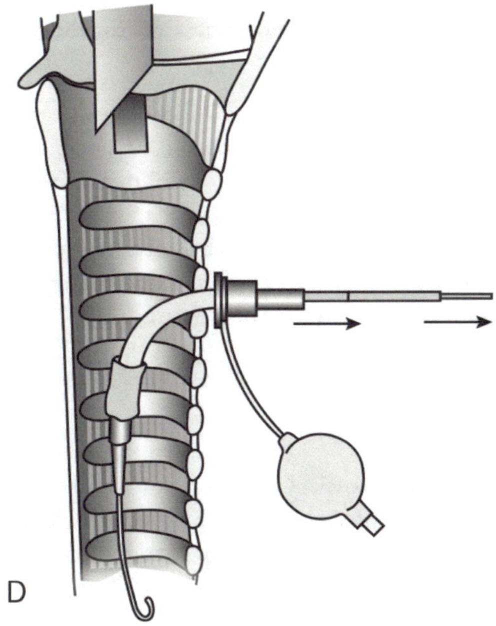

A) Insertion of tracheostomy tube over dilator. B) Bronchoscopic view of tracheostomy tube placed over dilator. (Bronchoscopic image courtesy of Alberto de Hoyos, MD)

Figure 2.10B Bronchoscopic View: Tracheostomy tube in place

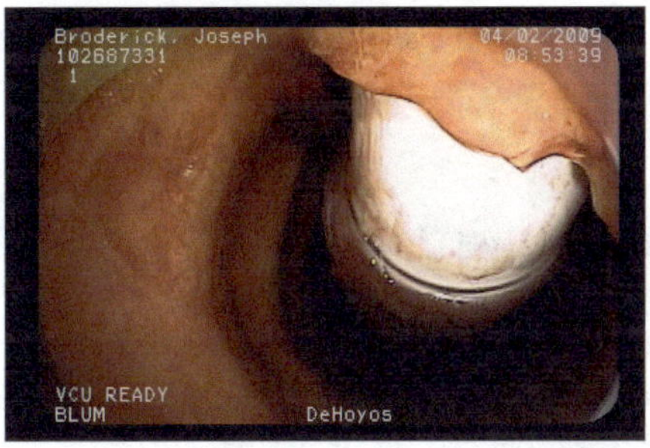

Proper placement is then confirmed by viewing the tracheobronchial tree through the tracheostomy tube, and the tube is secured into place with sutures and ties.

Pediatric Tracheotomy

As in adult tracheotomy, identifiable landmarks—including hyoid bone, thyroid notch, cricoid cartilage, thyroid isthmus, and sternal notch—are identified, and a skin incision is marked accordingly. It should be noted that these laryngotracheal landmarks are located relatively superiorly within the neck in the pediatric age group. Dissection then proceeds as in adults. Particular attention should be paid to avoid straying laterally due to the presence of the pulmonary apices within the cervical compartment in the younger age groups, which increases the risk of pleural puncture and resultant pneumothorax.

At the level of the trachea, the incision is generally made vertically through two or three tracheal rings, usually within the second to fifth tracheal rings. As in adults, an incision too close to the cricoid should be avoided, as it is associated with higher rates of subglottic stenosis.

Nylon traction sutures are placed in the trachea on either side of the incision line before the incision is made. Historically, these sutures serve to place traction on the tracheal rings during cannulation of the airway and are crucial in locating the tracheal window in cases of accidental tracheal displacement in the early postoperative period.[42] This portion of the procedure is still commonly utilized.

The vertical trans-tracheal incision should be long enough to easily allow passage of the tracheostomy tube in order to prevent undue damage to the integrity of the cartilage framework. Too small of an incision or a horizontal intra-cartilaginous incision may lead to the collapse of the suprastomal tracheal ring as the curved tube exerts backward pressure on the ring above the incision.

After the tracheostomy tube is placed, it is secured in a similar fashion to adults. The traction sutures are tied loosely and taped to the skin of the anterior chest wall. Tape labels are used to clearly identify the right and left traction sutures so they are not reversed when used to recannulate the trachea. Reversal of these labels would have the opposite undesired effect of approximating the edges of the tracheal window.

The position of the tracheostomy tube with respect to the carina and tracheal wall can be determined via either passing a pediatric flexible endoscope through the tube or obtaining a postoperative chest radiograph. The tip of the tracheostomy tube should be 5 to 20 mm above the carina. The tube should not be so short that the lumen faces posteriorly or is at risk for exiting the tracheal window and entering a false pretracheal passage. Certain patients, such as obese children or those with metabolic storage diseases, may have excessively long tracts between the skin and trachea, requiring custom tracheostomy tubes with extra-long proximal, extra-tracheal portion.

Postoperative Care

The post-operative care and teaching of a patient and family is crucial for the patient to adapt to the new way of breathing. Family counseling is also important in order to optimize postoperative patient support for those able to be discharged. Highly skilled nursing care is crucial for success in this area.

In the initial postoperative period, the patient is usually placed in an intensive care setting in order to continuously monitor vital signs. Indeed, subtle changes in the patient's behavior, pulse, blood pressure, or respiratory rate may herald an obstruction of the tracheotomy tube with dried blood or secretions, which requires immediate attention. Tracheal suctioning must be performed as frequently as needed—often more frequently than would be possible outside of an ICU setting. The humidification of inhaled air is important for the mucociliary transport of secretions and to prevent the obstruction of the airway with dried secretions. The inner cannula must be removed frequently for cleaning and to avoid the accumulation of obstructing crusts. The tracheostomy tube is rarely changed before the third postoperative day, and it is common to wait until at least the fifth postoperative day to allow the tract to mature and to avoid tissue collapse that would seal off the airway.

A general recommendation is to have the first tracheostomy tube change be done on post-operative day 5-7 after an open procedure versus days 10-14 after a percutaneous procedure. The rationale behind this is the tighter fit of the percutaneous tracheostomy tube is at a high risk of recoiling to a smaller size if the earlier the change is done. Therefore, it is reasonable to delay longer than after an open procedure.[43] Initial tube replacement within the first 72 hours postoperatively should be done in the same conditions as the original procedure and requires adequate headlights, suction, cricoid hook, and assistance. This may be required if the cuff of the tracheostomy tube fails in a patient continuing to need positive-pressure ventilation after the procedure.

Summary

The surgical technique of tracheotomy should be adapted to the situation at hand, especially for patients with complicated neck anatomy, those with previous tracheotomies, or pediatric patients. Attention to detail during the procedure will help avoid the pitfalls and complications that can plague tracheostomy patients during the postoperative period. There continues to be controversy between open and percutaneous dilatational tracheotomy, but both have long track records, and application of one versus the other depends on the established practice patterns of individual clinicians.

Regardless of the quality of intervention at the time of the procedure, long-term success and the prevention of complications depends on meticulous care during the postoperative period.

Key Points

- Indications for tracheotomy depend on multiple factors, including risk of the procedure, the patient's respiratory anatomy and physiology, specific pathologic processes, and available resources.
- The optimal timing for tracheotomy differs among patient indications and practitioner preferences. Evidence indicates favorable morbidity, mortality, duration of mechanical ventilation, and length of stay with earlier timing of tracheotomy.
- Safe conduct of tracheotomy procedures requires detailed preoperative patient evaluation, preparation of appropriate monitors, institution of safety guidelines, and availability of standardized equipment and adequate video-assisted devices.

- Open surgical tracheotomy can be performed in the OR or the ICU, with bedside tracheotomies having the advantage of decreased patient transport risk, OR cost, and schedule burden.
- PDT is a popular approach and is performed under bronchoscopic guidance to identify immediate complications and confirm tube placement.
- After the procedure, patients require close monitoring of vital signs in an ICU.

Acknowledgment

Bronchoscopic images of percutaneous dilatational tracheotomy were provided by Alberto de Hoyos, MD.

REVIEW QUESTIONS

1. At what post-operative day is it recommended to perform the first tracheostomy tube change after a PDT?
    a. 1 day
    b. 3 days
    c. 10 days
    d. 15 days

    ANSWER: C. The recommended time to change the tracheostomy tube after a PDT is approximately post-operative days 10-12. This is later than the 5 days recommended for the open tracheostomy procedure due to the tightness of the stoma around the tracheostomy and risk of recoil and stenosis of the tissues if the change is done earlier.[43]

2. A patient with an underlying neurological disorder is admitted to the hospital in respiratory failure. He has remained intubated in the ICU for several days secondary to pulmonary insufficiency. The possibility of tracheotomy is discussed. Which benefit would this patient likely have if a tracheotomy is performed prior to the 10th hospital day?
    a. Improved overall survival
    b. Decreased cardiac risk
    c. Immediate improvement in communication
    d. Improved neurological status

    ANSWER: A. The evidence suggests that patients who receive early tracheotomy in a prolonged ICU stay are likely to have a survival benefit with early tracheotomy.[9] There is no direct evidence that suggests patients with tracheotomies would have decreased cardiac risk or improved neurological status. Vocal communication would not be possible in the immediate post-operative period because the inflated cuff prevents air from passing through the vocal cords.

3. A 63-year-old man with a BMI of 42, extensive cardiac history, and a history of radiation to the head and neck is intubated due to progressive laryngeal squamous cell carcinoma occluding the airway. What is the most important factor to consider regarding possible tracheotomy?
    a. BMI
    b. Cardiac history
    c. Anticipated duration of mechanical ventilation
    d. History of radiation therapy

    ANSWER: C. The literature states that the most important factor in evaluating a patient for tracheotomy is to consider the anticipated duration of mechanical.[17,18,19] In this patient with laryngeal cancer blocking the airway, it is reasonable to assume that the need for an artificial airway will not resolve without bypassing this blockage.

4. What step should be taken prior to making an incision of the trachea during tracheotomy?
    a. Placement of traction sutures on either side of the incision line
    b. Marking of the tracheal incision
    c. Increase the fraction of inspired oxygen
    d. Utilize topical lidocaine with epinephrine on the surgical field

    ANSWER: A. The placement of traction sutures in the trachea and taping to the skin is a crucial step for later post-operative management, especially in obese patients. The risk of loss of airway if the trachea were to pull away from the skin could result in catastrophic results.[42] There is no evidence that marking the tracheal incision would be helpful and the use of topical lidocaine with epinephrine on the field is not indicated. The increase in FiO_2 would increase the risk of airway fire and is not recommended.

5. A patient is brought to the operating room for an open surgical tracheotomy. The patient is positioned correctly, landmarks are palpated and marked, and the patient is prepped using sterile technique with DuraPrep. An incision is made, and electro-cautery is utilized when a fire erupts on the surgical table. What is the likely culprit?
    a. High FiO_2 delivered via the endotracheal tube
    b. Oxygen accumulation under the drapes
    c. Use of an alcohol-based prep solution
    d. Poor surgical technique

    ANSWER: C. There are many fire risks which must be identified before starting tracheotomy procedure. The use of alcohol-based preps is one such risk, and it is recommended that non-flammable preparation solutions be used, such as Povidone Iodine. The accumulation of oxygen underneath the drapes and a high FiO_2 (> 40%) delivered through the endotracheal tube would increase risk of fire but would present later in the case in different ways.

REFERENCES

1. Frost EA. Tracing the tracheostomy. *Ann Otol Rhinol Laryngol.* 1976;85(5, Pt.1):618-624.
2. American Academy of Otolaryngology-Head and Neck Surgery. Clinical Indicators Compendium: Tracheostomy. 2016. Retrieved June 9, 2020 from https://www.entnet.org/content/clinical-indicators.
3. Stone DJ, Bogdonoff DL. Airway considerations in the management of patients requiring long-term endotracheal intubation. *Anesth Analg.* 1992;74(2):276-287.
4. Plummer AL, Gracey DR. Consensus conference on artificial airways in patients requiring mechanical ventilation. *Chest.* 1989;96:178-180.
5. Heffner JE. Timing of tracheotomy in mechanically ventilated patients. *Am Rev Respir Dis.* 1993;147:768.
6. Durbin CG. Tracheostomy: Why, when, and how? *Respir Care.* 2010;55(8): 1056-68.
7. Bishop MJ. The timing of tracheotomy: An evolving consensus. *Chest.* 1989;96:712.
8. Esteban A, Anzueto A, Alia I, Gordo F, Apezteguia C, Palizas F, Cide D, Goldwaser R, Soto L, Bugedo G, Rodrigo C, Pimentel J, Raimondi G, Tobin MJ. How is mechanical ventilation employed in the intensive care unit? An international review. *Am J Respir Crit Care Med.* 2000;161(5):1450-1458.
9. Rumbak MJ, Newton M, Truncale T, Schwartz SW, Adams JW, Hazard PB. A prospective, randomized study comparing early percutaneous dilational tracheotomy to prolonged translaryngeal intubation (delayed tracheotomy) in critically ill medical patients. *Crit Care Med.* 2004;32(8):1689-1694.
10. Patel SA, Plowman EK, Halum S, Merati AL, Sardesai MG. Late tracheotomy is associated with higher morbidity and mortality in mechanically ventilated patients. *Laryngoscope.* 2015;125:2134-2138.
11. Griffiths J, Barber VS, Morgan L, Young JD. Systematic review and meta-analysis of studies of the timing of tracheostomy in adult patients undergoing artificial ventilation. *Brit Med J.* 2005;330:1243.
12. Scales DC, Thiruchelvam D, Kiss A, Redelmeier DA. The effect of tracheostomy timing during critical illness on long-term survival. *Crit Care Med.* 2008;36:254–2557.
13. Colice GL, Stukel TA, Dain B. Laryngeal complications of prolonged intubation. *Chest.* 1989;89:877.
14. Colton HJ, Noordzij JP, Murgia B, Langmore S. Laryngeal injury from prolonged intubation: A prospective analysis of contributing factors. *Laryngoscope.* 2011;121(3):596–600. http://doi.org/10.1002/lary.21403.
15. Young D, Harrison DA, Cuthbertson BH, Rowan K, TracMan Collaborators FT. Effect of early vs. late tracheostomy placement on survival in patients receiving mechanical ventilation-The TracMan randomized trial. *JAMA.* 2013;309(20):2121-2129.
16. Blot F, Similowski T, Trouillet JL, Chardon P, Korach JM, Costa MA, Juornois D, Thiéry G, Fartoukh M, Pipien I, Bruder N, Orlikowski D, Tankere F, Durand-Zaelski I, Auboyer C, Nitenberg G, Holzapfel L, Tenaillon A, Chastre J, Laplanche A. (2008). Early tracheotomy versus prolonged endotracheal intubation in unselected severely ill ICU patients. *Intensive Care Med.* 2008;34:1779-1787.
17. Cheung NH, Napolitano LM. Tracheostomy: epidemiology, indications, timing, technique and outcomes. *Respir Care.* 2014;59(6):895-915.

18. Cipriano A, Mao ML, Hon HH, Vazquez D, Stawicki S, Sharpe R, Evans D. An overview of complications associated with open and percutaneous tracheostomy procedures. *Int J Crit Illness Injury Sci.* 2015;5(3):179-188.
19. Puentes W, Jerath A, Djaiani G, Sanchez RC, Wąsowicz M. Early versus late tracheostomy in cardiovascular intensive care patients. *Anaesthesiol Intensive Ther.* 2016;48(2):89-94.
20. Nekhendzy V, Guta C, Champeau MW. Tracheotomy/tracheostomy and cricothyroidotomy: Anesthetic considerations. In Jaffe RA, Samuels SI. eds. *Anesthesiologist's Manual of Surgical Procedures.* Philadelphia: Lippincott Williams & Wilkins; 2009:187-189.
21. American Society of Anesthesiologists, Practice guidelines for preoperative fasting and the use of pharmacologic agents to reduce the risk of pulmonary aspiration: Application to healthy patients undergoing elective procedures: An Updated report by the American Society of Anesthesiologists task force on preoperative fasting and the use of pharmacologic agents to reduce the risk of pulmonary aspiration. *Anesthesiology.* 2017;126(3):376-393.
22. Grillo HC. Development of tracheal surgery: A historical review. Part 1: Techniques of tracheal surgery. *Ann of Thorac Surg.* 2003;75:610-619.
23. Weber SM, Hargunani CA, Wax MK. DuraPrep and the risk of fire during tracheostomy. *Head Neck.* 2006;28(7):649-652.
24. Jones EL, Overbey DM, Chapman BC, Jones TS, Hilton SA, Moore JT, Robinson TN. Operating room fires and surgical skin preparation. J Am Coll Surg. 2017;225(1):160-165.
25. Whitley R, Castillo N, Hassett JM, Banyas J, Luchette FA. Early tracheostomal healing in rabbits with use of various tracheal incisions. *Wound Repair & Regeneration.* 1997;5(4):323-328.
26. Natvig K, Olving JH. Tracheal changes in relation to different tracheostomy techniques (An experimental study on rabbits). *J Laryngol Otol.* 1981;95(1):61-68.
27. Malata CM, Foo IT, Simpson KH, Batchelor AG. An audit of Bjork flap tracheostomies in head and neck plastic surgery. *Br J of Oral Maxillofac Surg.* 1996;34(1):42-46.
28. Dukes H. (1970). Tracheostomy. *Thorax.* 1970;25:573-576.
29. Sarper A, Ayten A, Eser I, Ozbudak O, Demircan A. Tracheal stenosis after tracheostomy or intubation: Review with special regard to cause and management. *Tex Heart Inst J.* 2005;32(2):154-158.
30. Seldinger ST. Catheter replacement of the needle in percutaneous arteriography. *Acta Radiol.* 1953;39:368-376.
31. Shelden CH, Pudenz RH, Freshwater DB, Crue BL. New method for tracheotomy. *J Neurosurg.* 1955;12:428-431.
32. Toy FJ, Weinstein JD. A percutaneous tracheotomy device. *Surg.* 1969;65:384-389.
33. Schachner A, Ovil Y, Sidi J, Rogev M, Heilbronn Y, Levy MJ. Percutaneous tracheotomy: A new method. *Crit Care Med.* 1989;17:1052-1056.
34. Griggs WM, Worthley LIG, Gilligan JE, Thomas PD, Myburg JA. A simple percutaneous tracheotomy technique. *Surg Gynecol Obstet.* 1990;170:543-546.
35. Couch ME, Bhatti N. The current status of percutaneous tracheotomy. *Adv Surg.* 2002;36:275-296.
36. Kost KM. Endoscopic percutaneous dilatational tracheotomy: A prospective evaluation of 500 consecutive cases. *Laryngoscope.* 2005;115:1-30.
37. El A, Solh AA, Jaafar W. A comparative study of the complications of surgical tracheostomy in morbidly obese critically ill patients. *Crit Care Med.* 2006;34(12)Suppl:A95.

38. Abouzgheib W, Meena N, Jagtap P, Schorr C, Boujaoude Z, Bartter T. Percutaneous dilational tracheostomy in patients receiving antiplatelet therapy: is it safe? *J Bronchology Interv Pulmonol.* 2013;20:322-325.
39. Patel D, Devulapally K, Islam S. Safety of percutaneous tracheostomy in patients with coagulopathy and high ventilatory demand. *Chest.* 2009;136(4):50S
40. Mayberry JC, Wu IC, Goldman RK, Chesnut RM. Cervical spine clearance and neck extension during percutaneous tracheostomy in trauma patients. *Crit Care Med.* 2000;28:3436-3440.
41. Meyer M, Critchlow J, Mansharamani N, Angel L, Garland R, Ernst A. Repeat bedside percutaneous dilational tracheostomy is a safe procedure. *Crit Care Med.* 2002;30(5):986-988.
42. Parnes SM, Myers EN. Traction sutures in a tracheostomy using a ligature passer. *Trans Sect Opthalmol Am Acad Ophthalmol Otolaryngol.* 1976;82(4):ORL479–485.
43. Morris L, Whitmer A, McIntosh E. Tracheostomy care and complications in the intensive care unit. *Crit Care Nurs.* 2013;33(5):18-22, 24-31.

3

Types of Tracheostomy Tubes and Related Appliances

by Linda L. Morris

Objectives

- Identify the components of a tracheostomy tube
- Provide general indications for specific tubes
- Pair features of specific tracheostomy tubes with selective applications
- Summarize an array of tracheostomy tubes from an expansive list of manufacturers

Introduction

Each tracheostomy tube has a variety of features, and there are many different tracheostomy tubes to choose from. There are many manufacturers, and all offer different features, materials, lengths, inner and outer diameters, and so forth. Some have a single cannula, while others have dual cannulas—that is, both inner and outer cannulas. Some have low-pressure cuffs, and a few have high-pressure cuffs. Still others are cuffless. The choices are abundant.

Early tracheostomy tubes were composed of metal, either silver or stainless steel. Most modern tracheostomy tubes are composed of medical-grade plastics such as polyvinyl chloride, polyurethane, silicone, or a combination. Although metal tubes are still in use today, softer materials are much more widespread. Plastic tubes have the advantages of being cheaper, lighter, easier to modify for special needs, and, depending on the material, more pliable. These softer materials have allowed for cuffs at the distal end of the tube. Metal tracheostomy tubes have the advantage of thinner walls, but they usually cannot be connected to a ventilator because they do not have cuffs.[1,2]

It is important for the clinician to be aware of the many tube choices available. Because of this variety and the specific features of each tracheostomy tube, most hospitals choose one line of tracheostomies for primary use by all clinicians, supplemented with others as the need arises. This is done primarily for safety reasons so that clinical staff can become familiar with the primary features of one particular line of tubes.

An effort will be made here to discuss the major characteristics of most of the tracheostomy tubes currently on the market in the United States, as well as many tubes from manufacturers in other countries. While the list is not complete, the information will illustrate the tubes' structure with some guided purpose for their use.

PARTS OF A TRACHEOSTOMY TUBE

Most tracheostomy tubes are composed of only a few standard parts, as shown in **Figure 3.1**. For clarity, it is important to be familiar with the names of the major parts of a tracheostomy tube. The shaft of the tracheostomy tube fits, usually entirely, within the trachea. It may be constructed of plastic, silicone, or metal, and may be rigid or flexible. The outer diameter of the tracheostomy tube refers to the widest diameter of the tube itself, excluding the cuff. This diameter varies based on the materials used and the presence of an inner cannula. The outer cannula of each line of tracheostomies varies in terms of materials, length, diameter, angle of curvature, and presence of a cuff.

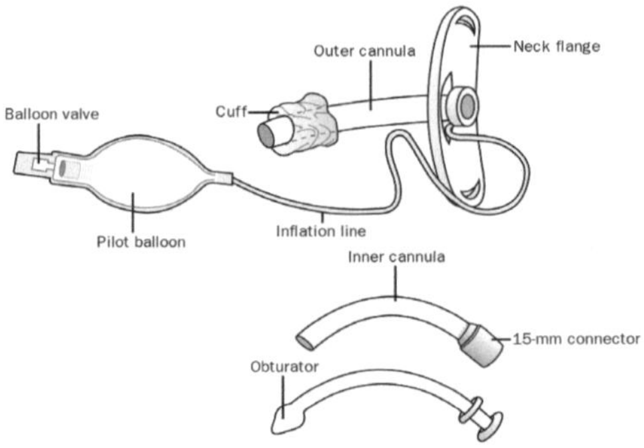

Figure 3.1 Parts of a tracheostomy tube

The curvature of the shaft can be angled differently from one type of tube to another. **Figure 3.2** shows the varied curvatures of tracheostomy tubes. Some tubes have a 90-degree angle, or an angle like the arc of a circle, and others have a narrower angle.

The neck plate, or neck flange, fits directly against the neck and allows the tracheostomy tube to be anchored to the neck. The outer cannula may or may not have a cuff. There may or may not be an inner cannula. Decisions about when and why to place a cuffed versus an uncuffed tracheostomy tube will be discussed in chapter 4. If a cuff is present, it is connected to the pilot balloon by means of an inflation line. The inflation port, or inflation valve, at the distal end of the pilot balloon allows for the attachment of a syringe to inflate the cuff. Only a syringe or pressure measurement device should be connected to the inflation port.

Figure 3.2 Curvature of shafts on different tracheostomy tubes

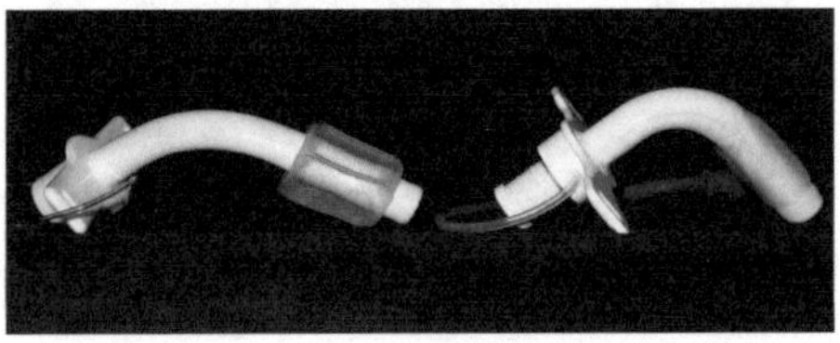

Curvature of shafts on different tracheostomy tubes. Note the relatively narrow angle of the tube on the left (Shiley SCT), compared to the wide angle of the tube on the right Arcadia Air Cuff (no longer manufactured).

Sizing of a Tracheostomy Tube

The size of the tracheostomy tube usually refers to the inner diameter of the inner cannula. In other words, the inner diameter reflects the narrowest diameter of each specific tracheostomy tube. However, there are two sizing systems for tracheostomies: the Jackson sizing system and the International Standards Organization (ISO) sizing system. The Jackson sizing system was initially used with metal tracheostomy tubes and is still used with the Jackson and the legacy Shiley brands. It is important to note that the two largest tracheostomy manufacturers in the United States (Portex and Shiley) use different sizing systems. The Shiley tracheostomies and all of the metal tracheostomy tubes use the Jackson sizing system, while most all other tracheostomy tubes are sized using the ISO system. Shiley has launched a newer line of tracheostomies (the Shiley Flexible) that includes both ISO and Jackson sizing. The ISO sizing system refers to the inner diameter of the outer cannula; however, the Jackson sizing system does not directly refer to the inner diameter.[1,2] For example, the inner diameter of a size 6 Portex cuffed tracheostomy tube is 6.0 mm; however, the inner diameter of a comparable Shiley 6 cuffed tracheostomy tube is 6.4 mm.

St. John and Malen[2] point out that one must consider the inner diameter of the tracheostomy both with and without the inner cannula in place. It is important to take note of these two different inner diameters because they may impact fitting a tracheostomy tube. When the inner cannula is in place, the functional diameter of the tube can decrease by up to 2 mm. These 1 or 2 mm can sometimes make a surprising difference in a patient's ability to breathe comfortably.

The Inner Cannula

The inner cannula, when present, nests within the outer cannula and is secured to it. The primary purpose of the inner cannula is to clear secretions through cleaning or replacement at regular intervals. The standard inner cannula is used most often in the hospital setting because it frequently provides a 15-mm adapter—the standard connection for a manual resuscitation bag, ventilator circuit tubing, and other respiratory and airway appliances. Cosmetic inner cannulas lack this adapter and give a low-profile appearance to the tracheostomy. Therefore, cosmetic or low-profile inner cannulas should probably not be used in the hospital to avoid confusion in case of an emergency. Outside of a hospital, the cosmetic inner cannula may be used when a low-profile appearance is desired.

It is important to ensure that the inner cannula, when present, is locked in place at all times. Different manufacturers provide different locking mechanisms for their tracheostomy tubes, and they are not interchangeable from one manufacturer to another, from one model to another, or from one size to another. Failure to lock the inner cannula can result in inadvertent dislodgement, as it may be easily coughed out.

The Obturator

The sole purpose of the obturator, sometimes called a pilot, is to assist with the insertion of the tracheostomy tube. It is important to note that the obturator cannot be ordered separately and is packaged as part of each separate tube. Depending on the tube, it may be necessary to remove the inner cannula in order for the obturator to fit within the outer cannula. The blunted tip of the obturator cushions the distal tip of the tube as it is inserted, avoiding potential tissue damage as it is advanced into the trachea. Immediately following placement, the obturator should be removed and replaced with the inner cannula (when present). The obturator should then be securely placed in full view, allowing rapid visualization and access in the event of an emergency, such as inadvertent decannulation.

The Neck Flange or Neck Plate

The purpose of the neck flange is to stabilize the tracheostomy tube, seating it against the neck and preventing it from migrating inward. The neck flange contains an opening at its lateral ends so it can be secured to the neck, typically by means of cloth tape, a soft collar, sutures, or sometimes a chain. The neck flange can be fixed to the shaft of the tube, or it can be adjustable and adaptable to a variety of needs.

The neck flange can be rigid or flexible. If rigid, it may tilt on the horizontal plane, the vertical plane, or both. This tilting mechanism is designed to provide comfort as well as adjust for patient movement; however, it can also be a source of inward traction against the stoma. The neck flange should lie flush against the neck and usually lies directly over the stoma, or it can be angled for a better fit in specific patients.

The neck flange is an important source of clinical information. The specifications of each tube are usually imprinted or embossed on it. One can usually find the manufacturer's name, the model name or code, the inner diameter, the outer diameter, and sometimes the length or serial number.

The Pilot Balloon and the Inflation Line

The inflation line is used to inflate or deflate the cuff. At the distal end of the inflation line is the cuff. At the proximal end of the inflation line are the pilot balloon and the inflation valve. The shape of the pilot balloon indicates whether or not there is air within the cuff. A completely flat pilot balloon indicates there is no air in the cuff, and an inflated pilot balloon indicates there is some air in the cuff. Many experienced clinicians believe they can accurately estimate cuff pressure by palpating the pilot balloon; however, one study showed that cuff pressure was accurately estimated by palpation only 61% of the time.[3]

The Cuff

One of the primary purposes of the cuff is to seal the airway, especially with positive-pressure ventilation. When the cuff is inflated, there is no admixture of room air with inspired gases, and the patient breathes entirely through the tracheostomy tube. Deflation of the cuff allows for the admixture of room air as part of the inspired tidal volume.

Cuffs have evolved over time. Early tracheostomy tubes were made of metal, and early cuffs were detachable and often made of rubber. These rubber cuffs created high pressures against the trachea and resulted in numerous complications, including airway obstruction from detached cuffs. Over the years, these high-pressure cuffs have been almost totally replaced by high-volume, low-pressure cuffs.[4]

Cuffs come in different shapes, sizes, and types, some of which are illustrated in **Figure 3.3**. There are barrel-shaped cuffs, teardrop-shaped cuffs, and foam-type cuffs. There are cuffs that are filled with air and others that are filled with fluid. There are still some high-pressure cuffs, but today, most are low-pressure. Each of these cuffs has different characteristics.

Figure 3.3 Shape of cuffs on different tracheostomy tubes

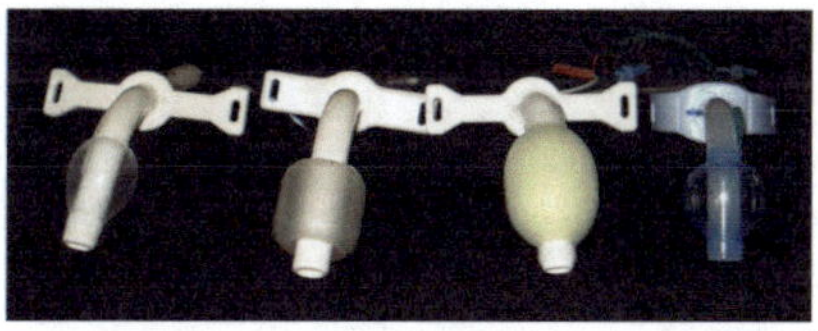

Shape of cuffs on different tracheostomy tubes. From left to right: Bivona TTS (low volume, high pressure). Shiley SCT (barrel shaped, low pressure, high volume). Bivona Fome-Cuf (low pressure, high volume). Portex Blue Line (teardrop shaped, low pressure, high volume).

The barrel-shaped cuff is designed to diffuse pressure along a wider surface area. Rather than creating specific pressure points with a circular balloon, the barrel-shaped cuff minimizes pressure points.

The teardrop-shaped cuff was designed to minimize the pistoning effect— the up-and-down movement of the cuff with positive-pressure breaths. Pistoning will be discussed in chapter 5.

The foam-type cuff tracheostomy tube has an extra-large cuff that naturally expands to fit the shape of the trachea. It was designed to overcome problems with continued leaks around the cuff, while minimizing pressure-related problems.

A deflated cuff that lies tight to the shaft of the tracheostomy tube allows laminar airflow around it, lessening resistance. This is in contrast to the cuffs of most tracheostomy tubes, which have some bulk when deflated. Decisions regarding the most appropriate type of cuff are discussed in chapter 4.

The inflated cuff is used to protect the airway when the patient is unable to do so. It also creates a seal in the airway when delivering positive-pressure ventilation. Inflation of the cuff can help prevent secretions, fluid, or food from entering the lungs, but its success depends on many factors and is not guaranteed. It is important to realize that inflation of the cuff does not prevent aspiration. For a patient who cannot protect his airway, aspiration precautions must be maintained even though the cuff is inflated. This includes elevation of the head of the bed, checking residuals for the patient with enteral feedings, optimizing cuff pressure, and so forth.

Capillary perfusion pressure is considered to be between 20–30 cm H_2O (conversion factor to kPa: 1 cm water = 0.098 kPa).[5,6] The challenge is to maintain a cuff pressure high enough to ensure an adequate seal to provide optimal delivery of positive-pressure breaths and prevent the seepage of secretions around the cuff, yet low enough to minimize pressure against the trachea.

Another purpose of the cuff is to seat the tube squarely in the center of the trachea and protect it from creating erosion against the trachea. Lateralization of the tube can result from herniation of the cuff and/or additional pressure against the trachea. Lateralization can interfere with optimal delivery of positive pressure breaths, which can result in increased airway pressures.

General Types of Tracheostomy Tubes

Tracheostomy tubes can be classified into four major groups: dual-cannula, cuffed; dual-cannula, uncuffed; single-cannula, cuffed; and single-cannula, uncuffed. However, there are certain types of tracheostomy tubes that, while they fit into one of these general categories, have other unique features that require further discussion. These unique tubes include metal tracheostomy tubes, fenestrated tubes, and extra-length tubes. The following is a discussion of the wide variety of tracheostomy tubes available today, with some explanation of their strengths, weaknesses, and indications for use.

Standard Dual-Cannula Cuffed Tracheostomy Tubes

The standard dual-cannula cuffed tracheostomy tube is often the first choice for a patient who requires positive-pressure ventilation or otherwise cannot protect the airway. The inner cannula provides added protection for patients with copious secretions, as it can be easily removed and cleaned or replaced. It is locked in place to the outer cannula, and the method of securing the inner cannula varies by model. The features of different types of dual-cannula tracheostomy tubes are described in the following (**Figures 3.4** through **Figure 3.13** below).

Figure 3.4 DURACUFF®

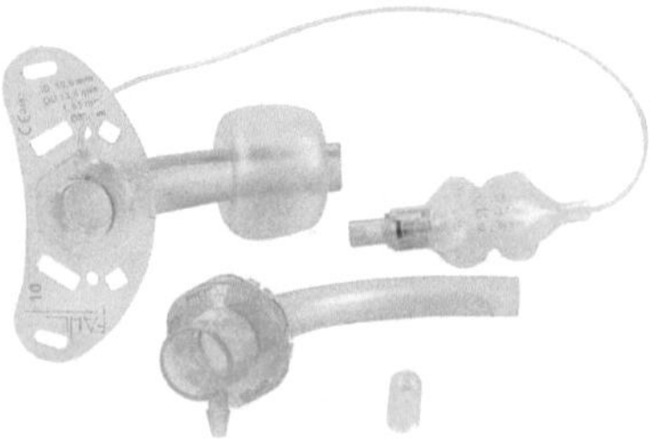

Structure: Cuffed, dual-cannula or single cannula

Material: Medical-grade PVC-DEHP (Di 2-ethylhyxyl phthalate) free

Manufacturer: Andreas Fahl Medizintechnik-Vertrieb GmbH

Unique Features: Has radiopaque contrast strip; comes in three lengths

Use: Patients who require a cuffed tube for positive pressure ventilation, airway protection, or when secretions are a concern

With friendly permission of Andreas Fahl Medizintechnik-Vertrieb GmbH, Cologne, Germany

The DURACUFF® tube is manufactured of medical grade PVC and adapts to the shape of the trachea at body temperature. There is a radiopaque strip along the shaft to allow radiological visualization. The manufacturer recommends using a special cuff pressure gauge to inflate the cuff and suggests that use of a syringe presents a risk of overinflation and subsequent damage to the tracheal wall. The DURACUFF® tracheostomy tube comes in several different models: The DURACUFF® VARIO does not have an inner cannula. The DURACUFF®VARIO-KOMBI LINGO is a "sieved" tube with the addition of a combi-adapter to accommodate a 22-mm adapter (rather than the standard 15-mm connector). The DURACUFF®UNI-VARIO is a tracheostomy tube with two inner cannulas: one with a standard 15-mm connector, and the other with a rotating 15-mm swivel connector. The DURACUFF®VARIO SUCTION has an additional line that ends above the cuff to allow for removal of secretions when connected to suction. The DURACUFF®VARIO-KOMBI

LINGO-PHON is the speaking version of the tube. It is a fenestrated tube with a detachable silicone speaking valve (COMBIPHON®). The DURACUFF®VARIO-KOMBI LINGO-PHON SUCTION is also a fenestrated tube with an additional suction line and a silicone speaking (COMBIPHONE®) valve. The Duracuff O_2 provides an additional oxygen line through a port on the inner cannula.

Figure 3.5 Fahl DURATWIX® UNI VARIO

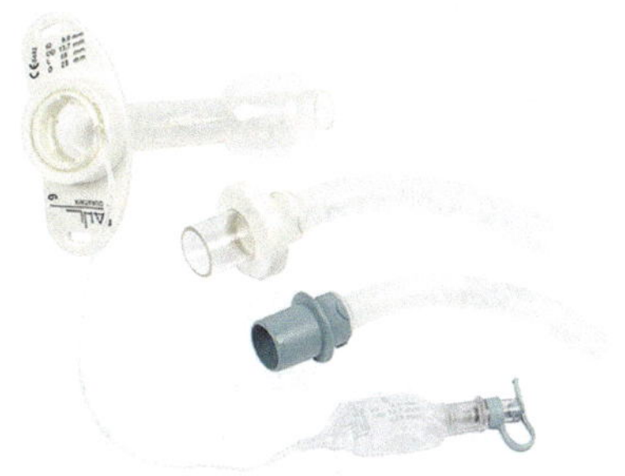

Structure: Cuffed, dual-cannula

Material: Soft, medical grade polyurethane, thermosensitive

Manufacturer: Andreas Fahl Medizintechnik-Vertrieb GmbH

Unique Features: Soft double swivel neck flange, allows 360° rotation for improved neck mobility; available in two lengths

Use: For the patient who requires a cuffed tube for positive pressure ventilation, airway protection, or when secretions may be a concern

With friendly permission of Andreas Fahl Medizintechnik-Vertrieb GmbH, Cologne, Germany

The DURATWIX® tracheostomy tubes have a modular design and are compatible with different adapters and accessories. Cannula surfaces are very smooth, allowing easy glide. Like the DURACUFF®, the DURATWIX® also comes in several versions. The DURATWIX® UNI-VARIO LINGO CUFF is a fenestrated "sieved" tube with single or dual cannulas, with both cuffed and cuffless versions. The manufacturer reports that the special placement of the sieve reduces risk of aspiration. The DURATWIX® UNI CUFF is a single-cannula cuffed tracheostomy tube, and the DURATWIX® UNI is an uncuffed tube with dual or single cannulas.

Figure 3.6 Rüsch CrystalClear Plus

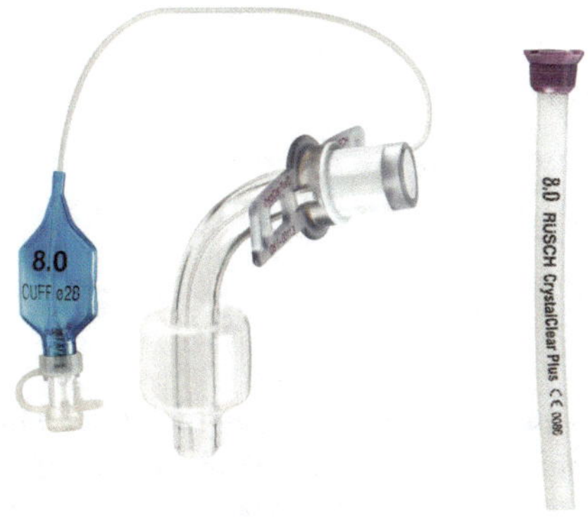

Structure: Cuffed, dual cannula

Material: Thermosensitive PVC

Manufacturer: Teleflex

Unique Features: Transparent neck flange and rotating connector; color-coded hub on inner cannula; comes in a PDT version for use with percutaneous insertion

Use: Patients who require a cuffed tube for positive pressure ventilation, airway protection, or when secretions are a concern

Image courtesy of Teleflex Incorporated. © 2019 Teleflex Incorporated. All rights reserved.

Rüsch Trachflex Plus (no image available)

Structure: Cuffed, dual cannula

Material: Thermosensitive PVC, DEHP-free

Manufacturer: Teleflex

Unique Features: Armored (wire-reinforced) shaft; color-coded hub on inner cannula; there are models of this tube with extended proximal length and extended distal length; comes in a PDT version for use with percutaneous insertion

Use: Patients who require a cuffed tube for positive pressure ventilation, airway protection, or when secretions are a concern

Figure 3.7 Shiley Flexible

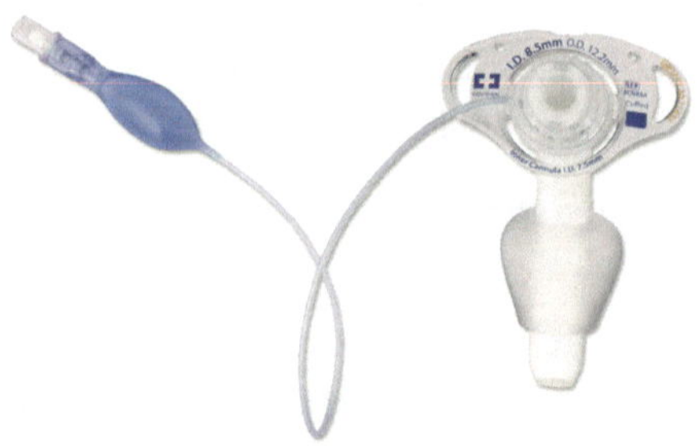

Structure: Dual cannula, cuffed or cuffless tube

Material: Soft, thermosensitive polyvinyl chloride

Manufacturer: Medtronic

Unique Features: less bulky cuff compared to standard Shiley tracheotomy tubes, TaperGuard™ cuff that reduces leakage around it, and transparent flange with window to increase airflow

Use: Patients who require a cuffed tube for positive pressure ventilation, airway protection, or when secretions are a concern

Figure 3.8 Shiley LPC (without inner cannula)

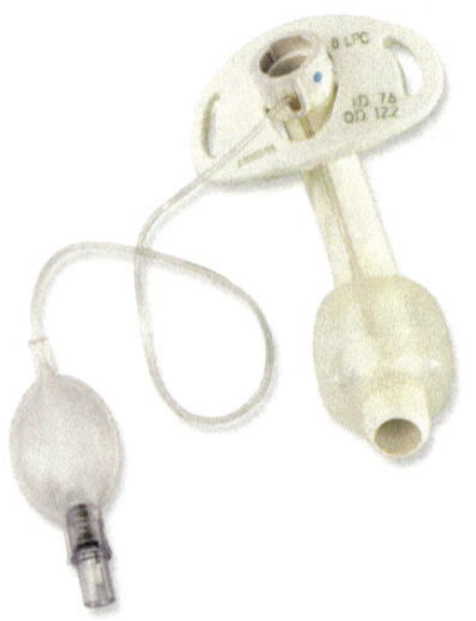

Structure: Cuffed, dual-cannula, arc of circle curvature

Material: Rigid polyvinyl chloride

Manufacturer: Medtronic

Unique Features: Non-disposable inner cannula, rigid neck flange that tilts on horizontal plane

Use: Patients who require a cuffed tube for positive pressure ventilation, airway protection, or when secretions are a concern

The Shiley LPC dual-cannula tracheostomy tube is made of a rigid polyvinyl chloride. The neck flange has a horizontal swivel mechanism that can accommodate some patient movement. The inner cannula locks in place with a twist-lock mechanism. When the blue dot on the outer cannula aligns with the blue dot on the inner cannula, it is locked in place. Unless the blue dots are aligned, the inner cannula can be easily dislodged or coughed out.

The 15-mm connector is built into the inner cannula of all Shiley dual-cannula tracheostomy tubes. Therefore, an inner cannula must be with the patient at all times because respiratory and anesthesia equipment can only be attached when the inner cannula is in place. On the neck flange is printed the size, type, and inner and outer diameter of the tube. The lateral edges of the neck flange have openings of a somewhat softer material so it is easier to attach tracheostomy ties.

Figure 3.9 Shiley DCT (disposable inner cannula)

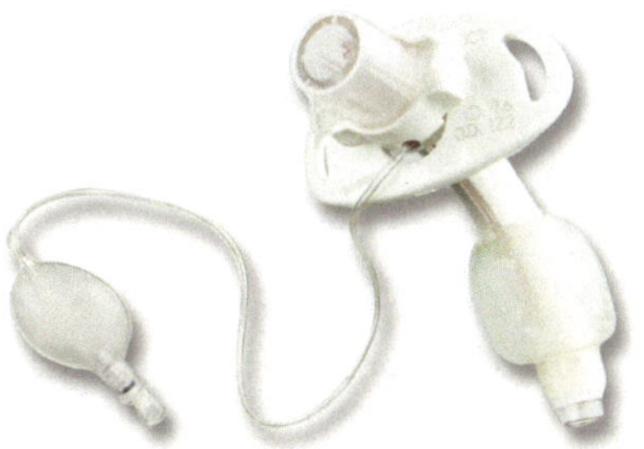

Structure: Cuffed, dual-cannula, arc of circle curvature

Material: Rigid polyvinyl chloride

Manufacturer: Medtronic

Unique Features: Disposable inner cannula, rigid neck flange that tilts on horizontal plane

Use: Patients who require a cuffed tube for positive pressure ventilation, airway protection, or when secretions are a concern

Medtronic makes two standard-sized dual-cannula cuffed tracheostomy tubes. The Shiley LPC provides a non-disposable rigid inner cannula, and the Shiley DCT provides a somewhat softer, disposable inner cannula. The outer cannulas of the Shiley LPC and DCT tracheostomies are almost identical and are constructed of rigid polyvinyl chloride. The primary difference between these two tubes is their locking mechanisms and that the inner cannulas are not interchangeable. With the Shiley DCT, "wings" on each side are pinched together and provide a clipping mechanism (not unlike a telephone jack) when the inner cannula is locked in place. This is in contrast to the twist-lock mechanism of the LPC. The inner cannula of the Shiley DCT is constructed of a softer and more flexible material than the inner cannula of the LPC, and it is intended for limited-time use.

Another difference between the Shiley LPC and DCT tubes is the neck flange. The neck flange of the LPC is rounded and semiflexible; however, the neck flange of the DCT can be rectangular and rigid. For both the Shiley LPC and DCT, the inflation line lies on the shaft of the outer cannula. With all Shiley dual-cannula tracheostomy tubes, the attachment of a manual resuscitation bag or ventilator is possible only when the inner cannula is locked in place.

Figure 3.10 Shiley PERC (percutaneous)

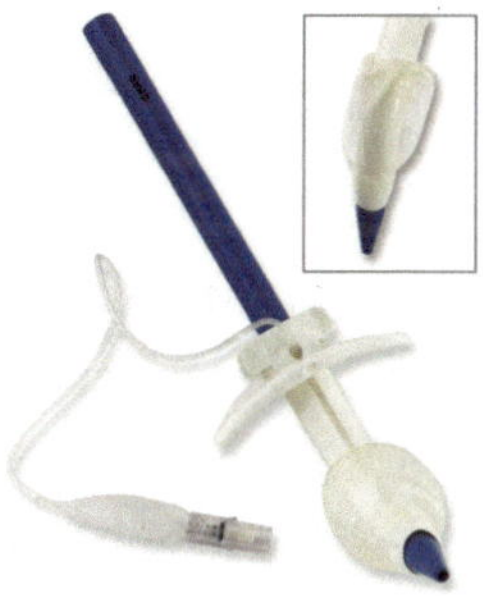

Structure: Cuffed, dual-cannula, arc of circle curvature

Material: Rigid polyvinyl chloride

Manufacturer: Medtronic

Unique Features: Tapered distal tip and inverted cuff shoulder allow ease of insertion when loaded on dilator

Use: For placement with percutaneous tracheostomy procedure

The Shiley percutaneous tracheostomy tube, PERC, is included in a kit manufactured by Cook Medical in their line of percutaneous tracheostomy introducer sets and trays. The tube itself is very similar to the Shiley DCT tube; however, the distal tip is tapered and the cuff has an inverted shoulder to facilitate its placement with an introducer. With the PERC, the introducer is also a dilator. Using the modified Ciaglia technique, the PERC is advanced into place while it is loaded on the dilator—called the Blue Rhino or the newer, fluid-filled Blue Dolphin. The percutaneous technique of tracheostomy placement is discussed in chapter 2.

Portex Per-fit (no image available)

Structure: Cuffed, dual-cannula

Material: Rigid polyvinyl chloride

Manufacturer: Smiths Medical

Unique Features: Tapered distal tip and inverted cuff shoulder allow ease of insertion when loaded on dilator

Use: For use with percutaneous procedure

The Portex version of the percutaneous tracheostomy is called the Portex Per-fit. The tube itself is made of flexible polyvinyl chloride with a tapered distal tip and low-profile cuff. The percutaneous tracheostomy kit has a series of dilators for use with the Ciaglia technique. The tapered distal tips of both the Shiley PERC and the Portex Per-fit are designed for an easier fit over a dilator, facilitating easier insertion.

Figure 3.11 Cook VersaTube

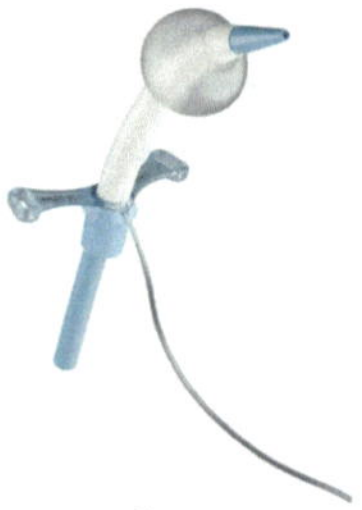

Structure: Dual cannula, cuffed tube

Material: Soft polyvinyl chloride

Manufacturer: Cook Medical

Unique Features: Tapered distal tip for fit on a dilator, color-coded inner cannula

Use: For use with percutaneous procedure

Permission for use granted by Cook Medical, Bloomington, Indiana

Figure 3.12 Portex DIC

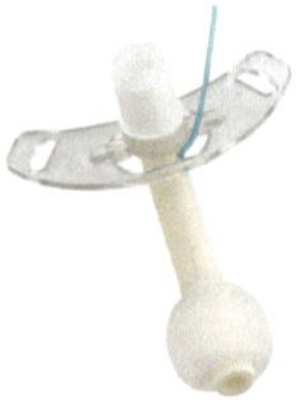

Structure: Cuffed, dual-cannula, arched curve

Material: Rigid polyvinyl chloride

Manufacturer: Smiths Medical

Unique Features: Color-coded inner cannula to identify size; the 15-mm connector is fused with the outer cannula so that a manual resuscitation bag can be used without the inner cannula in place

Use: Patients who require a cuffed tube for positive pressure ventilation, airway protection, or when secretions are a concern

Photo courtesy of Smiths Medical

Portex also makes two dual-cannula cuffed tracheostomy tubes. Made of polyethylene, the Portex DIC cuffed tracheostomy tube provides a rigid structure to the tube. The 15-mm adapter of the Portex DIC is color coded based on size. **Table 3.1** shows the colors related to size.

Table 3.1. Color-coded Inner Cannulas for Portex DIC

Color of 15-mm Connector	**Size (Inner Diameter)**
Orange	6
Green	7
White	8
Blue	9
Yellow	10

The neck flange of the Portex tracheostomy tube is soft and pliable and may offer more comfort than a rigid neck flange. The inner cannula of the Portex DIC is removed by lifting up on the ring and pulling it out or pushing it in until it snaps in place. In contrast to the Shiley LPC or DCT, patients with a Portex DIC or Portex Flex DIC tracheostomy can be ventilated with or without the inner cannula in place.

Portex Flex DIC (no image available)

Structure: Cuffed, dual-cannula, arched curve

Material: Flexible polyvinyl chloride with silicone coating

Manufacturer: Smiths Medical

Unique Features: Color-coded inner cannula to identify size

Use: Patients who require a cuffed tube for positive pressure ventilation, airway protection, or when secretions are a concern

The Portex Flex DIC cuffed tracheostomy tube is made of a softer thermosensitive polyvinyl chloride with a silicone coating. Because of the difference in material, the outer diameters are different than the standard Portex DIC; however, the color-coding system for the inner cannula is the same (**Table 3.1**). The Portex DIC and Flex DIC tubes have an arched curve to the shaft, similar to the Shiley LPC and DCT. The Portex DIC and Flex DIC both have a barrel-shaped cuff.

Figure 3.13 TRACOE Twist Series

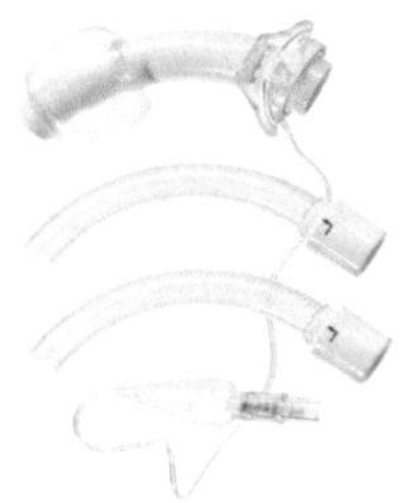

Structure: Cuffed, dual-cannula

Material: Flexible thermoelastic polyurethane

Manufacturer: TRACOE

Unique Features: Neck flange that rotates on two planes

Use: Patients who require a cuffed tube for positive pressure ventilation, airway protection, or when secretions are a concern

The TRACOE Twist series of tracheostomy tubes is similar to the Shiley LPC in that they have a cuff and consist of an inner cannula nested into an outer cannula with a twist-lock mechanism. However, they are made of a more flexible material—polyurethane—that becomes more pliable at body temperature. Another difference is that the neck flange moves on two planes, both vertically and horizontally, accommodating more patient movement.

The TRACOE Twist line of tubes comes in a wide variety of features. There are dual-cannula cuffed tubes, dual-cannula cuffless tubes, cuffed tubes with suction lines, fenestrated cuffed tubes, fenestrated cuffless tubes, cuffed tubes with oxygen supply lines, and cuffed tubes with air supply lines. All these tracheostomy tubes have the same dimensions of inner diameter, outer diameter, and length.

Portex Lo-Profile Cuffed Tube (no image available)

Structure: Cuffed, dual-cannula

Material: Polyvinyl chloride

Manufacturer: Smiths Medical

Unique Features: Clear neck flange and 15-mm connector, low profile, semi-reusable inner cannula

Use: For the patient who requires a cuffed tube but desires a less conspicuous appearance

The Portex Lo-Profile series of tracheostomy tubes are designed "for the active patient." They have a clear neck flange and a clear, low-profile inner cannula. They are also packaged with a standard inner cannula with a clear 15-mm connector. They come in cuffed and cuffless versions. The inner cannula is semi-reusable, meaning it can be cleaned and reused up to 21 times. As opposed to the Portex Blue Line series, DIC series, and Flex DIC series of tracheostomy tubes, the inflation line and pilot balloon of the Portex Lo-Profile tubes are clear.

Dual-Cannula Cuffless Tracheostomy Tubes

Cuffless dual-cannula tracheostomy tubes **(Figure 3.14** through **Figure 3.21)** should be used only in those patients who can protect their airway and are best used for those who also have thick or large quantities of secretions. In this circumstance, the inner cannula can be removed and cleaned or replaced to prevent obstruction of the tube. This type of tube is ideally suited for the patient who can protect the airway, who does not require positive-pressure ventilation, and who wishes to speak; however, secretions may be an issue.

The Portex versions of dual-cannula cuffless tracheostomy tubes are the Portex DIC uncuffed and the Portex Flex DIC uncuffed tubes. Both tubes have color-coded inner cannulas.

Figure 3.14 Fahl DURATWIX® UNI

Structure: Cuffless, dual-cannula

Material: Soft, medical grade polymer

Manufacturer: Andreas Fahl Medizintechnik-Vertrieb GmbH

Unique Features: The soft double-swivel neck flange allows free movement of the neck flange in all directions; available in two lengths

Use: For the patient who can protect the airway, yet secretions may be a concern

With friendly permission of Andreas Fahl Medizintechnik-Vertrieb GmbH, Cologne, Germany

Figure 3.15 Fahl DURAVENT®®

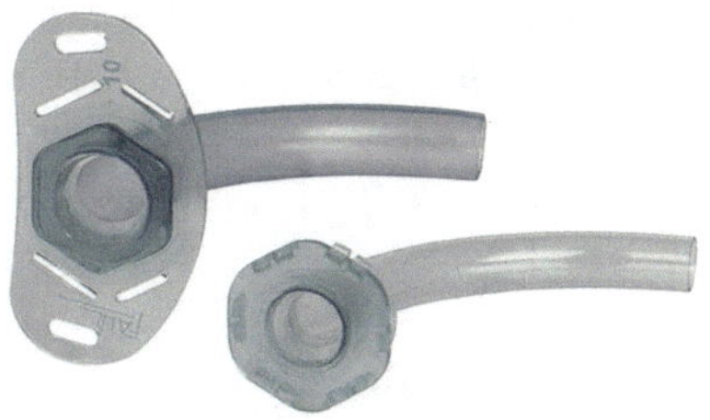

Structure: Uncuffed, dual-cannula

Material: Medical grade polymer

Manufacturer: Andreas Fahl Medizintechnik-Vertrieb GmbH

Unique Features: Radiolucent contrast strip for radiological visualization; easy-lock that secures inner cannula and other accessories to outer cannula

Use: For the patient who can protect the airway, yet secretions may be a concern

With friendly permission of Andreas Fahl Medizintechnik-Vertrieb GmbH, Cologne, Germany

The DURAVENT® tube has several versions. The DURAVENT® LINGO has a fenestrated inner cannula and a "sieved" outer cannula and can also accommodate a speaking valve. The DURAVENT® KOMBI is also a fenestrated tube with the addition of a combi-adapter to accommodate a 22-mm adapter (rather than the standard 15-mm connector). The DURAVENT® UNI has inner cannulas with 15-mm connector. The DURAVENT® UNI-KOMBI has two inner cannulas: one with a 15-mm connector and one with a 22-mm connector. The DURAVENT® UNI LINGO-PHON also has a fenestrated model with a low-profile silver speaking valve, and another model with a silicone speaking valve.

Figure 3.16 Portex DIC Uncuffed

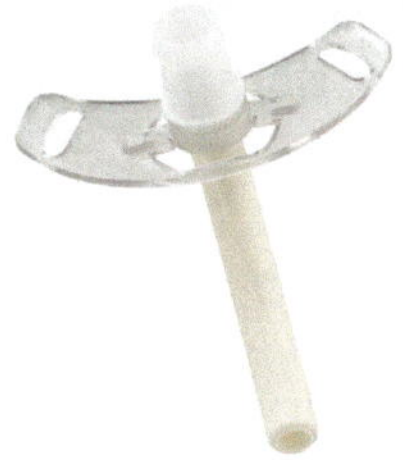

Structure: Dual-cannula, cuffless, curved arch to the shaft

Material: Rigid polyvinyl chloride

Manufacturer: Smiths Medical

Unique Features: Disposable and color-coded inner cannula

Use: For the patient who can protect the airway, yet secretions may be a concern

Photo courtesy of Smiths Medical

The Portex DIC uncuffed tracheostomy tube is identical to the Portex DIC except that it is cuffless. The inner cannula is color coded based on size (**Table 3.1**). It includes a locking ring that secures the inner cannula to the outer cannula. The disposable inner cannula is removed and replaced on a regular basis—usually every eight hours—to prevent the accumulation of secretions. The disposable inner cannula is often preferred by nurses because it saves cleaning time (see chapter 7).

Portex Flex DIC Uncuffed (no image available)

Structure: Dual-cannula, cuffless, curved arch to the shaft

Material: Flexible thermosensitive polyvinyl chloride with silicone coating

Manufacturer: Smiths Medical

Unique Features: Color-coded inner cannula to identify size

Use: For the patient who can protect the airway, yet secretions may be a concern

The materials for these uncuffed tubes are the same as the cuffed versions. The Portex Flex DIC tracheostomy tube is made of a softer thermosensitive polyvinyl chloride with a silicone coating, and the Portex DIC is made of a rigid polyvinyl chloride. The color-coding system for the inner cannula is also the same (**Table 3.1**). The Portex DIC and Portex Flex DIC tracheostomy tubes have an arched curve to the shaft, similar to the Shiley LPC and DCT.

Figure 3.17 Shiley CFS (without inner cannula)

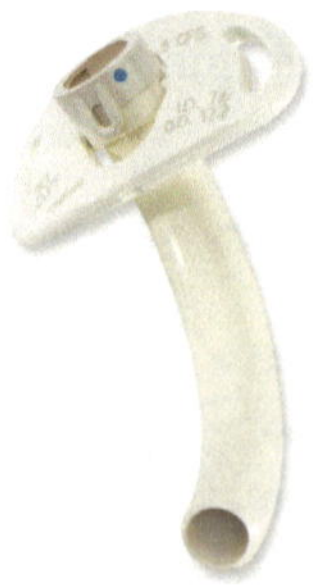

Structure: Dual-cannula, cuffless, arched curve to the shaft

Material: Rigid polyvinyl chloride

Manufacturer: Medtronic

Unique Features: Cosmetic inner cannula and capped inner cannula are included in kit

Use: For the patient who can protect the airway, yet secretions may be a concern

The Shiley CFS is identical to the LPC except that it is cuffless. It is constructed of rigid polyvinyl chloride. The CFS is packaged with a standard inner cannula, a capped inner cannula, a cosmetic inner cannula, and an obturator. The cosmetic inner cannula may be used to provide a low-profile appearance; however, its use should be restricted in the hospital because it does not provide a 15-mm connector, so it is impossible to connect to a manual resuscitation bag or ventilator. The capped inner cannula is used to provide a low-profile appearance when a cap is in place. The outer tip of the capped inner cannula is red for clear visibility.

Figure 3.18 Shiley DCFS (without inner cannula)

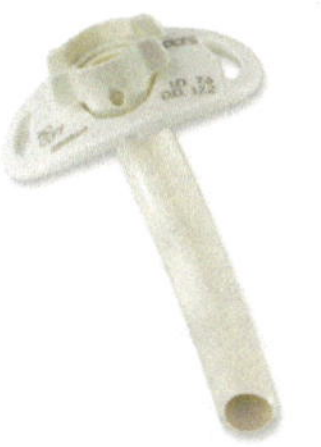

Structure: Dual-cannula, cuffless

Material: Rigid polyvinyl chloride

Manufacturer: Medtronic

Unique Features: Disposable inner cannula

Use: For the patient who can protect the airway, yet secretions may be a concern

The Shiley DCFS tracheostomy tube is identical to the Shiley DCT tube except that it is cuffless. Like the DCT, the inner cannula is disposable and locks in place with a clipping mechanism.

Figure 3.19 Shiley Flexible Cuffless

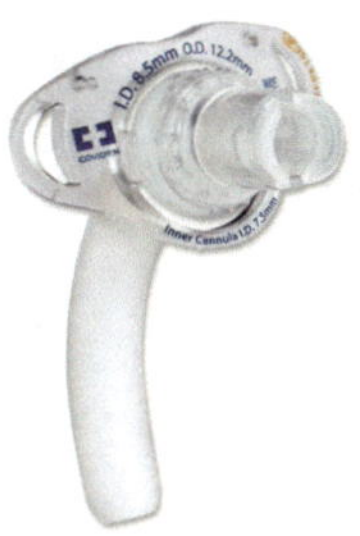

Structure: Dual cannula, cuffed or cuffless tube

Material: Soft thermosensitive PVC

Manufacturer: Medtronic

Unique Features: Less bulky cuff compared to standard Shiley tracheotomy tubes, TaperGuard™ cuff that reduces leakage around it, and transparent flange with window to increase airflow

Use: For the patient who can protect his airway, yet secretions may be a concern

Figure 3.20 TRACOE Twist Cuffless

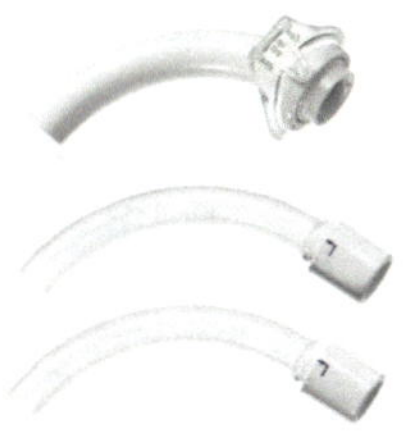

Structure: Dual-cannula, cuffless

Material: Flexible thermoelastic polyurethane

Manufacturer: TRACOE

Unique Features: Packaged with two inner cannulas

Use: For the patient who can protect the airway, yet secretions may be a concern

The TRACOE Twist cuffless tracheostomy tubes are made of medical-grade polyurethane and are identical to the TRACOE Twist cuffed tubes, but without the cuff. They are packaged with two individual inner cannulas with 15-mm connectors.

Figure 3.21 TRACOE Comfort

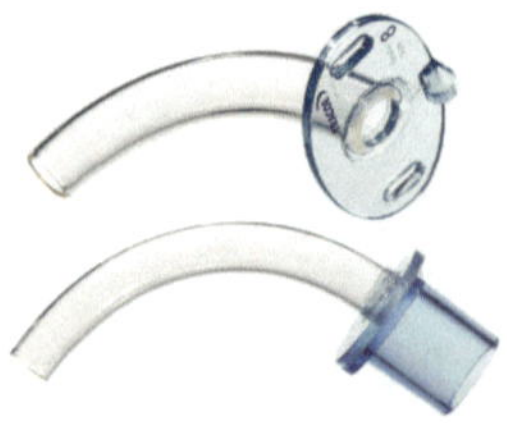

Structure: Uncuffed, single- or dual-cannula

Material: Flexible polyvinyl chloride

Manufacturer: TRACOE

Unique Features: Clear, flexible, lightweight, and soft material

Use: When positive pressure ventilation is not required and secretions are not a concern

The TRACOE Comfort line of tracheostomy tubes is made of a very soft, flexible, clear, and lightweight medical polymer. They are always cuffless and come with or without an inner cannula. Most of the models are low profile in nature and do not have 15-mm adapters; however, one of the models (103 A) comes with a 15-mm adapter on the inner cannula, so positive pressure ventilation can be applied. Model 104 comes with a swivel speaking valve. Model 103 comes with a silver speaking valve and can also be ordered with an oxygen supply port. The manufacturer recommends that paraffin oil be used with the dual-cannula tracheostomy tubes. It should be used at least every other day to lubricate the inner cannula, and ensure it is easy to insert and remove.

Portex Lo-Profile Uncuffed Tube (no image available)

Structure: Dual-cannula, cuffless

Material: Polyvinyl chloride

Manufacturer: Smiths Medical

Unique Features: Clear neck flange and 15-mm connector; clear, low-profile, semi-resuable inner cannula

Use: For the patient who can protect their airway, yet secretions may be a concern and who desires a less conspicuous appearance

The Portex Lo-Profile tracheostomy tubes also come in cuffless versions. For specific information about this tube, refer to the earlier section describing the Portex Lo-Profile cuffed tracheostomy tube.

Single-Cannula Cuffed Tracheostomy Tubes

Single-cannula cuffed tracheostomy tubes **(Figure 3.22** through **Figure 3.34)** are used for patients who require a cuffed tube for airway protection or positive-pressure ventilation but for whom secretions are not a major concern. Because there is no inner cannula, single-cannula tracheostomy tubes have a narrower outer diameter than comparably sized dual-cannula tubes.

Figure 3.22 Angiplast Cuffed Tube

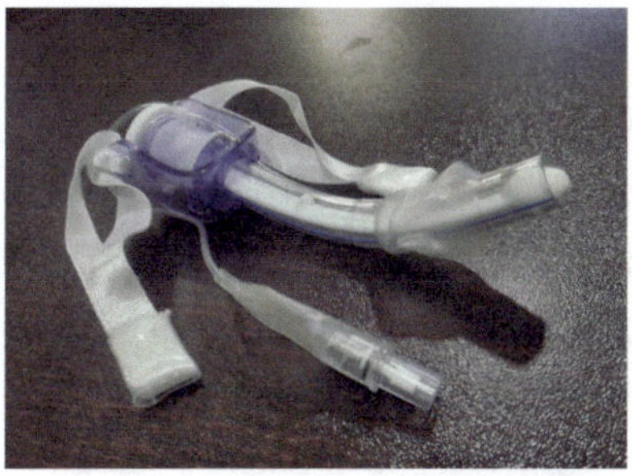

Structure: Cuffed, single-cannula

Material: Siliconized polyvinyl chloride

Manufacturer: Angiplast

Unique Features: Cuffed sizes in 5.0 to 10.0 mm; cuffless sizes 4.0 to 10.0 mm

Use: For the patient who requires a cuff, yet for whom secretions are not a concern

Photo courtesy of Angiplast

Figure 3.23 Fahl DURACUFF® Cuffed Tube

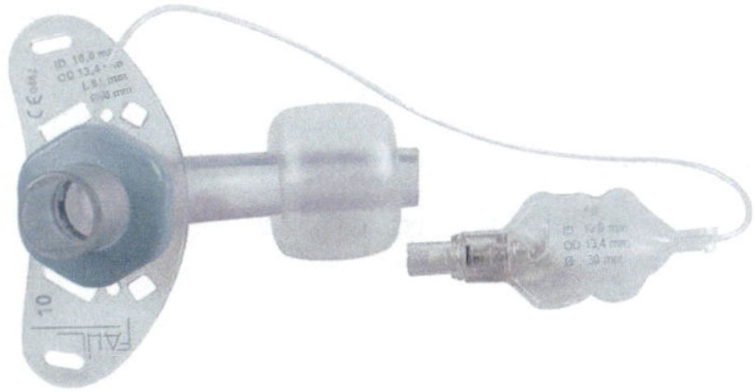

Structure: Cuffed, dual-cannula or single cannula

Material: Medical-grade PVC-DEHP free

Manufacturer: Andreas Fahl Medizintechnik-Vertrieb GmbH

Unique Features: Has radiopaque contrast strip; comes in three lengths

Use: Patients who require a cuffed tube for positive pressure ventilation, airway protection, or when secretions are a concern; the Duracuff UNI also comes in a version with an additional suction line to remove secretions above the cuff

With friendly permission of Andreas Fahl Medizintechnik-Vertrieb GmbH, Cologne, Germany

Fahl DURACUFF® VARIO (no image available)

Structure: Cuffed, single-cannula

Material: Medical grade PVC-DEHP free

Manufacturer: Andreas Fahl Medizintechnik-Vertrieb GmbH

Unique Features: There is a radiopaque strip along the shaft to allow visualization, and there are several models with different features

Use: For the patient who requires a cuffed tube for positive pressure ventilation or airway protection, yet secretions may not be a concern

Figure 3.24 Fahl DURATWIX UNI CUFF

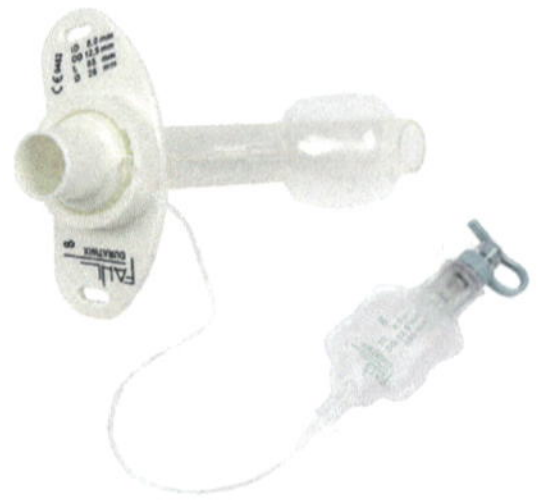

Structure: Cuffed, single-cannula

Material: Soft, medical grade polyurethane

Manufacturer: Andreas Fahl Medizintechnik-Vertrieb GmbH

Unique Features: Ball joint between neck flange and tube allows free movement of the neck flange in all directions; available in two lengths

Use: For the patient who requires a cuffed tube for positive pressure ventilation or airway protection, yet secretions may not be a concern

With friendly permission of Andreas Fahl Medizintechnik-Vertrieb GmbH, Cologne, Germany

Figure 3.25 Fahl SPIRAFLEX® UNI CUFF

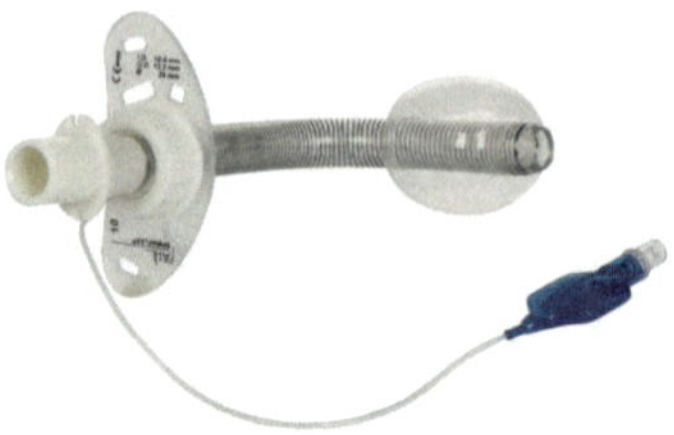

Structure: Cuffed, single-cannula

Material: Soft, medical grade polymer with wire reinforcement

Manufacturer: Andreas Fahl Medizintechnik-Vertrieb GmbH

Unique Features: Adjustable neck flange; wire reinforced

Use: For the patient who requires a cuffed tube for positive pressure ventilation or airway protection, yet secretions may not be a concern

With friendly permission of Andreas Fahl Medizintechnik-Vertrieb GmbH, Cologne, Germany

Figure 3.26 Fahl TRACHEOTEC® VARIO CUFF

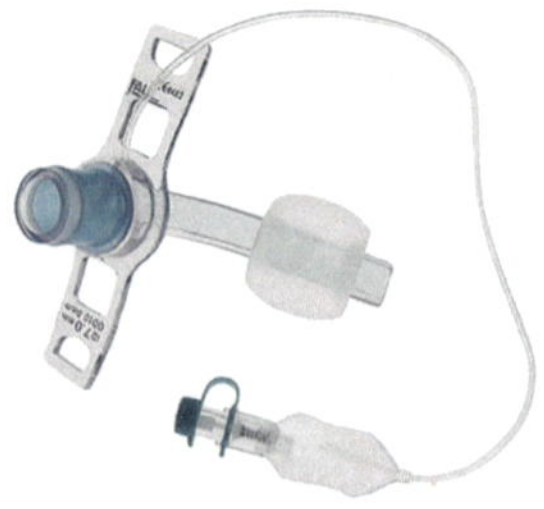

Structure: Cuffed, single-cannula

Material: Soft, medical grade polymer

Manufacturer: Andreas Fahl Medizintechnik-Vertrieb GmbH

Unique Features: Clear and transparent tube shaft with x-ray contrast strip

Use: For the patient who requires a cuffed tube for positive pressure ventilation or airway protection, yet secretions may not be a concern

With friendly permission of Andreas Fahl Medizintechnik-Vertrieb GmbH, Cologne, Germany

There are three additional models of the TRACHEOTEC®. The TRACHEOTEC® VARIO has a 15-mm swivel adapter and the TRACHEOTEC® VARIO CUFF is a cuffed tube, and the TRACHEOTEC® VARIO CUFF-SUCTION has an additional suction line to remove secretions above the cuff.

Figure 3.27 Rüsch CrystalClear Plus

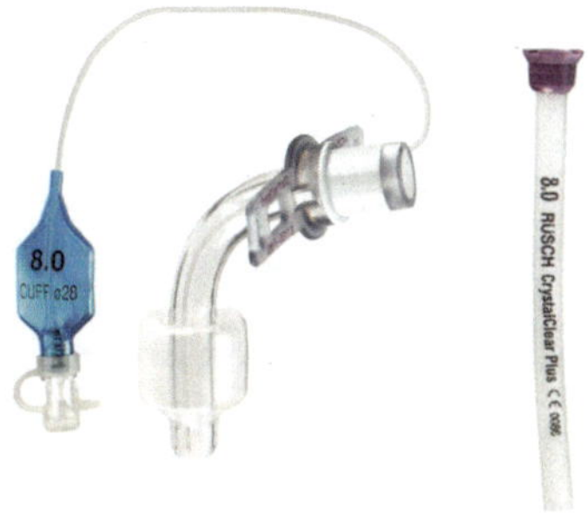

Structure: Cuffed, single cannula (with optional inner cannula)

Material: Thermosensitive PVC

Manufacturer: Teleflex

Unique Features: Transparent neck flange and rotating connector; color-coded hub on inner cannula; blue pilot balloon

Use: For the patient who requires a cuffed tube for positive pressure ventilation or airway protection, yet secretions may not be a concern

Rüsch SafetyClear (no image available)

Structure: Cuffed, single cannula

Material: Thermosensitive PVC

Manufacturer: Teleflex

Unique Features: Blue pilot balloon

Use: For the patient who requires a cuffed tube for positive pressure ventilation or airway protection, yet secretions may not be a concern

Figure 3.28 Shiley SCT

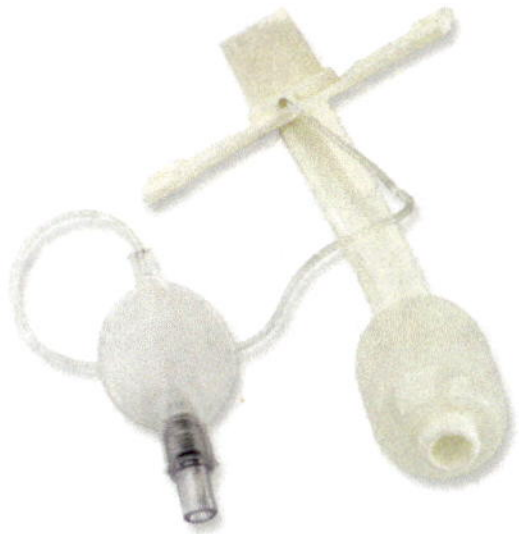

Structure: Cuffed, single-cannula

Material: Flexible polyvinyl chloride

Manufacturer: Medtronic

Unique Features: Longer shaft than comparably sized tube

Use: For the patient who requires a cuff, yet for whom secretions are not a concern; can also be used when a longer tube is desired

The Shiley SCT is constructed of polyvinyl chloride but is more flexible than standard Shiley tubes. It is the only Shiley tracheostomy tube without an inner cannula, and as such, the outer diameter is narrower than a comparable dual-cannula tracheostomy tube. It is also distinctly longer than a comparably sized Shiley DCT or LPC. As opposed to the standard Shiley tubes, the SCT uses the ISO sizing system. The manufacturer recommends that no solution other than saline be used to clean any part of the tube.

Portex Blue Line (no image available)

Structure: Cuffed, single-cannula, 90-degree curvature to the shaft

Material: Siliconized polyvinyl chloride

Manufacturer: Smiths Medical

Unique Features: Identifiable by its blue neck flange, inflation line, and pilot balloon

Use: For the patient who requires a cuff, yet for whom secretions are not a concern; however, a separate inner cannula can be used when necessary

Figure 3.29 Portex Blue Line Ultra

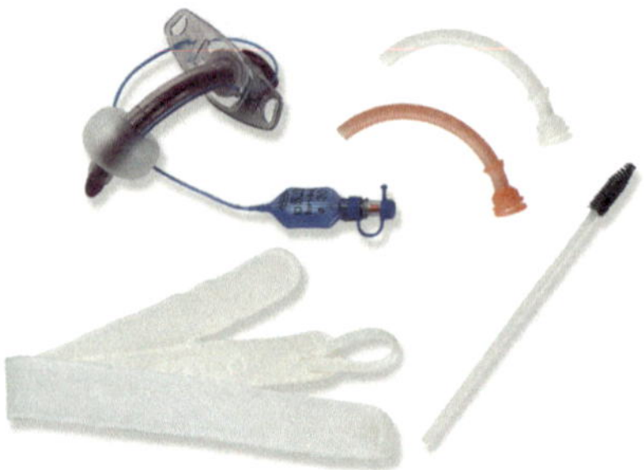

Structure: Cuffed, single-cannula

Material: Siliconized polyvinyl chloride

Manufacturer: Smiths Medical

Unique Features: Presence of a central channel to accommodate guidewire; larger curvature than standard Blue Line tube

Use: For the patient who requires a cuff, yet for whom secretions are not a concern

Photo courtesy of Smiths Medical

The Portex Blue Line Ultra series of tracheostomy tubes is very similar to the standard Portex Blue Line tubes but with a larger curvature. This feature theoretically allows the cuff to be more centrally placed within the airway. The inner cannula of the Blue Line Ultra decreases the diameter of the airway by 1 mm, as opposed to 2 mm for the other Portex tracheostomy tubes.

There is also a type of Blue Line Ultra tracheostomy tube that provides an extra port for subglottic suctioning of secretions that accumulate above the cuff (Suctionaid). One of the most unique features of the Blue Line Ultra is the presence of a central channel through the obturator that can accommodate a guidewire for insertion.

Figure 3.30 Bivona Mid-Range Aire-Cuf

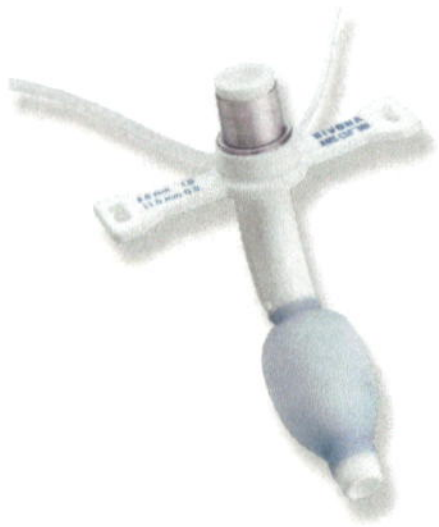

Structure: Cuffed, single-cannula

Material: Silicone

Manufacturer: Smiths Medical

Unique Features: 360-degree swivel adapter; soft, "low-trauma" tip

Use: For the patient who requires a cuff, yet for whom secretions are not a concern

Photo courtesy of Smiths Medical

The Bivona Mid-Range Aire-Cuf tracheostomy tube has a flexible neck flange, a white inflation line, and a blue pilot balloon.

All of the Bivona tracheostomy tubes, regardless of the line, are constructed entirely of silicone and are more flexible. The theoretical advantage to silicone is that secretions are less likely to adhere to the material; however, no studies have been conducted to verify this claim. All Bivona tracheostomy tubes are single cannula tubes and have 360-degree swivel adapters to accommodate some patient movement. Bivona tracheostomy tubes also come with a disconnect wedge, which is helpful because the single-molded 15-mm swivel connector can sometimes get wedged into the adaptor of a manual resuscitation bag or ventilator tubing. The forceful removal of any device from a Bivona tracheostomy tube can result in permanent damage to the tube, so the use of the disconnect wedge is advised whenever removing any device from this tube. In addition, the obturators have been redesigned to be hollow, supporting the use of a guidewire as a tube exchanger.

Figure 3.31 Bivona Fome-Cuf

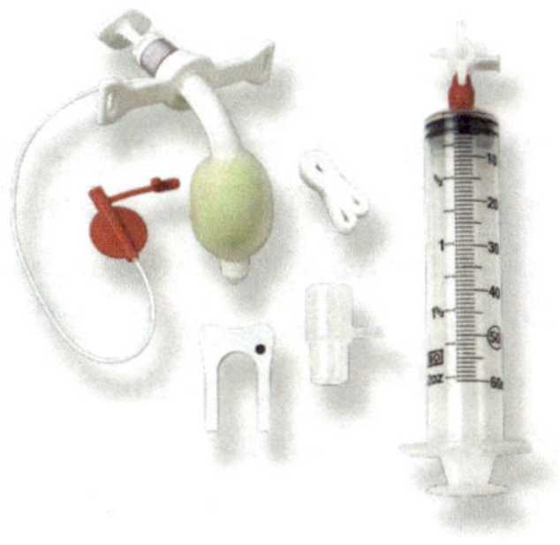

Photo courtesy of Smiths Medical

Structure: Cuffed, single-cannula

Material: Silicone

Manufacturer: Smiths Medical

Unique Features: Default-inflated, foam-filled cuff that expands automatically to fit tracheal diameter

Use: For the patient who has repeated cuff leaks and does not desire to speak

The Bivona Fome-Cuf tracheostomy tube is constructed entirely of silicone. The Fome-Cuf tube is unique in that it provides a large, self-inflating cuff that adjusts itself to the patient's trachea. Once in place, the pilot balloon should remain open to air at all times, and no additional air should be injected into this cuff. This tracheostomy tube is inserted by first deflating the cuff completely. Because of the extra-large cuff, this is best done with the large syringe and three-way stopcock that comes in the tracheostomy kit. The deflated cuff is particularly bulky; however, when inflated, it is usually able to provide a complete seal within the airway.

The Fome-Cuf tracheostomy tube may be chosen when positive-pressure ventilation is required. Over time, however, moisture may collect within the cuff, especially when using the ventilator adapter. Consequently, routine cuff deflation is recommended every eight hours. It is also recommended that this tracheostomy tube be routinely changed at least every month to minimize the collection of moisture and debris and prevent solidification within the cuff.

If the ventilator circuit attachment should become difficult to remove from the 15-mm connector of the tube, the Fome-Cuf tube has a disconnect wedge that can be used as a lever to simplify removal. Forceful attempts to remove the circuit can result in damage to the tracheostomy tube itself. The manufacturer's recommendations state that these tracheostomy tubes should not be used with lasers or electrosurgical devices.

Figure 3.32 Bivona TTS (Tight-to-Shaft)

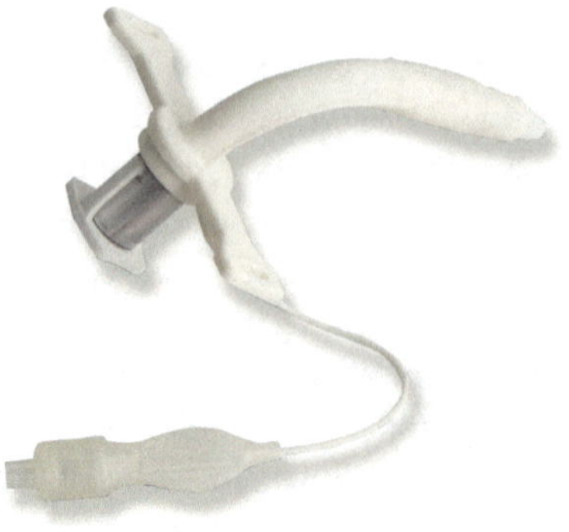

Structure: Cuffed, single-cannula

Material: Silicone

Manufacturer: Smiths Medical

Unique Features: When this high-pressure cuff is deflated, it lies tight to the shaft, minimizing resistance when breathing around the tube; when prolonged cuff inflation is desired, it should be inflated with sterile water; because the cuff essentially disappears upon deflation, this tube is the only cuffed tube that may be safely capped when deflated

Use: Ideal for the patient who requires intermittent positive-pressure ventilation, yet who also desires to speak

Photo courtesy of Smiths Medical

The Bivona Tight-to-Shaft, or TTS, tracheostomy tube is constructed of silicone material and provides some flexibility. It is a single-cannula tracheostomy tube whose most notable feature is its cuff, which, when deflated, lies tight to the shaft of the tube—hence its name. The TTS is ideally suited for the patient who may require intermittent cuff inflation (such as for nocturnal ventilation) yet who wishes to speak at intervals when the cuff is deflated. The TTS design provides laminar flow around the outside of the tube, so it can be capped to allow phonation. (The details of phonation will be discussed in chapter 6.) It is important to note that the cuff of the TTS is a high-pressure cuff, so precautions must be taken to minimize pressure against the tracheal wall. This is best done using minimal leak technique.

The cuff of the TTS tracheostomy tube is inflated with sterile water (not saline) in order to minimize gas permeability across the cuff that might otherwise result when air is used for cuff inflation. This gas permeability manifests as cuff deflation over time. The TTS tracheostomy tube is packaged with a disconnection wedge to be used in case the ventilator circuit becomes difficult to remove from the 15-mm connector. If force is used, the TTS tracheostomy tube can become damaged.

Figure 3.33 Rüsch Trachflex Plus

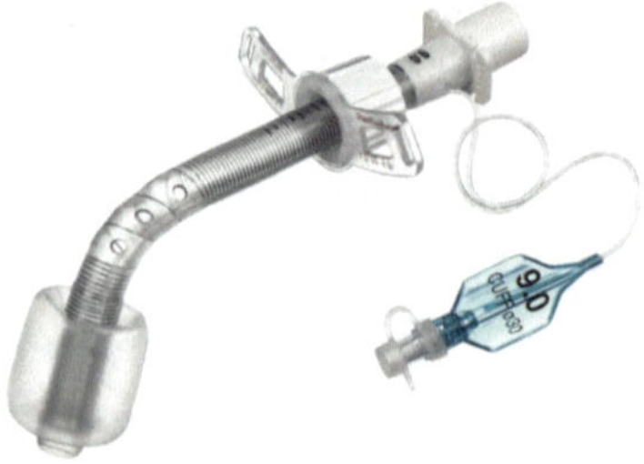

Structure: Cuffed, single cannula (with optional inner cannula)

Material: Thermosensitive PVC, DEHP-free

Manufacturer: Teleflex

Unique Features: Armored shaft; adjustable neck flange with locking system, optional color-coded inner cannula

Use: Patients who require a cuffed tube for positive pressure ventilation, airway protection, or when secretions are a concern; one model has fenestrations on the shaft to allow phonation

Image courtesy of Teleflex Incorporated.

Figure 3.34 Rüsch Ultra Tracheoflex

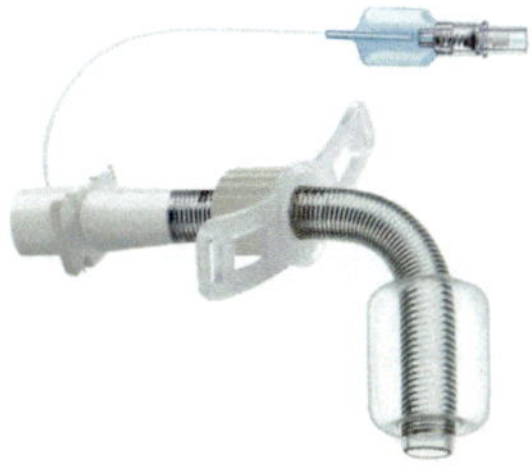

Structure: Cuffed, single cannula

Material: Thermosensitive PVC

Manufacturer: Teleflex

Unique Features: Armored (wire-reinforced) shaft; adjustable neck flange; there are models of this tube with extended proximal length and extended distal length

Use: Patients who require a cuffed tube for positive pressure ventilation, airway protection, or when secretions are a concern

Image courtesy of Teleflex Incorporated.

Suru Cuffed (no image available)

Structure: Cuffed, single-cannula

Material: Siliconized polyvinyl chloride

Manufacturer: Suru

Unique Features: Soft and flexible flange

Use: For the patient who requires a cuff, yet for whom secretions are not a concern

Single-Cannula Cuffless Tracheostomy Tubes

Single-cannula cuffless tracheostomy tubes **(Figure 3.35** through **Figure 3.45)** are used when exclusive breathing through the tube is not necessary (or not desired) and secretions are not a concern.

Figure 3.35 Angiplast Tube Cuffless

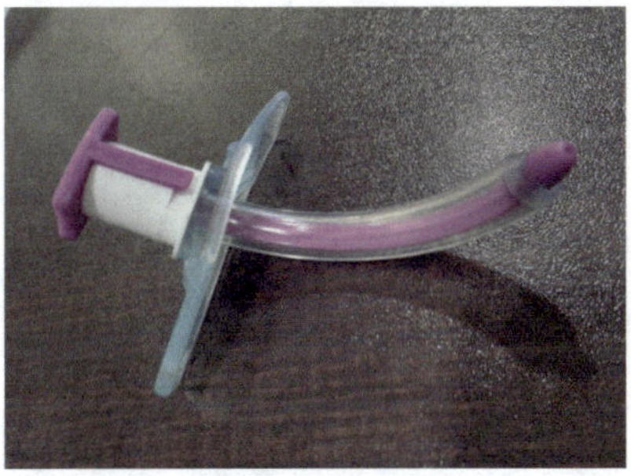

Structure: Cuffless, single-cannula

Material: Siliconized polyvinyl chloride

Manufacturer: Angiplast

Unique Features: Cuffed sizes in 5.0 mm to 10.0 mm; cuffless sizes 4.0 mm to 10.0 mm

Use: When positive-pressure ventilation is not required and secretions are not a concern

Photo courtesy of Angiplast

Figure 3.36 Bivona Uncuffed

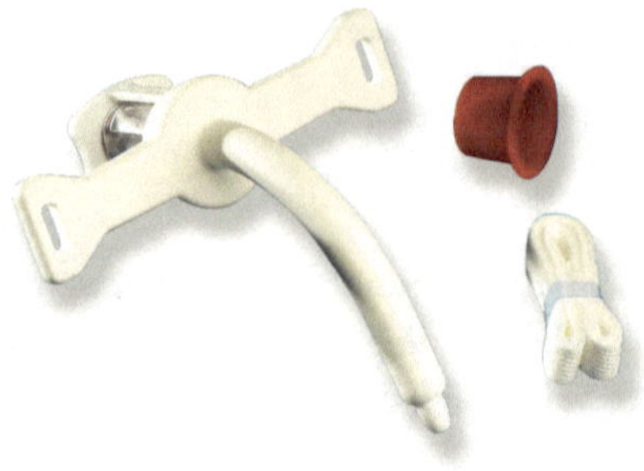

Structure: Cuffless, single-cannula

Material: Silicone

Manufacturer: Smiths Medical

Unique Features: Swivel mechanism of 15-mm adapter

Use: When positive-pressure ventilation is not required and secretions are not a concern

Photo courtesy of Smiths Medical

The Bivona uncuffed tracheostomy tube is a single-cannula tube and is composed of silicone. The neck flange is flexible, and the 15-mm connector has a swivel mechanism that accommodates some patient movement.

Figure 3.37 Air-Lon Tracheostomy Tube and Inhalation Set

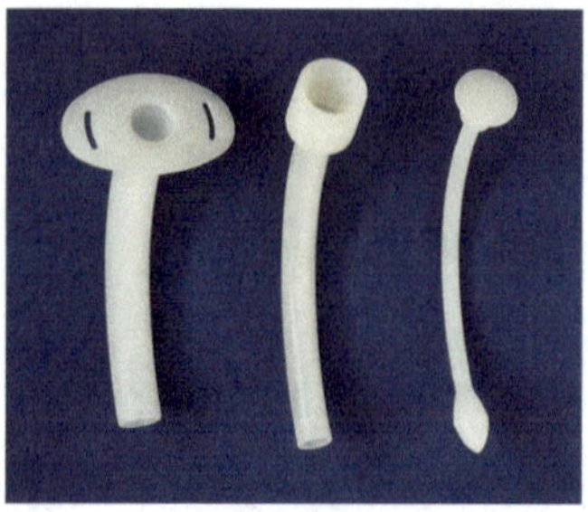

Structure: Cuffless, single-cannula, 90-degree curvature to the shaft

Material: Nylon

Manufacturer: Smiths Medical

Unique Features: Swivel mechanism of 15-mm adapter

Use: When positive-pressure ventilation is not required, and secretions are not a concern

Photo courtesy of Smiths Medical

The Air-Lon™ tracheostomy tube is cuffless and made of nylon. The outer cannula has a 90-degree arc. It comes with an obturator and low-profile inner cannula. If positive-pressure ventilation is desired, the Air-Lon™ Inhalation Set can be used.

Figure 3.38 Fahl DURATWIX Uncuffed

Structure: Uncuffed, single-cannula

Material: Soft, medical grade polymer

Manufacturer: Andreas Fahl Medizintechnik-Vertrieb GmbH

Unique Features: Ball joint between neck flange and tube allows free movement of the neck flange in all directions; available in two lengths

Use: When positive pressure ventilation is not required and secretions are not a concern

With friendly permission of Andreas Fahl Medizintechnik-Vertrieb GmbH, Cologne, Germany

Figure 3.39 Fahl DURAVENT

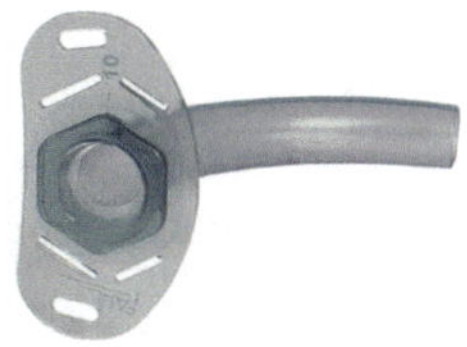

Structure: Uncuffed, single-cannula

Material: Medical grade polymer

Manufacturer: Andreas Fahl Medizintechnik-Vertrieb GmbH

Unique Features: Radiolucent contrast strip for radiological visualization; hexagonal lock that secures inner cannula to outer cannula; comes in standard and extra length

Use: When positive pressure ventilation is not required and secretions are not a concern

With friendly permission of Andreas Fahl Medizintechnik-Vertrieb GmbH, Cologne, Germany

Figure 3.40 Fahl SPIRAFLEX Uncuffed

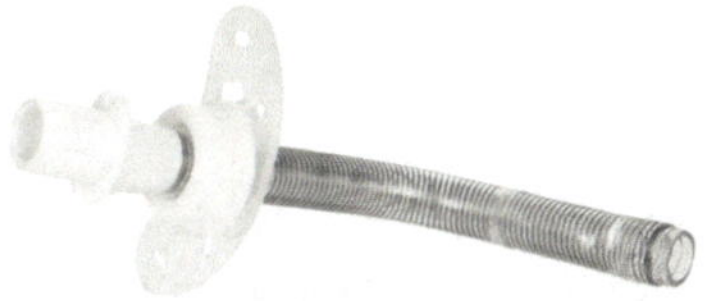

Structure: Uncuffed, single-cannula

Material: Soft, medical grade polymer with wire reinforcement

Manufacturer: Andreas Fahl Medizintechnik-Vertrieb GmbH

Unique Features: Adjustable neck flange; wire reinforced

Use: When positive pressure ventilation is not required and secretions are not a concern

With friendly permission of Andreas Fahl Medizintechnik-Vertrieb GmbH, Cologne, Germany

Figure 3.41 Fahl TRACHEOTEC VARIO

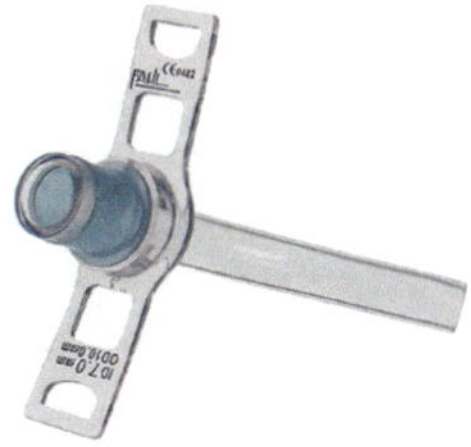

Structure: Uncuffed, single-cannula

Material: Soft, medical grade polymer

Manufacturer: Andreas Fahl Medizintechnik-Vertrieb GmbH

Unique Features: Contrast strip for radiological visualization

Use: When positive pressure ventilation is not required and secretions are not a concern

With friendly permission of Andreas Fahl Medizintechnik-Vertrieb GmbH, Cologne, Germany

Figure 3.42 TRACOE Comfort

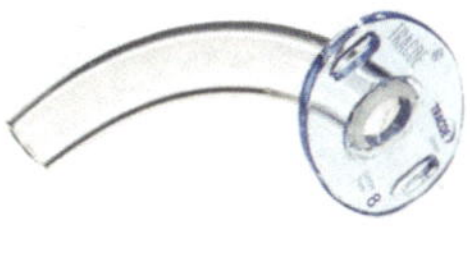

Structure: Uncuffed, single- or dual-cannula

Material: Flexible polyvinyl chloride

Manufacturer: TRACOE

Unique *Features:* Clear, flexible material; low-profile appearance

Use: When positive pressure ventilation is not required and secretions are not a concern

Courtesy of TRACOE medical GmbH, Germany.

The TRACOE Comfort line of tracheostomy tubes is made of a very soft, flexible, clear, and lightweight medical polymer. They are always cuffless and come with or without an inner cannula. The TRACOE Comfort single cannula (Model 101) is a single-cannula tube that is low profile in nature. Paraffin oil should be used to lubricate the inner cannula within the outer cannula.

Figure 3.43 Portex Blue-Line Ultra Uncuffed

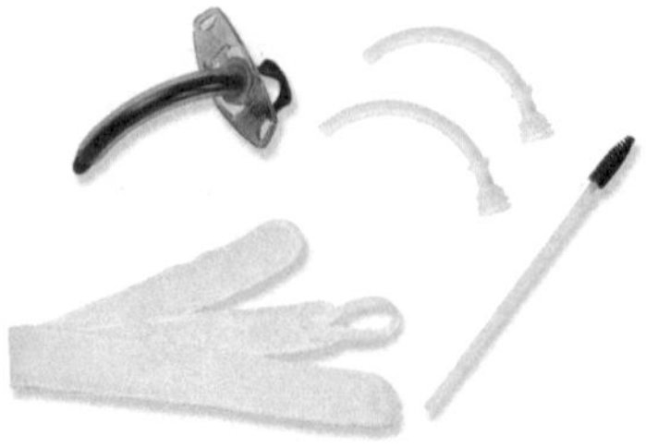

Structure: Uncuffed, single-cannula, with optional inner cannula

Material: Siliconized polyvinyl chloride

Manufacturer: Smiths Medical

Unique Features: Presence of a central channel to accommodate guide wire; larger curvature than standard Blue Line tube

Use: When positive-pressure ventilation is not required and secretions are not a concern

Photo courtesy of Smiths Medical

The Portex Blue Line Ultra series of tracheostomy tubes are very similar to the standard Portex Blue Line tubes but have a larger curvature. This feature theoretically allows the cuff to be more centrally placed within the airway. The inner cannula of the Blue Line Ultra decreases the diameter of the airway by 1 mm, as opposed to 2 mm for the other Portex tubes. One of the most unique features of the Blue Line Ultra is a central channel through the obturator, which can accommodate a guidewire for insertion.

Suru Uncuffed (no image available)

Structure: Uncuffed, single-cannula

Material: Siliconized polyvinyl chloride

Manufacturer: Suru

Unique Features: Soft and flexible flange

Use: When positive-pressure ventilation is not required and secretions are not a concern

Figure 3.44 Moore

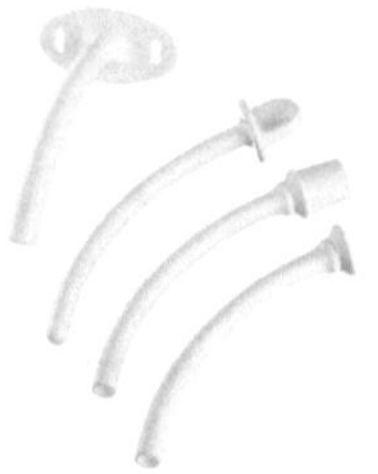

Structure: Uncuffed, single- or dual-cannula

Material: Silicone

Manufacturer: Boston Medical Products

Unique Features: Soft and flexible, conforms to shape of individual neck and trachea

Use: When positive-pressure ventilation is not required and comfort is desired

Photo courtesy of Boston Medical Products. All rights reserved.

The Moore tracheostomy tube is a flexible, single- or dual-cannula cuffless tube made of silicone. It comes in three sizes (6, 8, 10), and all have a standard length of 109.2 mm. The manufacturer reports that the extra-long length can be trimmed to fit. The outer cannula comes with a standard inner cannula, a low-profile inner cannula, and an obturator. The inner cannula can be soaked in warm soapy water for 10 minutes to loosen any crusts. If necessary, the inside of the inner cannula can be cleaned with a soft-bristle bottle brush.

Figure 3.45 Bivona Sleep Apnea

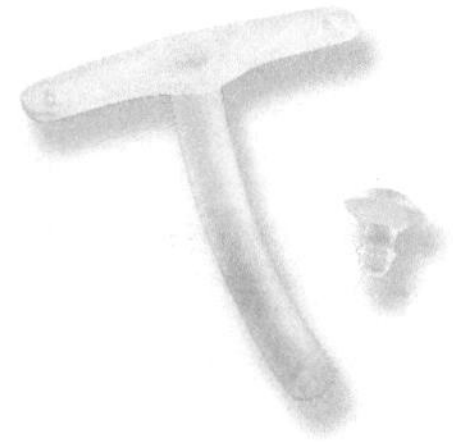

Structure: Uncuffed, single-cannula

Material: Flexible silicone

Manufacturer: Smiths Medical

Unique Features: Low-profile appearance; comes with two plugs

Use: When positive-pressure ventilation is not required and secretions are not a concern

Photo courtesy of Smiths Medical

The Bivona Sleep Apnea tubes are always cuffless and have a low profile. They are made of flexible silicone. Because of their low-profile nature, they are not recommended for patients who require ventilatory support or airway access for suctioning and pulmonary hygiene. Its low-profile design makes it easily capped and concealed during waking hours. The Bivona Sleep Apnea tracheostomy tube also comes in a version with an inner cannula with a 15-mm connector, which is called an "inhalation set."

Special Use Tracheostomy Tubes

There are several specialty tracheostomy tubes available for specific needs. These include talking tracheostomy tubes, extra-long tubes, fenestrated tubes, double-cuffed tubes, and custom-designed tubes.

Talking Tracheostomy Tubes

There are a few tracheostomy tubes available that are called "talking trachs." Talking tracheostomy tubes **(Figure 3.46** through **Figure 3.52)** are typically cuffed tubes with an additional lumen that terminates above the cuff and allows air to reach the vocal cords. When the tube is in the proper position and the proximal connector is attached to oxygen or an air-regulated gas source, air flows into the line. The patient or assistant must occlude the thumb port of this air supply line to direct the gas flow upward through the vocal cords. Gas flow usually starts at 4–6 liters per minute and can be adjusted upward until optimal voice quality is attained; however, a maximum of 10–15 liters per minute is recommended.

Another method of phonation with the talking tracheostomy tube is connecting the gas line to a suction source. When the thumb port is occluded, air is drawn in through the nose and mouth and passes through the vocal cords from the opposite direction. The product literature for the Portex

Blue Line Trach Talk recommends setting the initial negative pressure on the suction system to 80 mm Hg and adjusting to voice quality with a maximum of 180 mm Hg.

This suction port can also be used as a suction line to remove secretions produced above the cuff, rather than for phonation. By occluding the thumb port, these secretions are easily removed. The disadvantage, however, is that the suction line may become clogged with secretions and can be a source of infection. Because of this, its use as a suction line should be limited to a select group of patients.

Figure 3.46 Blom Tracheostomy Tube System

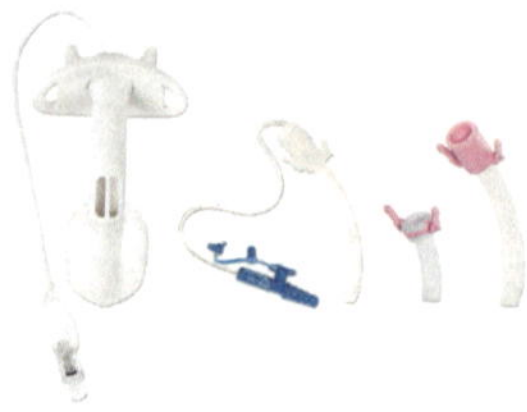

Structure: Cuffed, dual-cannula, fenestrated

Material: Outer cannula-kostrate and barium; cuff-polyvinyl chloride; neck flange-polycarbonate and polyvinyl chloride; standard cannula-polyurethane and polypropylene; speech cannula-silicone and polypropylene

Manufacturer: Pulmodyne

Unique Features: Speech cannula with two valves (flap and bubble valves), exhaled volume reservoir, subglottic suctioning cannula; fenestration is 1 mm above the cuff so the fenestration does not contact the tracheal mucosa when inflated

Use: For the ventilator-dependent patient who desires to speak

Reprinted with permission of Dr. Eric Blom

The Blom tracheostomy tube system was designed for the ventilator-dependent patient who desires to speak regardless of cuff inflation. It has a fenestrated shaft; however, the fenestration is only 1 mm above the cuff. When the cuff is fully inflated, the fenestration avoids contact with the tracheal mucosa. It also has two valves that redirect air. During inspiration, the flap valve opens, and the bubble valve expands into the fenestration and seals it. This allows all the air to be delivered to the patient's lungs and prevents air from escaping into the upper airway. On exhalation, the mechanism is reversed—the flap valve closes and the bubble valve collapses to unblock the fenestration and allow airflow up through the fenestration to the vocal cords.

Figure 3.47 Fahl DURACUFF KOMBI LINGO

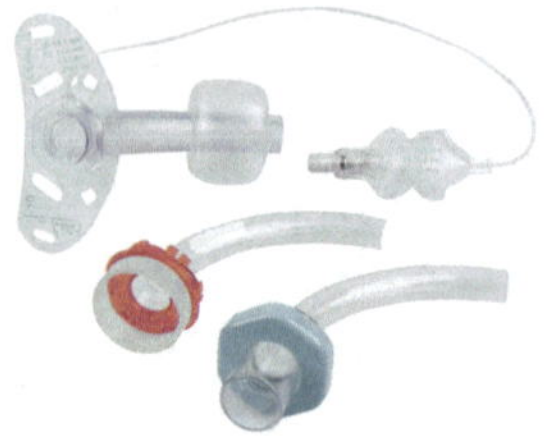

Structure: Cuffed, dual-cannula

Material: Medical grade polymer

Manufacturer: Andreas Fahl Medizintechnik-Vertrieb GmbH

Unique Features: "Sieved" fenestrations on outer cannula with single fenestration on inner cannula; comes in three lengths

Use: For the ventilator-dependent patient who desires to speak

With friendly permission of Andreas Fahl Medizintechnik-Vertrieb GmbH, Cologne, Germany

Fahl DURACUFF PHON (no image available)

Structure: Cuffed, dual-cannula

Material: Medical grade polymer

Manufacturer: Andreas Fahl Medizintechnik-Vertrieb GmbH

Unique Features: "Sieved" fenestrations on outer cannula with single fenestration on inner cannula; comes in three lengths

Use: For the ventilator-dependent patient who desires to speak

Fahl DURACUFF® SUCTION VOICE (no image available)

Structure: Cuffed, dual-cannula

Material: Medical grade polymer

Manufacturer: Andreas Fahl Medizintechnik-Vertrieb GmbH

Unique Features: "Sieved" fenestrations on outer cannula with single fenestration on inner cannula; comes in three lengths

Use: For the ventilator-dependent patient who desires to speak

Figure 3.48 Fahl DURACUFF® VARIO-KOMBI LINGO-PHON SUCTION

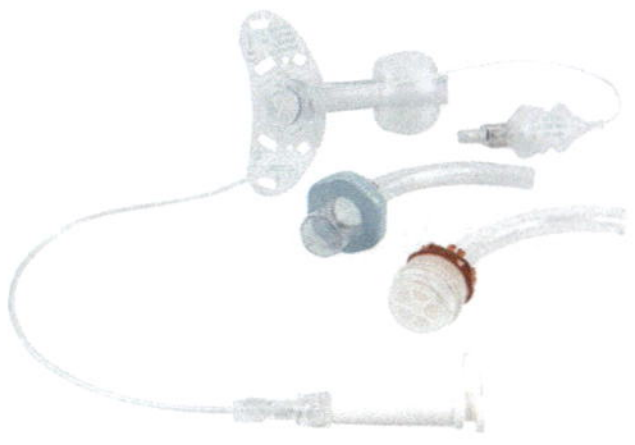

Structure: Cuffed, dual-cannula

Material: Medical grade polymer

Manufacturer: Andreas Fahl Medizintechnik-Vertrieb GmbH

Unique Features: "Sieved" fenestrations on outer cannula with single fenestration on inner cannula; comes in three lengths. Built-in speaking valve in inner cannula and integrated suction line

Use: For the ventilator-dependent patient who desires to speak

Figure 3.49 Fahl BIESALSKI®

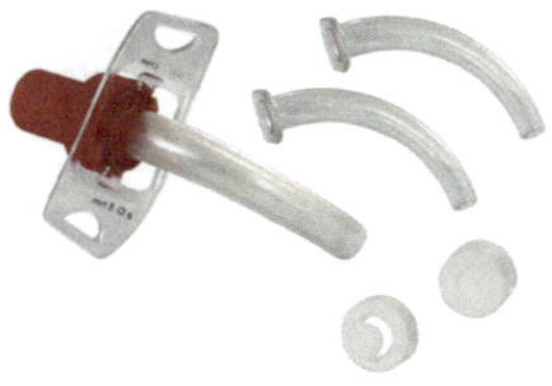

Structure: Uncuffed, dual cannula

Material: Medical grade polymer

Manufacturer: Andreas Fahl Medizintechnik-Vertrieb GmbH

Unique Features: The special shape of the tube allows generation of speech even though the tube is not fenestrated; phonation is facilitated because the outer diameter is tapered and exhaled air passes around the tube; it comes with its own speaking valve

Use: For the patient who is not on mechanical ventilation who desires to speak

With friendly permission of Andreas Fahl Medizintechnik-Vertrieb GmbH, Cologne, Germany

Portex Blue Line Trach Talk Suctionaid (no image available)

Structure: Cuffed, single-cannula

Material: Siliconized polyvinyl chloride

Manufacturer: Smiths Medical

Unique Features: Air supply line (green) with port that terminates above the cuff

Use: For the ventilator-dependent patient who desires to speak

The Portex Blue Line Trach Talk is similar to a Blue Line tracheostomy tube but has an additional lumen for gas flow. The distal port of the green gas line terminates just above the cuff of the tube.

Rüsch Biesalski * (no image available) *

Structure: Cuffed, dual cannula, or cuffless, dual cannula

Material: Thermosensitive PVC

Manufacturer: Teleflex

Unique Features: Set comes with bayonet fastener, speaking valve, and cap; special design of inner cannula allows speech without a fenestrated tube

Use: For the patient who desires to speak

Figure 3.50 Rüsch Tracheofix

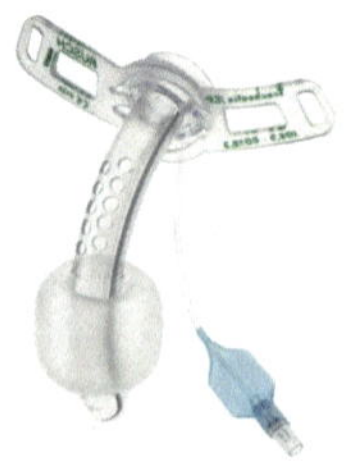

Structure: Cuffed, single cannula or cuffless, single cannula

Material: Thermosensitive PVC

Manufacturer: Teleflex

Unique Features: Fenestrated tube, clear shaft and neck flange; also comes in a PDT version for use with percutaneous insertion

Use: For the patient who desires to speak

Image courtesy of Teleflex Incorporated.

Rüsch Trachflex Plus Phonation * (no image available) *

Structure: Cuffed, single cannula (with optional inner cannula)

Material: Thermosensitive PVC, DEHP-free

Manufacturer: Teleflex

Unique Features: Armored shaft; adjustable neck flange with locking system, optional color-coded inner cannula

Use: Patients who require a cuffed tube for positive pressure ventilation, airway protection, or when secretions are a concern

Figure 3.51 TRACOE Twist with Air Supply Line®®

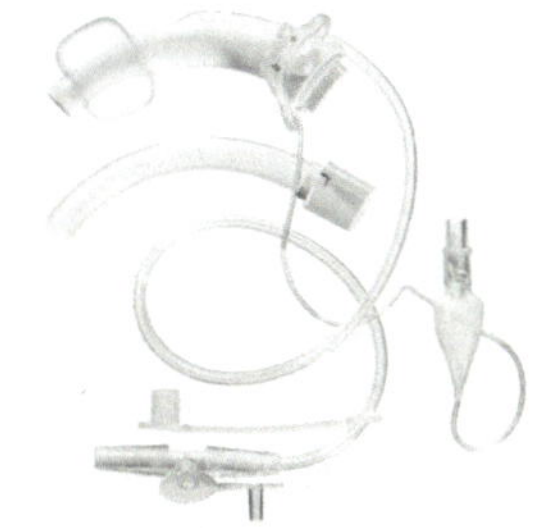

Structure: Cuffed, dual-cannula

Material: Flexible thermoelastic polyurethane

Manufacturer: TRACOE

Unique Features: Air supply line with port that terminates above the cuff

Use: For the ventilator-dependent patient who desires to speak

Courtesy of TRACOE medical GmbH, Germany. All rights reserved

The TRACOE Twist cuffed tracheostomy tube with air supply line is another version of the talking tracheostomy tube. It has all of the features of the TRACOE twist tubes previously discussed.

Figure 3.52 Bivona Fome-Cuf with Talk Attachment

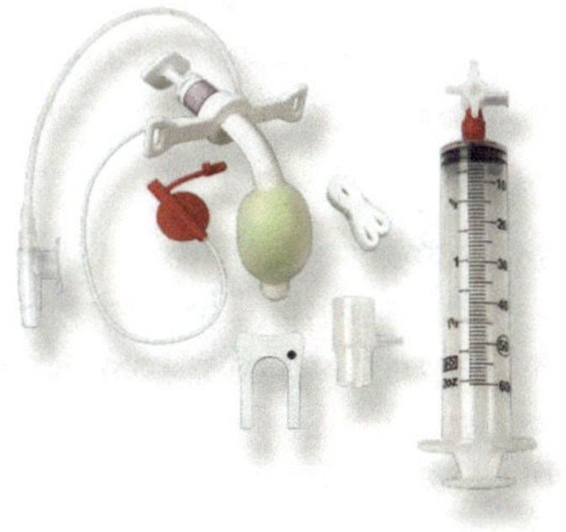

Structure: Cuffed, single-cannula

Material: Silicone

Manufacturer: Smiths Medical

Unique Features: Air supply line with port that terminates above the cuff

Use: For the ventilator-dependent patient who desires to speak

Photo courtesy of Smiths Medical

The Bivona Fome-Cuf with talk attachment is the only tube that allows a patient with a Fome-Cuf tracheostomy to talk. Otherwise, the bulkiness of this cuff, as well as its default-inflated position, does not allow any air to pass around the cuff

Extra-Long Tracheostomy Tubes

There are several circumstances in which an extra-long tracheostomy tube is beneficial. Extra-long tubes can be useful in cases of tracheomalacia, unusual anatomy, or morbid obesity. In the case of tracheomalacia, an extra-long tube will place the cuff in a more distal position within the trachea, which can allow the damaged area to heal. There are different types of extra-long tracheostomy tubes, and they all have different features (**Figure 3.53** through **Figure 3.57**).

Figure 3.53 Bivona Hyperflex

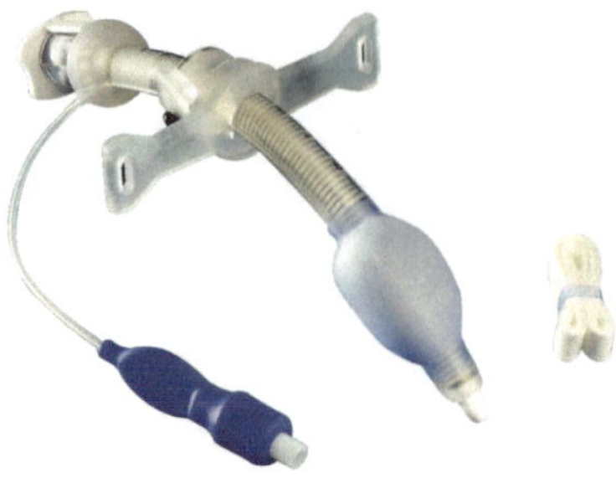

Structure: Cuffed, single-cannula, no curvature to the shaft

Material: Flexible silicone, wire reinforced

Manufacturer: Smiths Medical

Unique Features: There are two models: one with a fixed-neck flange and one with an adjustable neck flange to accommodate variable lengths; the shaft has no predetermined shape and can conform to a wide variety of anatomical variations, while wire reinforcement allows it to maintain its diameter without kinking, regardless of its position

Use: For the patient who requires an extra-long tracheostomy tube; ideal for the patient with unusual anatomy such as an extra-long or extra-wide neck

Photo courtesy of Smiths Medical

The Bivona Hyperflex tracheostomy tube is a single-cannula, extra-long tube with a silicone shaft reinforced with wire, allowing it to retain its shape regardless of its position. Because it is armored with wire, it is not compatible with magnetic resonance imaging (MRI). If the patient requires an MRI, this tube must be changed.

The Bivona Hyperflex was designed to provide extra length to accommodate patients with thick bull necks, anatomical airway anomalies, or other conditions such as tracheomalacia. The neck flange is manufactured with an adjustable or fixed neck. The adjustable-neck flange is designed as a temporary measure to accommodate individual needs. It is secured in place with a wrap-and-snap connection in which a band of silicone wraps around the shaft of the tube and hooks to itself. Even when locked in place, this adjustable-neck flange can move when traction is exerted on it, especially in a patient with a large amount of secretions. The manufacturer cautions that it is meant for temporary use until the proper length tube can be obtained. It should be replaced with a tracheostomy tube with a fixed-neck flange. The fixed-neck flange of the Hyperflex is flexible but fused to the shaft of the tube. The adjustable-neck flange model comes in two varieties of cuff: Aire-Cuf and TTS. The fixed-neck flange model used to be a custom order; however, it currently comes in standard lengths with three standard cuff varieties: Aire-Cuf, uncuffed, and TTS.

Figure 3.54 Fahl SPIRAFLEX® UNI CUFF XL

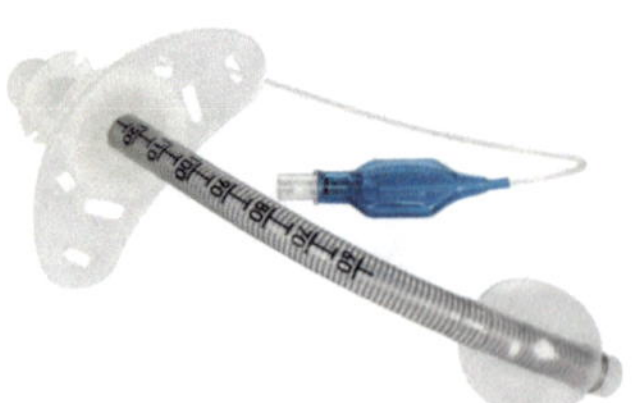

Structure: Cuffed, single cannula

Material: Soft, medical grade polymer with wire reinforcement

Manufacturer: Andreas Fahl Medizintechnik-Vertrieb GmbH

Unique Features: Adjustable neck flange, wire reinforced

Use: For the patient who requires an extra-long tracheostomy tube

With friendly permission of Andreas Fahl Medizintechnik-Vertrieb GmbH, Cologne, Germany

Rüsch Extra Tracheoflex (no image available)

Structure: Cuffed, single cannula

Material: Thermosensitive PVC

Manufacturer: Teleflex

Unique Features: Armored (wire-reinforced) shaft; adjustable neck flange

Use: For the patient who requires an extra-long tracheostomy tube

Figure 3.55 Shiley TracheoSoft XLT

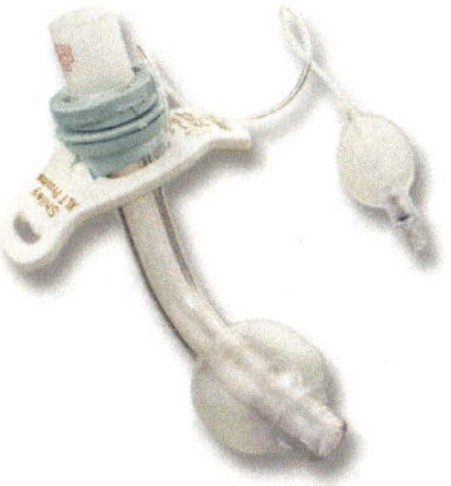

Structure: Cuffed, dual-cannula

Material: Semi-soft polyvinyl chloride

Manufacturer: Medtronic

Unique Features: Extra-long, dual-cannula tracheostomy tube, comes in either extra distal or extra proximal length

Use: For the patient who requires an extra-long tracheostomy tube, and for whom thick secretions are a concern

The Shiley TracheoSoft XLT tracheostomy tube is an extra-long tube constructed of semisoft polyvinyl chloride. It has a disposable inner cannula and comes in an extra distal as well as extra horizontal length. Its most valuable feature is that it is currently the only extra-length tracheostomy tube with an inner cannula. Because of its inner cannula and extra length, it is ideal for the patient with an extra-large or extra-long neck who also has a large amount of secretions.

Figure 3.56 TRACOE Vario

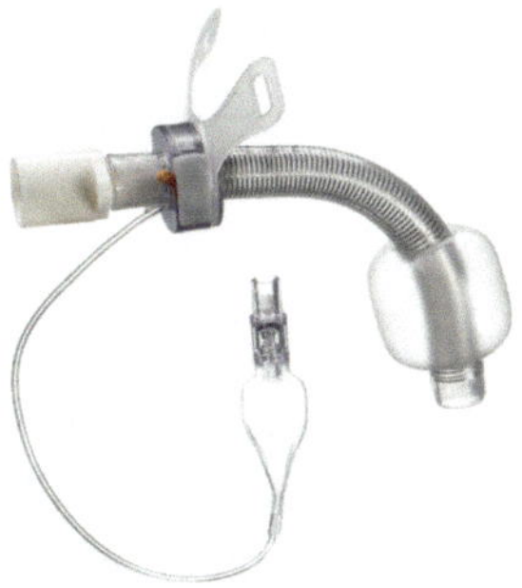

Structure: Cuffed or uncuffed, single-cannula

Material: Spiral reinforced polyvinyl chloride or clear polyvinyl chloride

Manufacturer: TRACOE

Unique Features: Extra length and adjustable wings on the neck flange, models include cuffed, cuffless, wire-reinforced, and one model with a suction port

Use: For the patient with unique anatomic needs

The TRACOE Vario tracheostomy tubes are extra-long, single-cannula tubes with adjustable-neck flanges. Two of the TRACOE Vario models are wire reinforced (models 450 and 455), and an MRI is contraindicated with these tubes in place. The TRACOE Vario tubes have a wide angle to the shaft and come in cuffed (models 450, 460, and 470) and cuffless (models 455 and 465) versions. In addition, one of the models also has a suction attachment port above the cuff for the patient with copious subglottic secretions (model 470). The wings of the neck flange can be placed in different positions.

TRACOE Comfort Extra Long (no image available)

Structure: Uncuffed, single- or dual-cannula, fenestrated or non-fenestrated

Material: Flexible polyvinyl chloride

Manufacturer: TRACOE

Unique Features: Clear, flexible material; low-profile appearance, extra length

Use: When positive pressure ventilation is not required, and secretions are not a concern

The TRACOE Comfort extra-length tracheostomy tubes are made of a very soft, flexible, clear, and lightweight medical polymer. They are always cuffless and come with or without an inner cannula. Most of the models are low profile in nature and do not have a 15-mm adapter; however, one of the models (205) comes with a 15-mm adapter on the inner cannula so positive pressure can be applied. Model 204 comes with a swivel speaking valve. Model 203 comes with a silver speaking valve and can also be ordered with an oxygen supply port. The manufacturer recommends that paraffin oil be used with the dual-cannula tracheostomy tubes at least every other day to lubricate the inner cannula and ensure it is easy to insert and remove.

Figure 3.57 Portex Uni-Perc

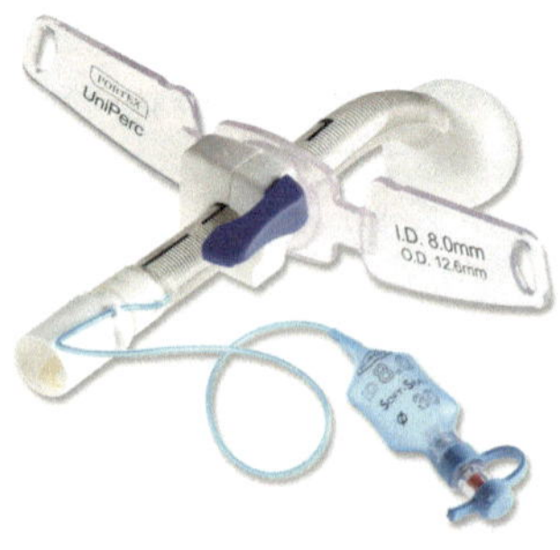

Photo courtesy of Smiths Medical

Structure: Cuffed, dual cannula, extra length.

Material: Reinforced PVC
Manufacturer: Smiths Medical

Unique Features: Extra length, locking clamp for individualized length

Use: Intended for patients with 50 mm pretracheal depth; components are longer than standard percutaneous tracheostomy kits

Tracheostomy Tubes with Additional Suction Channel

A few tracheostomy tubes on the market have specifically designed suction channels. The accumulation of secretions above the cuff has been implicated in the development of ventilator-associated pneumonia. Several tracheostomy tubes have been developed to meet that need. Tubes with specifically-designed suction ports include the Portex Blue Line Ultra Suctionaid tube **(Figure 3.58)**, TRACOE Twist and VARIO tubes, Fahl DURACUFF VARIO SUCTION, and TRACHEOTEC VARIO CUFF SUCTION **(Figure 3.59)** tubes. Any talking tracheostomy tubes or those with an additional air supply line have also been used successfully for intermittent or continuous suctioning above the cuff. The major problem with a suction channel of any kind is that it tends to get clogged with secretions.

Figure 3.58 Portex BlueLine Ultra Suctionaid

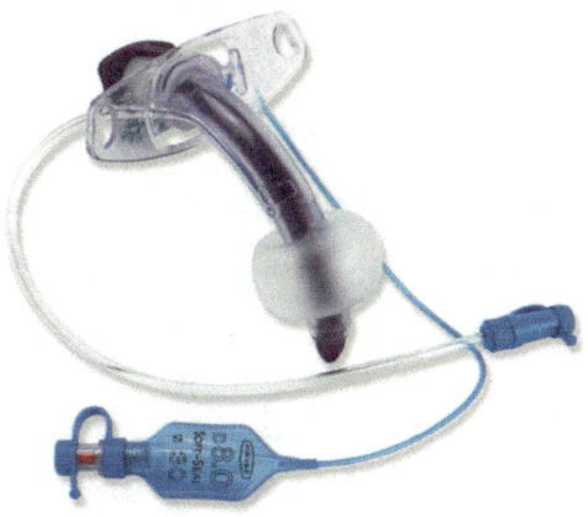

Structure: Cuffed, single cannula with optional inner cannula

Material: Thermosensitive PVC

Manufacturer: Smiths Medical

Unique Features: Additional suction channel for removal of secretions above the cuff

Use: For the patient who has oropharyngeal secretions

Photo courtesy of Smiths Medical

Fahl DURACUFF® VARIO SUCTION

Structure: Cuffed, dual cannula

Material: Medical-grade PVC-DEHP free

Manufacturer: Andreas Fahl Medizintechnik-Vertrieb GmbH

Unique Features: Additional suction channel for removal of secretions above the cuff; the fenestrated version of this tube is called the VARIO-KOMBI LINGO-PHON

Use: For the patient who has excessive pharyngeal secretions

Figure 3.59 Fahl TRACHEOTEC® VARIO CUFF-SUCTION

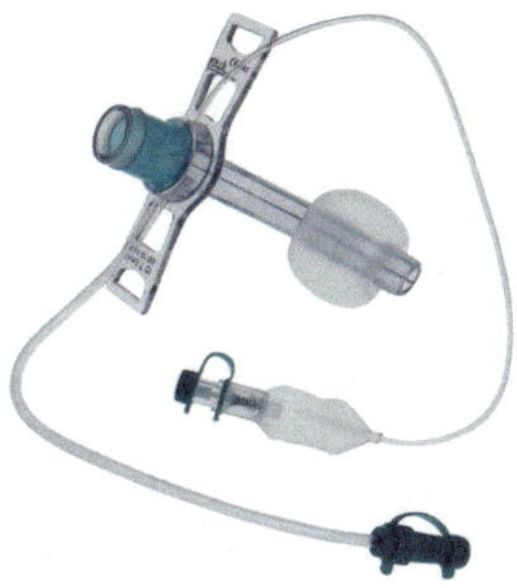

Structure: Cuffed, single cannula

Material: Soft medical grade polymer

Manufacturer: Andreas Fahl Medizintechnik-Vertrieb GmbH

Unique Features: Additional suction channel to remove secretions above the cuff

Use: For the patient who has excessive pharyngeal secretions

With friendly permission of Andreas Fahl Medizintechnik-Vertrieb GmbH, Cologne, Germany

Metal Tracheostomy Tubes

Metal tracheostomy tubes are always uncuffed. There are several types of metal tracheostomy tubes (**Figure 3.60** through **Figure 3.67**), but the Jackson tracheostomy is the oldest and probably best known. Metal tracheostomy tubes can be constructed of stainless steel or silver. They are heavier than plastic tubes and can reflect ambient temperature. The primary differences among these metal tubes are the design of the neck flange, the length, and the angle of tube curvature. A metal tracheostomy tube can last a lifetime, but it does require regular cleaning, as do tubes made of plastic and other softer materials. For this reason, a metal tracheostomy tube may be preferred in patients who pay out of pocket or those who will be returning to a country where plastic tubes are difficult to obtain.

Some medical centers frequently use metal tracheostomy tubes; in other centers, they are rarely seen. Metal tracheostomy tubes are sometimes preferred when it is known that the tube will be permanent, such as in head or neck cancer or trauma.

Metal tracheostomy tubes cannot be customized as easily as plastic tubes. For this reason, they often come in a variety of lengths. Many metal tubes are completely interchangeable within a size and style. One of the biggest advantages of metal tracheostomy tubes is that the walls of the tube are thinner. A unique advantage of silver tubes is that they are reported to have bactericidal properties.

One manufacturer recommends that metal tracheostomy tubes be cleaned daily. Chemical cleaners such as hydrogen peroxide, enzyme cleaners, or sodium peroxide should not be used with metal tubes because they can cause damage. More detailed instructions for cleaning metal tracheostomy tubes can be found in chapter 7.

Figure 3.60 Jackson Original

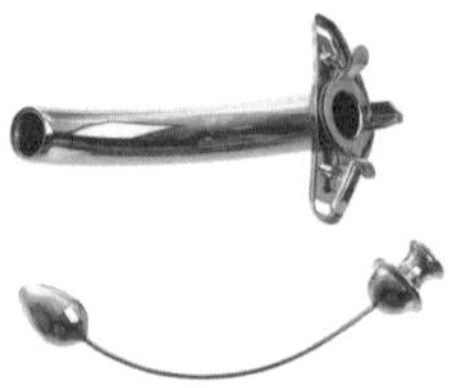

Structure: Uncuffed, dual-cannula

Material: Stainless steel or sterling silver

Manufacturer: Pilling (Teleflex Medical) or Premier Medical Products

Unique Features: Parts are completely adaptable within a size and style; sterling silver has a bactericidal effect

Use: For the patient who prefers a metal tracheostomy tube

Image courtesy of Teleflex Incorporated.

Figure 3.61 Jackson Improved

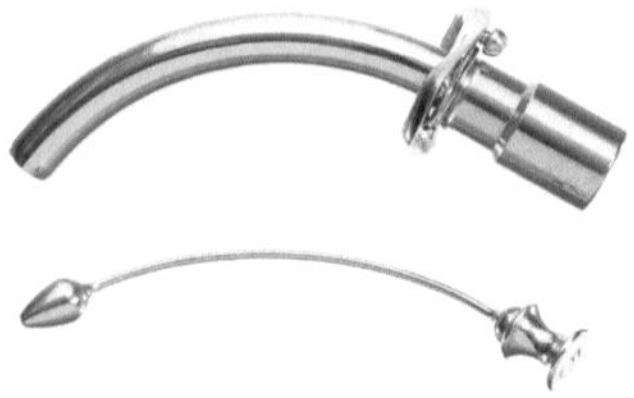

Structure: Uncuffed, dual-cannula

Material: Stainless steel or sterling silver

Manufacturer: Pilling (Teleflex Medical) or Premier Medical Products

Unique Features: Parts are completely adaptable within a size and style; sterling silver has a bactericidal effect

Use: For the patient who prefers a metal tracheostomy tube

Image courtesy of Teleflex Incorporated.

The Jackson tracheostomy tube was the original metal tube. The original Jackson tracheostomy tubes came in stainless steel, but there is also a model in sterling silver. This sterling silver model has a rotating lock to hold the low-profile inner cannula in place, and this swivel-locking ring is also found on the Jackson Improved models. The original Jackson tracheostomy tubes have a swivel lock to hold the inner cannula in place and as such are low profile, but they can be fitted with 15-mm adapters for use with positive-pressure ventilation. There are currently two manufacturers of the Jackson tracheostomy tube in the US: Pilling (Teleflex Medical) and Premier Medical Products. At Premier, the 15-mm adapter is permanently attached to the Improved pattern tube. The neck flange may have different shapes depending on the size of the tube. With Premier tubes, sizes 00 to 8 have a small rectangular shape, while sizes 9 and 10 have a larger oval neck flange (personal communication, Toni Banet, Premier Medical Products, May 2009).

Figure 3.62 Fahl SILVERVENT

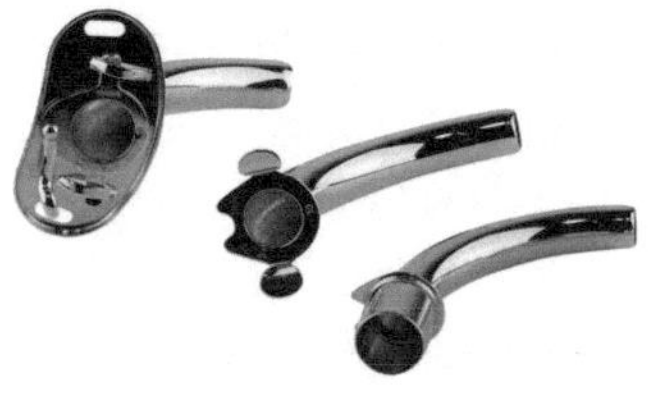

Structure: Cuffless, dual-cannula

Material: Sterling silver

Manufacturer: Andreas Fahl Medizintechnik-Vertrieb GmbH

Unique Features: Conical designed tube, with decreasing diameter from neck flange to the tip of the tube; standard version is ¼ radius, but the Jatho version is 1/8 radius (narrower angle); can include low-profile inner cannula as well as one that provides a 15-mm connector; sterling silver has a bactericidal effect

Use: For the patient who can protect his airway and prefers a metal tracheostomy tube

Figure 3.63 Fahl SILVERVENT LINGO PHON (with speaking valve on inner cannula)

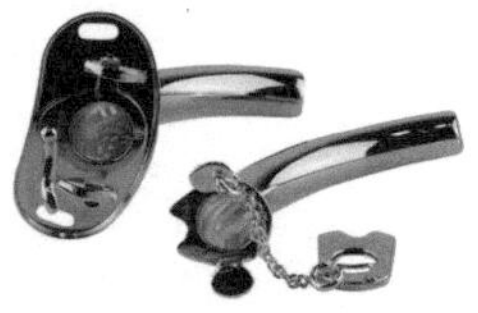

Structure: Cuffless, dual-cannula

Material: Sterling silver

Manufacturer: Andreas Fahl Medizintechnik-Vertrieb GmbH

Unique Features: Conical designed tube, with decreasing diameter from neck flange to the tip of the tube; standard version is ¼ radius, but the Jatho version is 1/8 radius (narrower angle); can include low-profile inner cannula as well as one that provides a 15-mm connector; one model also comes with a silver speaking valve; sterling silver has a bactericidal effect

Use: For the patient who can protect his airway and prefers a metal tracheostomy tube

With friendly permission of Andreas Fahl Medizintechnik-Vertrieb GmbH, Cologne, Germany

Holinger (no image available)

Structure: Uncuffed, dual-cannula

Material: Sterling silver

Manufacturer: Pilling (Teleflex Medical)

Unique Features: Tube is attached to the neck flange at a 65-degree, acute downward angle; sterling silver has bactericidal effect

Use: For the patient who prefers a metal tracheostomy tube

Holinger tracheostomy tubes are made of sterling silver with a rectangular neck flange. Sizes vary from 000 to 8. The Holinger tube is attached to the neck flange at an acute downward angle of 65 degrees, rather than the usual alignment of 90 degrees. Holinger tracheostomy tubes are low-profile tubes, with an inner cannula but without a 15-mm connector.

Figure 3.64 Tucker

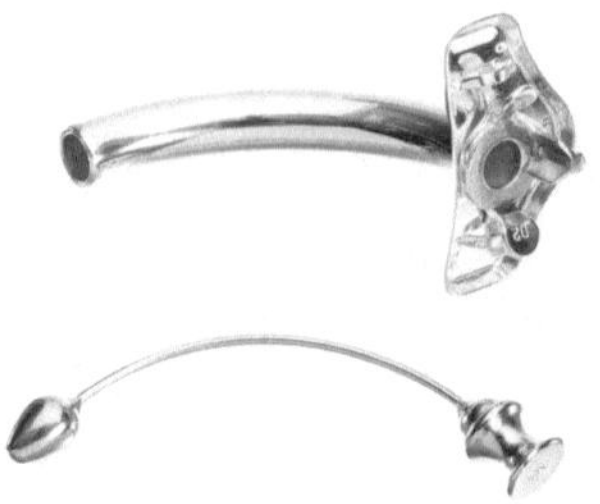

Structure: Uncuffed, dual-cannula

Material: Sterling silver

Manufacturer: Pilling (Teleflex Medical)

Unique Features: Valved inner cannula allows speech without digital occlusion; sterling silver has a bactericidal effect

Use: For the patient who prefers a metal tracheostomy tube

Image courtesy of Teleflex Incorporated.

Tucker tracheostomy tubes are made of sterling silver and may or may not have a Tucker valve along the shaft of the inner cannula. The Tucker valve bulges outward during inspiration, allowing the patient to speak without finger occlusion of the tube. This internal valve is quite different than other types of speaking valves, which are connected to the outside of the tube. The Tucker valve is for use with sterling silver tubes only. See chapter 6 for further discussion of phonation.

Mayo Clinic (no image available)

Structure: Uncuffed, dual-cannula

Material: Stainless steel

Manufacturer: Pilling (Teleflex Medical)

Unique Features: Holinger-style neck flange on Jackson stainless steel shaft

Use: For the patient who prefers a metal tracheostomy tube

The Mayo Clinic tube is a metal tracheostomy tube with a Holinger-style neck flange (rectangular) on a Jackson stainless steel shaft.

Figure 3.65 Luer

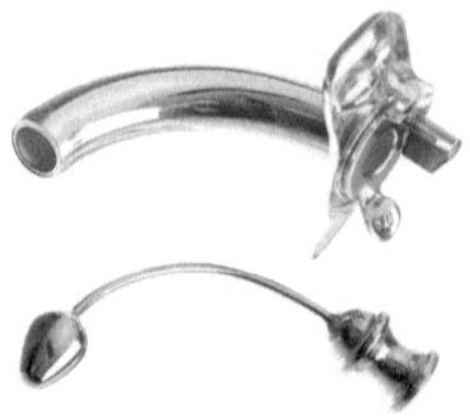

Structure: Uncuffed, dual-cannula

Material: Sterling silver

Manufacturer: Pilling (Teleflex Medical)

Unique Features: Shorter and more acute curve than Jackson tracheostomy tube. Sterling silver has a bactericidal effect

Use: For the patient who prefers a metal tracheostomy tube

Image courtesy of Teleflex Incorporated.

The Luer tracheostomy tube is made of sterling silver and is shorter in length than the comparable Jackson tube. It has a more acute curve than the Jackson tracheostomy tubes, but it has the original Jackson-style neck flange. These are low-profile tubes without 15-mm connectors.

Figure 3.66 Negus Silver Tracheostomy Tube

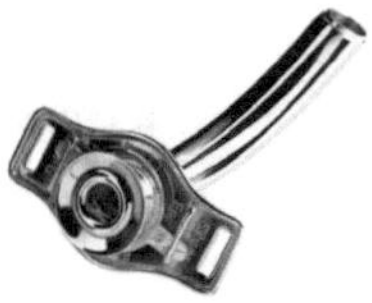

Structure: Cuffless, dual-cannula

Material: Sterling silver

Manufacturer: Kapitex

Unique Features: Speaking valve is incorporated into inner cannula, creating low profile, with spare non-valved inner cannula; sterling silver has a bactericidal effect

Use: For long-term tracheostomy use with phonation

Photo courtesy of Kapitex

Figure 3.67 Negus Silver Inner Cannula with Speaking Valve

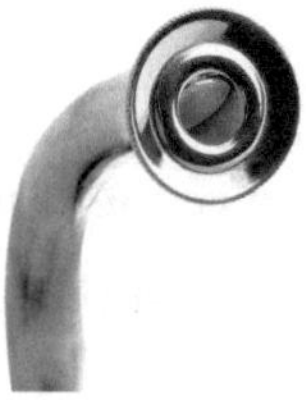

Photo courtesy of Kapitex

Chiner Silver Tracheostomy Tube (no image available)

Structure: Cuffless, dual-cannula

Material: Sterling silver

Manufacturer: Artesano Francisco Chiner

Unique Features: Comes in fenestrated and non-fenestrated models; some models also have a low-profile speaking valve; sterling silver has a bactericidal effect

Use: For long-term tracheostomy use

Laryngectomy Tubes

Laryngectomy tubes **(Figure 3.68** through **3.74)** are always cuffless because laryngectomy patients are neck breathers. The laryngectomy tube is typically shorter than the comparable tracheostomy tube and the angle of curvature is narrower. It can have either a single outer cannula or a dual cannula. Like tracheostomy tubes, laryngectomy tubes can be rigid or flexible. Because a laryngectomy necessitates a permanent stoma, the tube itself is often not required beyond a few months after initial placement.

Figure 3.68 Shiley LGT

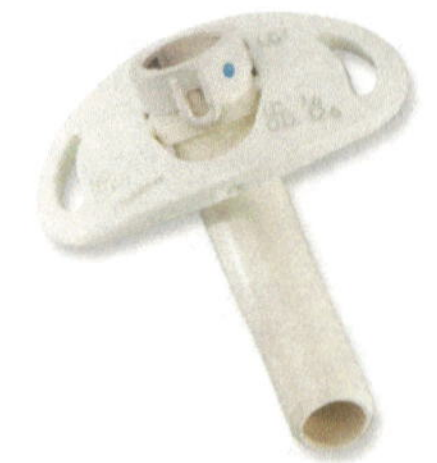

Structure: Uncuffed, dual-cannula, short, narrow curvature

Material: Rigid polyvinyl chloride

Manufacturer: Medtronic

Unique Features: Shorter length and narrower curvature than standard tracheostomy tube

Use: For the laryngectomy patient in whom secretions are a concern

The Shiley LGT tracheostomy tube is a rigid tube made of polyvinyl chloride. It has an inner cannula that nests within the outer cannula and, like the Shiley CFS and LPC, is attached by means of a twist lock. It also comes with a low-profile, cosmetic inner cannula.

Portex DIC Laryngectomy (no image available)

Structure: Uncuffed, dual-cannula, short, narrow curvature

Material: Silicone

Manufacturer: Smiths Medical

Unique Features: Shorter length and narrower curvature than standard tracheostomy tube

Use: For the laryngectomy patient in whom secretions may be a concern

The Portex DIC laryngectomy tube is a flexible silicone tube with an inner cannula.

Figure 3.69 TRACOE Twist Laryngectomy

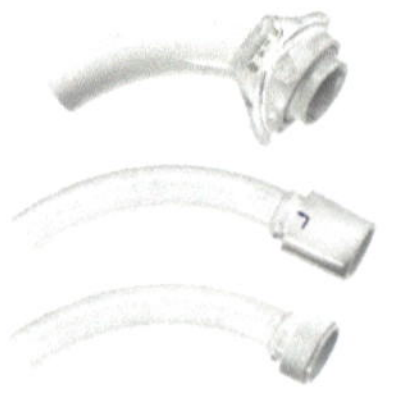

Structure: Uncuffed, dual-cannula, short, narrow curvature

Material: Flexible thermoelastic polyurethane

Manufacturer: TRACOE

Unique Features: Shorter length and narrower curvature than standard tracheostomy tube

Use: For the laryngectomy patient in whom secretions may be a concern

The TRACOE Twist laryngectomy tube is made of medical-grade polyurethane, similar to the TRACOE Twist tracheostomy tubes. It has a standard inner cannula with a 15-mm connector and a low-profile inner cannula.

Figure 3.70 TRACOE Comfort Laryngectomy

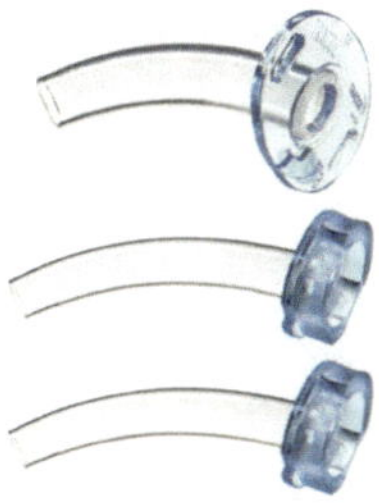

Structure: Uncuffed, dual-cannula, short, narrow curvature

Material: Flexible polyvinyl chloride

Manufacturer: TRACOE

Unique Features: Clear, flexible material; comes with one or two inner cannulas

Use: To maintain patency of the stoma following laryngectomy

The TRACOE Comfort laryngectomy tube is clear and flexible with an inner cannula that can be removed for cleaning.

Figure 3.71 Singer Laryngectomy

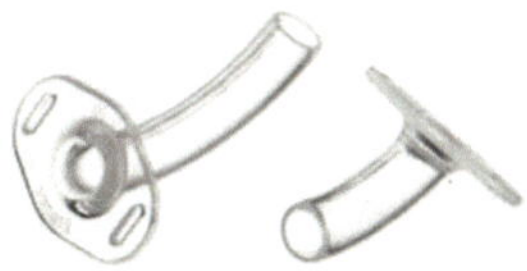

Structure: Uncuffed, single-cannula, short, narrow curvature

Material: Silicone

Manufacturer: Boston Medical Products

Unique Features: Clear and very flexible material

Use: To maintain patency of the stoma following laryngectomy

The Singer laryngectomy tube is clear, flexible, and made of silicone. It has a low-profile appearance and comes in 28 sizes. The flange is designed to cover a wide surface area to keep tracheostomy ties away from the healing stoma. The Singer tube should be rinsed under running water to clean. If crusts or mucous plugs are seen, it should be soaked in hot, soapy water for at least 10 minutes and cleaned with a nonabrasive brush. The manufacturer recommends it to be soaked overnight in a 3% hydrogen peroxide solution and then rinsed and air dried.

Figure 3.72 Provox LaryTube (with housing and HME) (

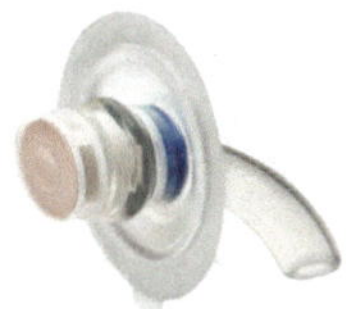

Structure: Uncuffed, single-cannula, short, narrow curvature

Material: Silicone

Manufacturer: Natus Medical

Unique Features: Fenestrated model is for use with voice prosthesis; can be used with its own heat moisture exchanger (HME) system

Use: For the laryngectomy patient in whom secretions are not a concern

The Provox LaryTube is made of flexible silicone and has a conical gradation from the short neck flange to the shaft. It comes in a standard model, a fenestrated model (for use with a voice prosthesis), and a model with a ring that attaches to an adhesive base plate for wear without ties around the neck. This tube can also be used with its own HME system.

Figure 3.73 Bivona Laryngectomy

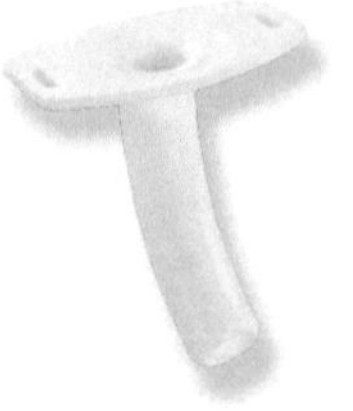

Structure: Uncuffed, single-cannula, short, narrow curvature

Material: Silicone

Manufacturer: Smiths Medical

Unique Features: Wider neck flange; short and long lengths for three different sizes

Use: For the laryngectomy patient in whom secretions are not a concern

Photo courtesy of Smiths Medical

The Bivona laryngectomy tube comes in three different sizes (9.5, 11, and 13) in three different lengths (55, 85, and 105 mm).

Figure 3.74 Fahl LARYNGOTEC®

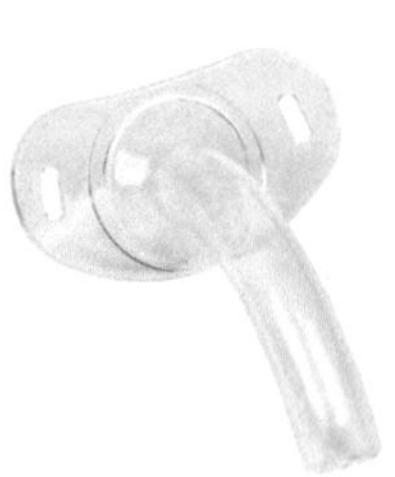

Structure: Uncuffed, single-cannula, short, narrow curvature

Material: Silicone

Manufacturer: Andreas Fahl Medizintechnik-Vertrieb GmbH

Unique Features: Available in three different lengths; custom sieved fenestration is possible

Use: For the laryngectomy patient in whom secretions are not a concern

With friendly permission of Andreas Fahl Medizintechnik-Vertrieb GmbH, Cologne, Germany

Fenestrated Tracheostomy Tubes

Fenestrated tracheostomy tubes can be cuffed or uncuffed (**Figure 3.75** through **Figure 3.81**). The term comes from the French word *fenêtre,* meaning window. The shaft of the fenestrated tube has an opening on the dorsal aspect that allows for an added boost of air to the vocal cords. The standard placement of the fenestration is at a point on the shaft one-third of its length as measured from the neck flange. Many clinicians do not realize that this fenestration must be measured to fit so that it aligns centrally within the airway. A failure to precisely fit this tracheostomy tube can result in the abutment of the fenestration with the anterior or posterior wall of the trachea, resulting in the growth of granulation tissue within the fenestration. The removal of a tracheostomy tube with a growth of this granulation tissue can be a surgical challenge. Manipulation of a fenestrated tracheostomy tube should be preceded by a thorough assessment of its placement within the airway. Initially, this can be done by shining a light within the opening of the tracheostomy and looking through the tube, with the patient's head in different positions. If a pale pink color is seen, it may be granulation tissue within the fenestration, and a consultation with an otolaryngologist should be done immediately. One can also attempt to gently move the tracheostomy tube within the stoma to assess for the mobility of the tube itself. The forceful removal of a fenestrated tracheostomy tube with an unrecognized growth of granulation tissue can result in hemorrhage and an airway catastrophe. For these reasons, many centers do not routinely place fenestrated tracheostomies. If a fenestrated tracheostomy remains the best option for the patient, the procedure to fit this tracheostomy tube is discussed in chapter 4.

Figure 3.75 Fahl DURAVENT® LINGO

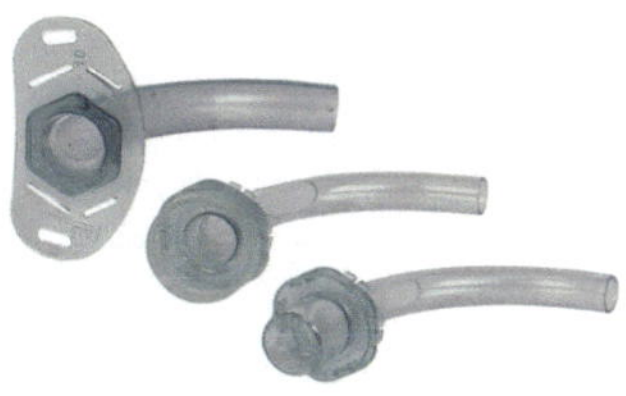

Structure: Uncuffed, dual-cannula

Material: Medical grade polymer

Manufacturer: Andreas Fahl Medizintechnik-Vertrieb GmbH

Unique Features: Fenestrated inner cannula and sieved outer cannula, that can also accommodate a speaking valve; the UNI LINGO-PHON version of the tube has one model with a low-profile silver speaking valve and another model with a silicone speaking valve

Use: For the patient who desires to speak

With friendly permission of Andreas Fahl Medizintechnik-Vertrieb GmbH, Cologne, Germany

Shiley Fenestrated FEN, CFN, DFEN, DCFN

Figure 3.76 Shiley FEN

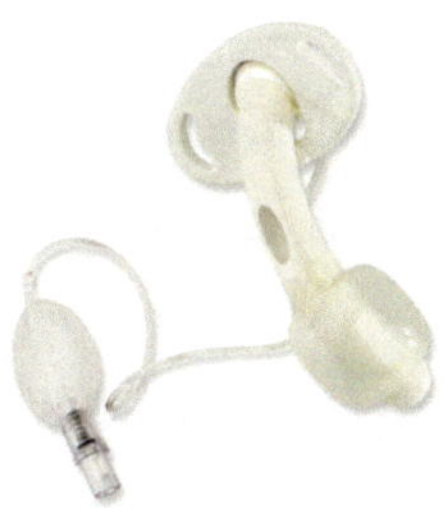

Structure: Cuffed (FEN, DFEN) or uncuffed (CFN, DCFN), dual-cannula

Material: Rigid polyvinyl chloride

Manufacturer: Medtronic

Unique Features: FEN and DFEN tubes have one large oval fenestration; CFN and DCFN tubes have narrower fenestrated slits

Use: For the patient who desires to speak

Figure 3.77 Shiley DFEN

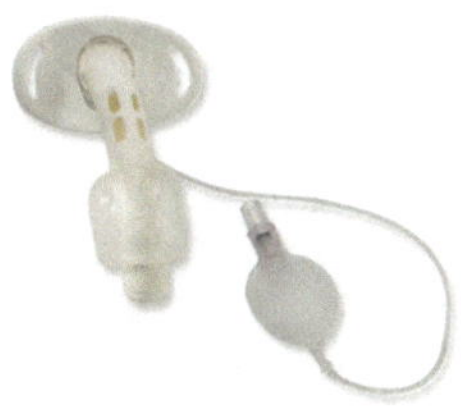

Structure: Cuffed (FEN, DFEN) or uncuffed (CFN, DCFN), dual-cannula

Material: Rigid polyvinyl chloride

Manufacturer: Medtronic

Unique Features: FEN and DFEN tubes have one large oval fenestration; CFN and DCFN tubes have narrower fenestrated slits

Use: For the patient who desires to speak

Shiley manufactures four types of fenestrated tracheostomy tubes—the FEN, CFN, DFEN, and DCFN—which are all made of rigid polyvinyl chloride. The Shiley FEN and DFEN are cuffed tubes; the CFN and the DCFN are cuffless tubes. Both the FEN and the CFN have a standard, nondisposable inner cannula and a fenestrated, nondisposable inner cannula. The DFEN and the DCFN have only a standard (non-fenestrated) disposable inner cannula. The fenestration of the FEN and the CFN is a large oval aperture on the dorsal aspect of the shaft. The fenestration of the DFEN and the DCFN is a set of linear slits along the dorsal aspect of the tube. Because the DFEN and DCFN have only a standard (non-fenestrated) inner cannula, they can only be used as a fenestrated tube without the inner cannula in place.

Portex DIC Fenestrated (no image available)

Structure: Cuffed or uncuffed, fenestrated

Material: Rigid polyvinyl chloride

Manufacturer: Smiths Medical

Unique Features: Color-coded disposable inner cannula

Use: For the patient who desires to speak, but for whom secretions may be a concern

The Portex DIC fenestrated tube has all the features of the other DIC tubes, including a color-coded inner cannula based on size (see **Table 3.1**). The fenestration is composed of two slits along the shaft of the tube to allow air to move up to the vocal cords.

Figure 3.78 Portex Flex DIC Fenestrated

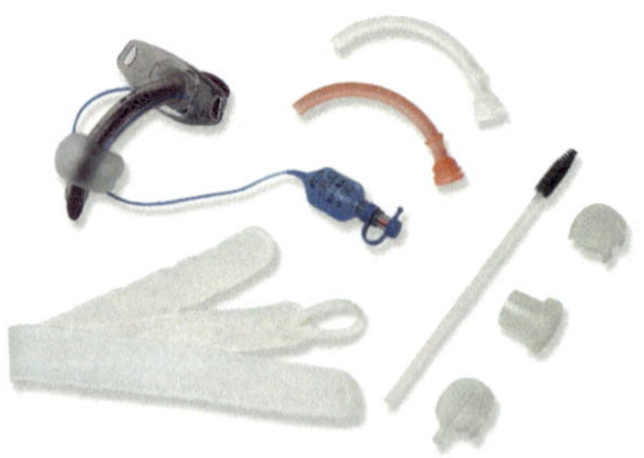

Photo courtesy of Smiths Medical

Structure: Cuffed or uncuffed, dual-cannula, fenestrated

Material: Flexible polyvinyl chloride with silicone coating

Manufacturer: Smiths Medical

Unique Features: Color-coded disposable inner cannula

Use: For the patient who desires to speak, but for whom secretions may be a concern

The Portex Flex DIC fenestrated tube has all the features of the other Flex DIC tubes, including a color-coded inner cannula based on size.

Portex Lo-Profile Fenestrated (no image available)

Structure: Cuffed or uncuffed, dual-cannula, fenestrated

Material: Rigid polyvinyl chloride

Manufacturer: Smiths Medical

Unique Features: Low profile inner cannula (without 15-mm adapter) and standard inner cannula (with 15-mm adapter)

Use: For the patient who desires to speak, but for whom secretions may be a concern

Figure 3.79 TRACOE Twist Fenestrated

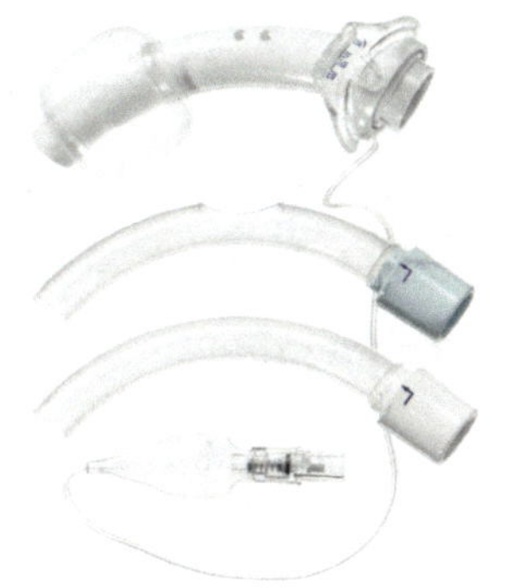

Structure: Cuffed or uncuffed, dual-cannula

Material: Flexible thermoelastic polyurethane

Manufacturer: TRACOE

Unique Features: Fenestrations consist of several small circular holes on dorsal aspect of shaft

Use: For the patient who desires to speak, but for whom secretions may be a concern

Courtesy of TRACOE medical GmbH, Germany. All rights reserved

The TRACOE Twist tracheostomy tubes also come in fenestrated versions. These fenestrated tubes come in cuffed and cuffless models. They have all the features of the standard TRACOE Twist tubes, with the addition of an oval-shaped fenestration. Unlike other fenestrated models, the fenestrations on this tube are a series of small circular holes on the dorsal aspect of the outer cannula and a large oval aperture on the inner cannula. Model numbers for the fenestrated versions of the TRACOE Twist tubes are 302 and 304. They are packaged with a standard inner cannula with a 15-mm connector, a fenestrated inner cannula, and an obturator.

Figure 3.80 TRACOE Comfort Fenestrated

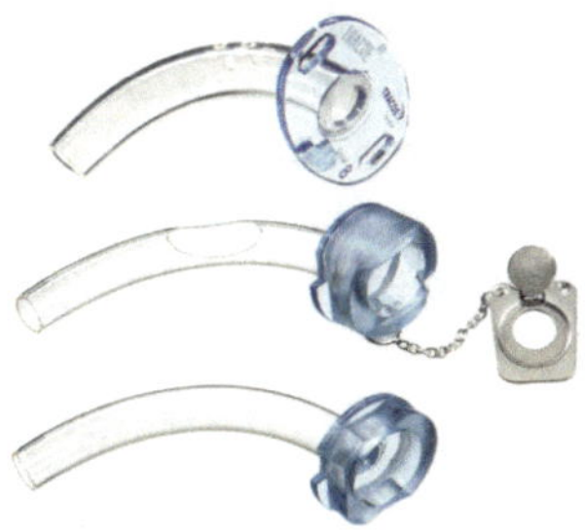

Structure: Uncuffed, dual-cannla

Material: Flexible polyvinyl chloride

Manufacturer: TRACOE

Unique Features: Clear, low-profile fenestrations are a series of round holes; one model comes with a silver speaking valve

Use: For the patient who desires to speak

Courtesy of TRACOE medical GmbH, Germany. All rights reserved

The TRACOE Comfort line of tracheostomy tubes also includes four models that are fenestrated: 103, 103A, 104, and 104A. This type of fenestration is unique to TRACOE tubes; the inner cannula has one large oval aperture while the outer cannula has a series of round holes on the dorsal aspect of the shaft. Two of the models (103 and 103A) also include a detachable silver speaking valve. Model 104 comes with a swivel speaking valve attached to the inner cannula.

Figure 3.81 Jackson Fenestrated

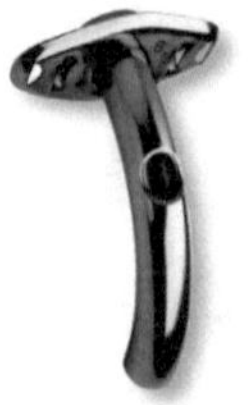

Structure: Uncuffed, dual-cannula

Material: Stainless steel or sterling silver

Manufacturer: Pilling (Teleflex Medical), Premier Medical Products

Unique Features: Large oval fenestration on dorsal aspect of shaft

Use: For the patient who prefers a metal tracheostomy tube and who desires to speak

The Jackson metal tracheostomy tube also comes in a fenestrated version. Unless otherwise ordered, the fenestration is placed one-third of the distance between the neck flange and the distal tip of the tube.

Fahl SILVERVENT LINGO PHON (see Figure 3.63)

Structure: Cuffless, dual-cannula

Material: Sterling silver

Manufacturer: Andreas Fahl Medizintechnik-Vertrieb GmbH

Unique Features: Conical designed tube, with decreasing diameter from neck flange to the tip of the tube; standard version is ¼ radius, but the Jatho version is 1/8 radius (narrower angle); can include low-profile inner cannula as well as one that provides a 15-mm connector; one model also comes with a silver speaking valve; sterling silver has a bactericidal effect

Use: For the patient who can protect his airway and prefers a metal tracheostomy tube

T-Tubes

T-tubes are tracheal stents designed to maintain an open airway for patients with tracheal stenosis or an airway reconstruction. First used in the mid-1960s, T-tubes were used for the repair of tracheal injuries and tracheomalacia.[7,8] The long limb is positioned within the trachea, and the short limb projects through the stoma. T-tubes are thought to be superior to silicone stents because they seldom migrate, can be suctioned, and are easily removable. They are well tolerated and have been reported to remain in place for up to 20 years.[9]

Figure 3.82 Montgomery Safe-T-Tube

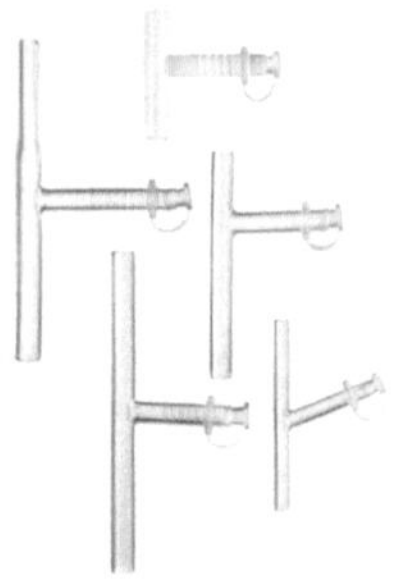

Structure: T-shaped airway stent

Material: Silicone

Manufacturer: Boston Medical Products

Unique Features: Clear or radiopaque; include plug/ring set; Hebeler model has internal balloon system to facilitate positive pressure ventilation

Use: To maintain adequate airway or to stent open a stenotic trachea during reconstruction

The Montgomery Safe-T-Tube **(Figure 3.82)** comes in adult sizes 4.5–16 mm in external diameter and pediatric sizes 4.5 to 8 mm in external diameter and has tapered ends to minimize trauma to the tracheal tissue.[8,10] It is made of silicone and is available in both clear and radiopaque models in five sizes: pediatric, standard, thoracic, extra-long, and tapered. In addition, a Hebeler model has an internal balloon to adjust airflow through the upper end of the tube. It can be inflated for intermittent closure of the upper limb in order to create a closed system between the tracheostomy tube and the lungs. When positive-pressure ventilation is no longer required, the balloon can be deflated, opening the upper limb for access to the upper respiratory tract.

Mini-Tracheostomy Tubes

Patients who have weak secretion clearance may benefit from a mini-tracheostomy. Indications for use of the mini-tracheostomy include patients after major thoracic or abdominal surgery at particular risk for pulmonary complications due to advanced age, chronic lung disease, or poor functional status. In this case, the mini-tracheostomy is a percutaneous procedure in the operating room. It can be considered a useful adjunct in the care of patients with sputum retention.

Wright[11] reported the success rate for the mini-tracheostomy at 96%–100%. The average duration of use is about one week, although cannulas are sometimes left in place for several months. When the patient has regained an adequate cough and no longer requires suctioning, the mini-tracheostomy can be removed. Swallowing is reported to be normal while the cannula is in place and complications are rare. Contraindications to the procedure include morbid obesity, neck mass, calcified cricothyroid membrane, coagulopathy, and impending respiratory failure.

The Portex Mini-Trach II is a small-bore cannula of 4 mm internal diameter. The kit also includes a scalpel, suction catheter, 15-mm connector, and cotton twill tape. **(Figure 3.83).**

Figure 3.83 Portex Mini-Trach II

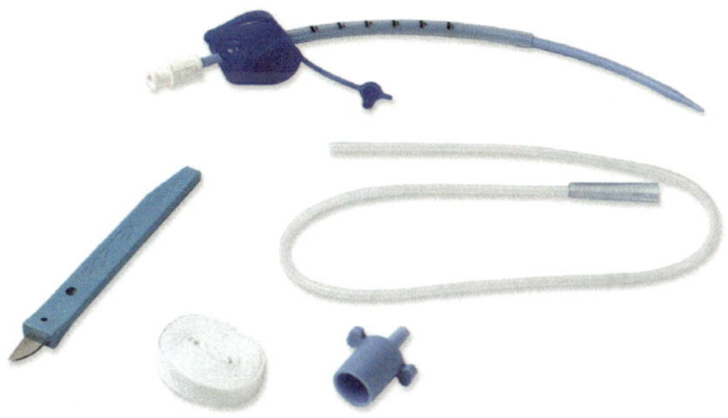

Photo courtesy of Smiths Medical

Pediatric Tubes

Compared to adult tubes, child and neonatal anatomy require differences not only in tube size (inner diameter, outer diameter, and length), but also in tube design. Because of the narrower diameter of the infant and child airway, their tracheostomy tubes do not have inner cannulas. Sometimes a child's chin can block the opening of a standard tracheostomy tube and result in tube obstruction because of their naturally very short necks. A Flextend tube **(Figure 3.84)** provides an extension of the proximal portion of the tracheostomy tube extending from the neck flange. The extension provided by the Flextend tube can promote optimal ventilation without the concern of anatomical tube obstruction by the chin or neck.

Another option on pediatric tubes is the design of the neck flange. Most adult tubes have standard horizontal neck flanges; however, a v-shaped neck flange **(Figure 3.85)** can sometimes allow better seating of the tube against the neck, which could prevent granulation tissue from forming because of the rubbing of the tube against the stoma.

Figure 3.84 Bivona Flextend

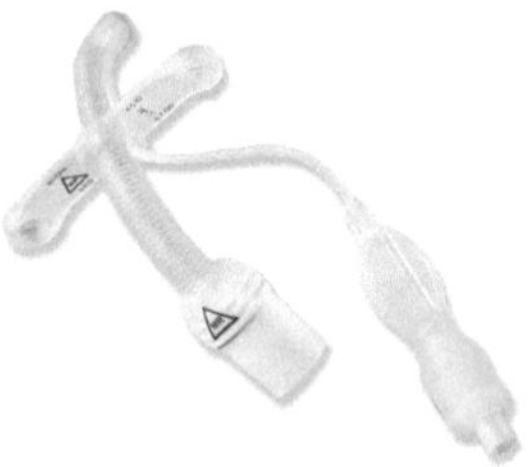

Structure: Single cannula, cuffless or with TTS cuff

Material: Silicone

Manufacturer: Smiths Medical

Unique Features: Extended length, allowing the 15 mm connector to protrude a distance from neck flange

Use: Children, neonates, and others with very short necks

Photo courtesy of Smiths Medical

Figure 3.85 Bivona TTS Neonatal (with v-shaped neck flange)

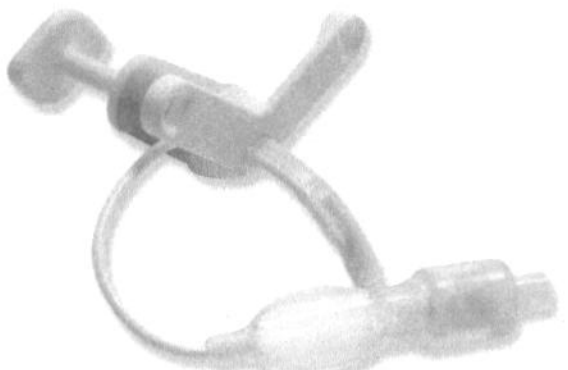

Structure: Single cannula, cuffless or with TTS cuff

Material: Silicone

Manufacturer: Smiths Medical

Unique Features: V-shaped neck flange for improved seating against the neck

Use: Children, neonates, and others with very short necks

Photo courtesy of Smiths Medical

Custom-Designed Tracheostomy Tubes

Occasionally, patients have special needs that cannot be met by available standard tracheostomy tubes. For these patients, it is possible to custom order a tracheostomy tube to meet their needs. A specific length or a specific curvature of tracheostomy tube can be ordered, often by sending CT scans to the manufacturer. Other options are the specific placement of a fenestration or a cuff. These custom tracheostomy tubes often come at a premium price. In addition, custom-designed tubes can take up to two weeks to manufacture, so some advance planning is necessary. Because of the time and expense required to manufacture these custom tubes, it is important that exact measurements be taken, and the goals of treatment be clearly discussed between the managing service, the tracheostomy specialist, and the manufacturer.

Tracheostomy Accessories and Appliances

There are many appliances and supplies available for the tracheostomy patient. These include speaking valves, disconnect wedges, HMEs, decannulation plugs, shower protection devices, and more. Some of these supplies and the conditions in which they may be helpful are discussed in this section.

Speaking Valves

Speaking valves are one-way valves used to facilitate phonation. Air enters the tracheostomy on inspiration but is diverted on expiration through the oropharynx. The variety of valves is discussed in detail in chapter 6.

Stoma Maintenance Devices

There are a variety of devices available that maintain stoma patency. Often these devices are employed during the rehabilitation phase or for patients who cannot otherwise be decannulated. Using these devices, patients can proceed through the rigors of rehabilitation; however, the airway can be immediately accessed if problems are encountered.

Tracheostomy Button/Tracheal Cannula

A tracheostomy button is used as a temporary stent to maintain the patency of the stoma. The Olympic tracheostomy button was the only device of its kind in the US and is no longer manufactured. Instead, patency of the stoma can be maintained with a capped tracheal cannula such as the Montgomery cannula (**Figure 3.86**) or the Fahl Tracheosafe (**Figure 3.87**). The benefit of these devices is that they can provide a low-profile appearance while allowing breathing through the upper airway. A tracheal cannula stents opens the stoma and does not interfere with airflow. However, the tracheal cannula is meant to allow direct access to the airway. The Montgomery cannula is a corrugated tube that is an open system, or a plug can be attached that closes off access to the airway. The Montgomery cannula is made of silicone and is very flexible. A ring washer holds it in place, and it comes with its own detachable plug/ring set to allow phonation. The Montgomery speaking valve was designed for use with the Montgomery cannula and comes in compatible sizes.

Figure 3.86 Montgomery Tracheal Cannula

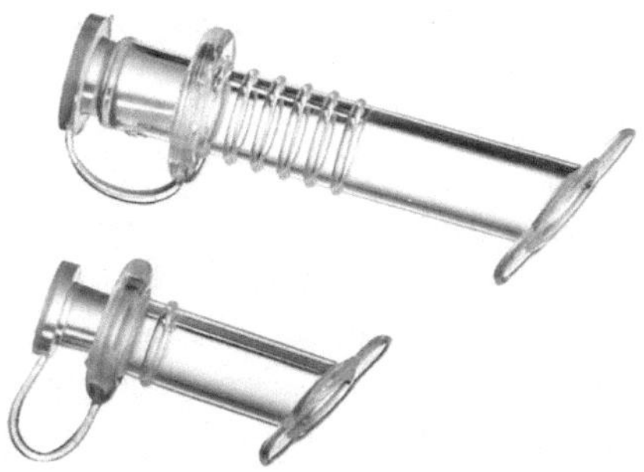

Photo courtesy of Boston Medical Products. All rights reserved.

Figure 3.87 Fahl Tracheosafe

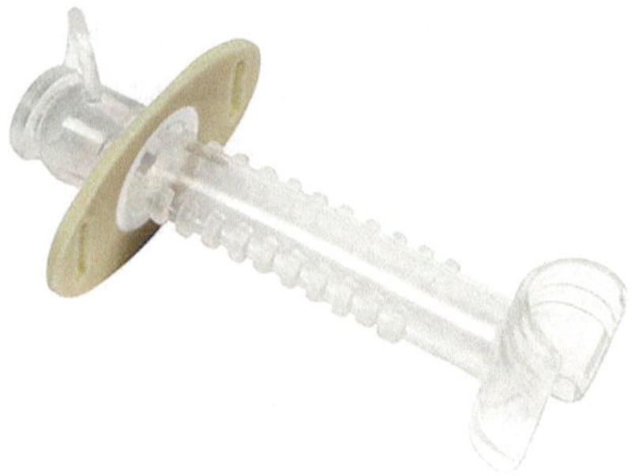

With friendly permission of Andreas Fahl Medizintechnik-Vertrieb GmbH, Cologne, Germany

Figure 3.88 Speak-EZ Tracheal Cannula

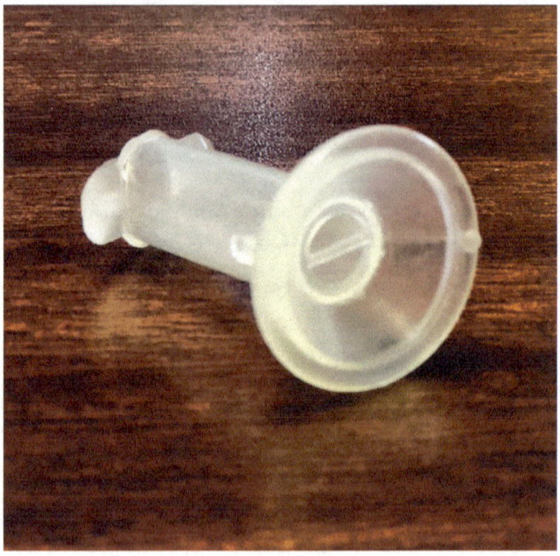

Photo courtesy of Technical Products Inc of Georgia, Lawrenceville, Georgia (www.tpi-ga.com).

The Speak EZ tracheal cannula **(Figure 3.88)** is a low-profile silicone stoma stent with the added benefit of a speaking valve. It is ideal for patients who have tracheal obstruction such as a paralyzed vocal cord. It comes in sizes 8, 11, 13, and 15 mm in multiple lengths.

Disconnect Wedges

A disconnect wedge (**Figure 3.89**) is used when airway equipment (e.g., ventilator circuit or a manual resuscitation bag) is difficult to remove from the 15-mm connector of the tracheostomy tube. Forceful removal should be avoided because the tube can become damaged. The wedge is used as a lever on the 15-mm connecter to disconnect the airway equipment from the tracheostomy tube. Disconnect wedges are packaged with the Bivona line of tracheostomy tubes.

Figure 3.89 Bivona Pediatric Fome-Cuf (with disconnect wedge)

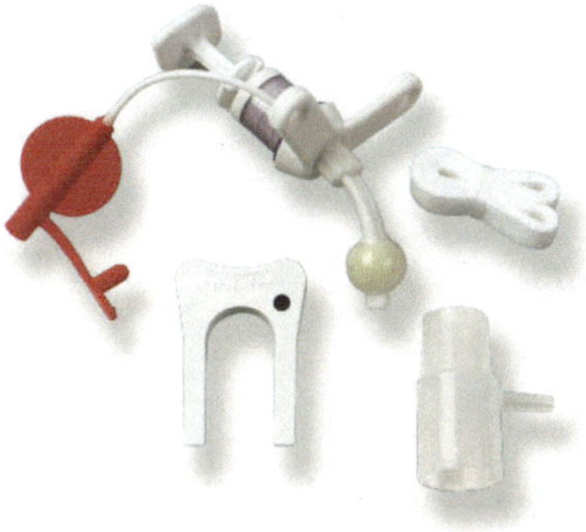

Bivona Pediatric Fome-Cuf tube with disconnect wedge (bottom left) and ventilator adapter (bottom right)

Photo courtesy of Smiths Medical

Caps

There are three primary types of tracheostomy tube caps **(Figure 3.90 through Figure 3.92)**: those applied to the tracheostomy tube, those that replace the inner cannula, and graded plugs. A standard cap is applied externally to the tracheostomy tube to "plug the hole." The Shiley CFS is the only tracheostomy tube with its own capped inner cannula. One must first remove the standard inner cannula and replace it with the capped inner cannula. Caps should never be used with standard (low-pressure, high-volume) cuffed tracheostomy tubes, even if the cuff is completely deflated. The proper use of caps is discussed in chapter 6.

Figure 3.90 Shiley CAP

Shiley CAP

Figure 3.91 TRACOE caps

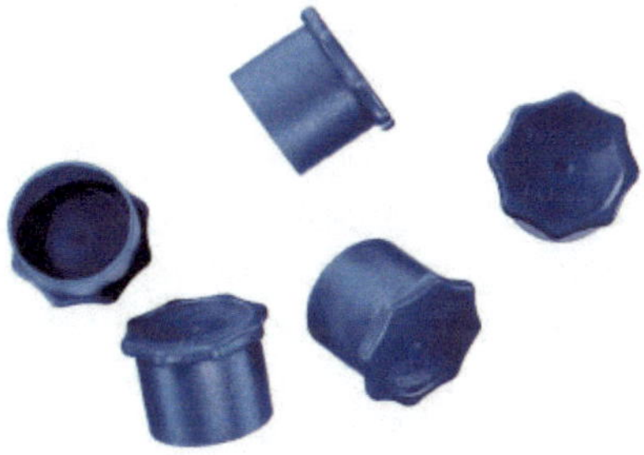

Figure 3.92 Bivona Cap

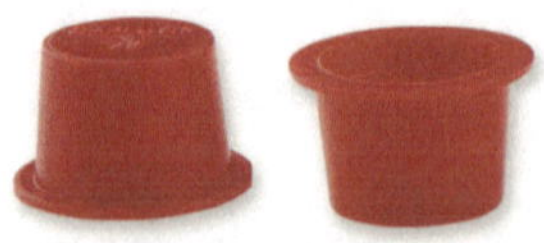

Photo courtesy of Smiths Medical

Decannulation Plugs

Rather than capping a tracheostomy tube, a decannulation plug can be used as a low-profile cap **(Figure 3.93** and **Figure 3.94)**. The use of a decannulation plug often requires the removal of the inner cannula and the attachment of the decannulation plug to the outer cannula. However, TRACOE provides red decannulation plugs for the outer cannulas of the TRACOE Twist tubes (Models 505–04, 505–10) or blue decannulation plugs for the inner cannulas (Models 504–04, 504–10).

Figure 3.93 Shiley DCP

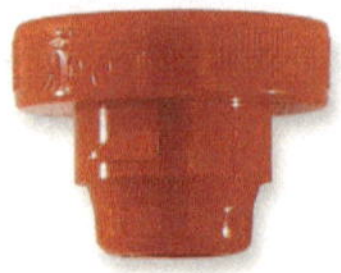

Shiley DCP (decannulation plug) for use with removal of inner cannula of CFS)

Figure 3.94 Shiley DDCP

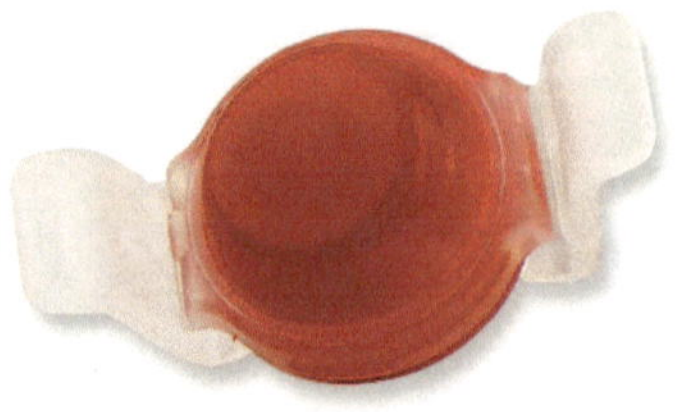

Shiley DDCP (decannulation plug) for use with removal of inner cannula of DCFS)

Corks, Plugs, or Stoppers

A cork, plug, or stopper is similar to a cap or decannulation plug; however, it fits within (rather than around) the inner or outer cannula of a tracheostomy tube **(Figure 3.95)**. These corks were previously made of cork but are now typically made of plastic. They are used for metal tracheostomy tubes and can be ordered to fit based on tube size. They can be ordered in gradations of occlusion in order to facilitate a gradual transition to full upper-airway breathing. For example, they can be ordered for one-fourth partial obstruction, one-half partial obstruction, three-fourths partial obstruction, or full obstruction.

Figure 3.95 Premier Decannulation Stopper

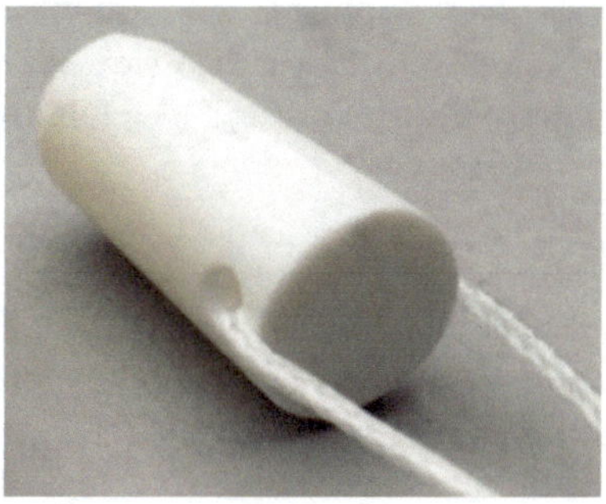

Photo courtesy of Premier Medical Products.

Spare Inner Cannula

Several tracheostomy manufacturers provide additional inner cannulas; however, because the inner cannula of most Shiley tracheostomy tubes must be in place in order to provide positive-pressure ventilation, one must have an extra inner cannula when cleaning the inner cannula of a Shiley tube. The Shiley SIC, or spare inner cannula (**Figure 3.96**), is identified by its red 15-mm connector and is a temporary inner cannula for use with the Shiley LPC, CFS, FEN, or CFN. It is not intended for long-term use and should be replaced with the permanent inner cannula as soon as possible.

Figure 3.96 Shiley SIC

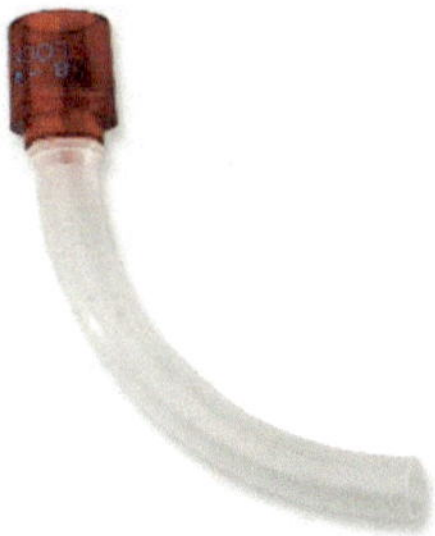

Shiley DIC

The Shiley DCT tracheostomy tube inner cannulas require regular replacement, rather than cleaning. The disposable inner cannula for these tubes is called the DIC.

Portex Per-Fit Inner Cannula

The Portex Per-Fit tracheostomy tube has a beveled distal tip for ease of insertion using the Seldinger technique over a dilator. The Per-Fit inner cannula has a beveled tip to match the outer cannula and its angled distal tip allows easier placement over a dilator during insertion.

Disposable Inner Cannulas for Portex DIC

Portex DIC tracheostomy tubes also have disposable inner cannulas that are color coded based on size. These inner cannulas must be replaced, rather than cleaned, on a regular basis. These inner cannulas are for use with all versions of Portex DIC and Flex DIC tracheostomy tubes.

Anti-disconnect Device

An anti-disconnect device, such as the Shiley Stronghold (Medtronic), helps to eliminate accidental disconnection of equipment from the tracheostomy tube. It is available in adult and pediatric sizes and is used to secure the tracheostomy tube to the ventilator circuit tubing.

Heat Moisture Exchanger

A HME is used to trap the moisture of exhaled gas, allowing the inspiration of added humidity. These devices are especially helpful when patients experience discomfort from dry mucous membranes. These devices can be used in-line with the ventilator circuit or attached separately onto the 15-mm connector of the tracheostomy tube.

Patients who prefer not to use an HME, but who have uncomfortably dry mucous membranes, can use a thin layer of damp gauze draped over the tracheostomy. Saline nasal mist can also be sprayed within the tracheostomy at intervals to moisten mucous membranes.

Ventilator Adapters

A ventilator adapter is available for use with the Bivona Fome-Cuf tracheostomy tube **(Figure 3.89)**. The ventilator adapter provides an additional inflation of air into the cuff with inhalation and a slight deflation of the cuff with exhalation. It is designed to be attached directly to the tracheostomy tube. The HME within the ventilator circuit normally collects exhaled moisture from the circuit and delivers it during inhalation. However, this ventilator adapter delivers moisturized air from the ventilator directly to the cuff. For this reason, an auto-control device is connected to the dry side of the ventilator circuit, and the port from the device is connected to the pilot balloon. This will inflate the cuff with dry gas.

Tracheostomy-Securing Devices

Tracheostomy tubes can be secured to the neck in a variety of ways, including cotton twill tape or soft collars with Velcro closures. Some patients prefer to secure their tracheostomy to their neck with a chain. There is no one recommended device; however, the priority is tube security, especially in the early postoperative period. It is recommended that no more than one finger fit under the securing device. If the securing device is too loose, the patient can easily cough out or otherwise dislodge the tracheostomy tube. If the device is too tight, it can erode into the skin of the neck.

Tracheostomy-Related Supplies

There are a variety of tracheostomy-related supplies and equipment available for the patient's convenience that are primarily for home use.

Tracheostomy Bibs, Dickies, and Scarves

Patients who have a large amount of secretions may find it helpful to wear a type of bib designed to protect their clothing or cover the device **(Figure 3.97** through **Figure 3.99)**. Bibs are also available that can filter and warm the environmental air. Scarves can also provide a method to camouflage the tracheostomy.

Figure 3.97 Fahl Tracheostomy Scarf

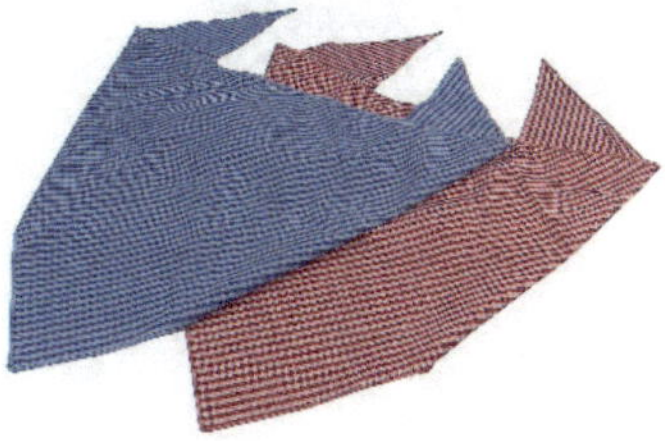

With friendly permission of Andreas Fahl Medizintechnik-Vertrieb GmbH, Cologne, Germany

Figure 3.98 Fahl Tracheostomy Scarf

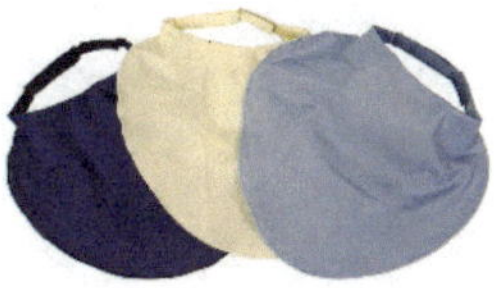

With friendly permission of Andreas Fahl Medizintechnik-Vertrieb GmbH, Cologne, Germany

Figure 3.99 Fahl Tracheostomy Dickies

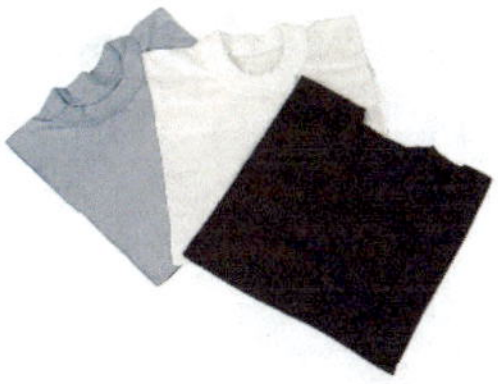

Photo courtesy of Kapitex

Patients who are concerned about the appearance of their tracheostomy may camouflage it by wearing decorative scarves or ascots, colored or beaded tracheostomy ties, or HME covers. Some of these are available in materials that resist staining and moisture.

Shower Protection Devices

Patients who are concerned that water may enter their tracheostomy or laryngectomy tube while showering can use a shower protection device **(Figure 3.100)**. Otherwise, patients should be taught to avoid facing the water flow.

Figure 3.100 Kapitex Shower Protection

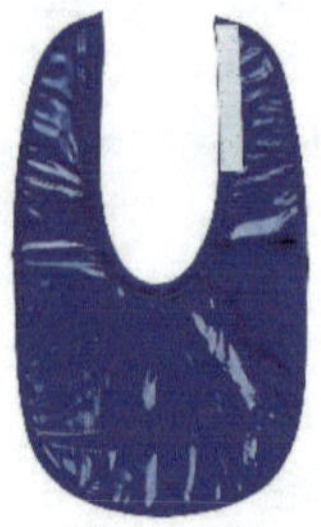

Photo courtesy of Kapitex

Tube Spacer

A tube spacer can be used to prevent blocking the aperture when the patient is wearing protective clothing around the stoma.

Grid or Mesh Screens

A mesh screen can be used to filter air in order to prevent inhalation and aspiration of particulate matter or foreign bodies.

SUMMARY

There are many choices of tracheostomy tubes. Each tube has its own characteristics with inherent strengths and precautions. The major categories of tracheostomy tubes include cuffed or cuffless and single- or dual-cannula. Many special-use tracheostomy tubes are also available, such as extra-length or talking tracheostomy tubes. One must have a clear understanding of the primary goals in order to choose the best tube for a particular patient.

KEY POINTS

- Tracheostomy tubes can be classified into four categories: dual-cannula, cuffed tubes; single-cannula, cuffed tubes; dual-cannula, cuffless tubes; and single-cannula, cuffless tubes.
- Tracheostomy tubes are constructed of a variety of materials, including polyvinyl chloride, silicone, nylon, stainless steel, or silver.
- Tracheostomy tubes with inner cannulas should be used in patients who have large amounts of secretions.
- Laryngectomy tubes are always cuffless and are usually shorter than a standard tube.
- Cuffless tracheostomy tubes are used in patients who can protect their airway.

REVIEW QUESTIONS

1. What is the purpose of the obturator?
    a. To cauterize a bleeding vessel
    b. To assist with insertion of a tracheostomy tube
    c. To replace the inner cannula in case of dislodgement
    d. To secure snugly against the neck

    ANSWER: B. The purpose of the obturator is to assist with insertion of a tracheostomy tube. The obturator cushions the tip of the tube, preventing tissue damage with insertion. All the other choices are distractors and incorrect.

2. Which type of tracheostomy tube is best used in a patient who can protect the airway but who also has very thick secretions?
    a. Single-cannula, cuffed tube
    b. Single-cannula, cuffless tube
    c. Dual-cannula, cuffed tube
    d. Dual-cannula, cuffless tube

    ANSWER: D. Since the patient can protect the airway, a cuffed tube is not needed. But since the patient has very thick secretions, an inner cannula is usually best to prevent tube obstruction.

3. A potential advantage of single-cannula tubes compared to dual cannula tubes of the same size is:
    a. They have narrower outer diameters
    b. They have extra length
    c. They have narrower inner diameters
    d. They have wider outer diameters

    ANSWER: A. A narrower outer diameter can be beneficial when attempting phonation as it allows more air around the outside of the tube. All the other choices are distractors and incorrect.

4. Which is the only tracheostomy tube that has a high-pressure cuff?
    a. Shiley DCT
    b. Fahl Duratwix
    c. Bivona TTS
    d. Rüsch Trachflex Plus

    ANSWER: C. The Bivona TTS is the only tracheostomy tube with a high-pressure, low-volume cuff, making it the only cuffed tube that is safe to cap. All the other choices have high-volume, low-pressure cuffs.

5. Compared to adult tubes, pediatric tracheostomy tubes do not have inner cannulas because:
    a. Pediatric tubes need additional humidity
    b. The internal diameter of the child's airway is much narrower
    c. The child's chin can block the opening of a tracheostomy tube
    d. The tube may require a different type of neck flange

ANSWER: B. Because of the narrower internal diameter of the airway, pediatric tubes do not have inner cannulas. Choice A is incorrect. Choices C and D are true but do not relate to the inner cannula.

Web Resources

Amy's Trach Ties, https://amystrachties.com/

Angiplast, manufacturer of Angiplast tracheostomy tubes, http://www.angiplast.com/

Atos Medical, manufacturer of Provox LaryTube and related laryngectomy products, https://www.atosmedical.com/

Boston Medical, manufacturer Montgomery, and Moore tracheostomy tubes and related devices, http://www.trachs.com

Adoracion Francisco Chiner, http://fchiner.es/our-products/?lang=en

Cook Medical Products, https://www.cookmedical.com/products/

Covidien, manufacturer of Shiley tracheostomy tubes, http://www.nellcor.com

Andreas Fahl Medizintechnik-Vertrieb Gmbh, manufacturer of Fahl tracheostomy tubes and related products https://www.fahl-medizintechnik.de/en/

Hood Labs, manufacturer of Hood stoma stent and Eliachar speaking valves, https://hoodlabs.com/

Kapitex, manufacturer of Kapitex tracheostomy tubes and related products, https://www.kapitex.com/

Premier Medical Products, manufacturer of Jackson original, Jackson Improved, and Air-Lon™ tracheostomy tubes, http://www.premusa.com

Pulmodyne, manufacturer of the Blom tracheostomy tube, http://www.pulmodyne.com

Smiths Medical, manufacturer of Bivona and Portex tracheostomies and related devices, http://www.smiths-medical.com

Suru, manufacturer of Suru tracheostomies and related devices, http://suru.com

Technical Products, Inc. of Georgia, manufacturer of Speak EZ tracheal cannula, http://www.techproductsga.com/

Teleflex Medical, Pilling, manufacturer of Teleflex, Pilling, and Rusch tracheostomy products, http://www.teleflexmedical.com

The Trach Shop, https://www.thetrachshop.com/

TRACOE Medical GmbH, manufacturer of TRACOE tracheostomy tubes and related products, https://www.tracoe.com

References

1. Dhand R, Johnson JC. Care of the chronic tracheostomy. *Respir Care.* 2006;*51*(9):984-1001.
2. St. John RE, Malen JF. Contemporary issues in adult tracheostomy management. *Crit Care Nurs Clin N Amer.* 2004;*16*(3):413-430.
3. Faris C, Koury E, Philpott J, Sharma S, Tolley N, Narula A. Estimation of tracheostomy tube cuff pressure by pilot balloon palpation. *J Laryngol Otol.* 2007;*121*(9):869-871.
4. Quigley RL. Tracheostomy—an overview. Management and complications. *Brit J Clin Pract.* 1988;*42*(10):430-434.
5. Bernhard WN, Yost L, Joynes D, Cothalis S, Turndorf H. Cuff pressures in endotracheal and tracheostomy tubes. Related cuff physical characteristics. *Chest.* 1985;*87:*720-725.
6. Duguet A, D'Amico L, Biondi G, Prodanovic H, Gonzalez-Bermejo J, Similowski T. Control of tracheal cuff pressure: A pilot study using a pneumatic device. Intens Care Med. 2007;33:128-132.
7. Huang C. Use of the silicone T-tube to treat tracheal stenosis or tracheal injury. *Ann Thorac Cardiovasc Surg.* 2001;*7*(4):192-196.
8. Wouters KMA, Byreddy R, Gleeson J, Morley AP. New approach to anaesthetizing a patient at risk of pulmonary aspiration with a Montgomery T-tube in situ. *Brit J Anaesth.* 2008;*101:*354–357.
9. Wahidi MM, Ernst A. The Montgomery T-tube tracheal stent. *Clin Chest Med.* 2003;*24:*437-443.
10. Guha Q, Mostafa SM, Kendall JB. The Montgomery T-tube: Anaesthetic problems and solutions. *Brit J Anaesth.* 2001;*87*(5):787-790.
11. Wright CD. Minitracheostomy. *Clin Chest Med.* 2003;*24*(3):431-435.

4

Fitting and Changing Tracheostomy Tubes

By Linda L. Morris

Objectives

- List goals when fitting a tracheostomy tube
- Match tube features with patient airway and clinical condition
- Detail step-by-step technique for tracheostomy tube changes
- Identify precautions when placing a fenestrated tube

Introduction

Fitting tracheostomy tubes is both a science and an art. One might believe it is a routine and straightforward procedure, but this is hardly the case. Fisher and colleagues[1] suggest that tracheostomy tubes are electively changed for a variety of reasons, including downsizing and facilitation of phonation and oral intake. There are numerous factors to consider when determining the optimal size and type of tracheostomy tube, particularly the patient's ability to protect his or her airway, the amount and thickness of secretions, if positive-pressure ventilation is required, anatomical considerations, a desire to speak, airway pressures, the size of the tracheostomy tube versus the size of the airway, and lung mechanics. Each of these factors must be taken into consideration in order to provide for the individual needs of each patient.

Considerations When Fitting a Tracheostomy Tube

Before Fitting a Tracheostomy Tube

There are numerous factors to consider when fitting a patient with a tracheostomy tube. Short-term and long-term goals should be identified and reviewed on a regular basis. Questions include the following:

- Will the patient require mechanical ventilation for the next week, next month, or some other time frame?
- Does the patient desire to speak?
- Is the patient able to manage airway secretions?
- Is the patient ready to be weaned from mechanical ventilation?
- Can the patient be managed with nocturnal positive-pressure ventilation and a tracheostomy collar during the day?
- Is the patient on a path to rehabilitation, or will the patient require long-term care?
- Does the family have the capability to safely manage the patient at home?

There are questions to ask at each point in the patient's hospitalization, discharge planning, rehabilitation, and outpatient settings because the goals often change as the patient progresses through each phase of treatment and recovery.

When fitting a tracheostomy tube, it is necessary to examine the inner diameter, outer diameter, and length of the tracheostomy tube in place, consider individual patient issues, and then determine the primary and secondary goals. If wishing to speak is a secondary goal, enough air must pass around the outside of the tube to easily reach the vocal cords. If a primary goal is to deliver positive-pressure ventilation, then an adequate seal would be the priority. The challenge comes when there are multiple or conflicting goals—for example, a patient who requires positive-pressure ventilation but who also desires to speak. Another challenging example is a patient who requires a longer tracheostomy tube but who also has copious thick secretions. One must constantly balance goals with priorities.

Clinical Scenario

Patient A received a tracheostomy after a long stay in the ICU following a motor vehicle accident, when a Shiley 8 LPC (cuffed, dual-cannula) tube was placed. He was liberated from ventilator support a few days after the tracheostomy was initially placed.

The tracheostomy specialist evaluates the patient, deflates the cuff, and recommends the patient be changed to a cuffless tube if he tolerates prolonged cuff deflation.

Assessing the Resistance of the Tracheostomy Tube

When fitting the optimal tracheostomy tube, one must first consider size. Poiseuille's Law states that flow is dependent upon the radius and length of the tube.

$$P = \frac{\dot{V}8L\eta}{\pi r^4}$$

In this equation, P is the pressure gradient across the tube, $\dot{V}$ represents gas flow, L represents tube length, η represents gas viscosity, r represents the tube radius, and 8 and π represent constants. In other words, when flow is laminar, resistance is directly proportional to the radius of the tube raised to the fourth power. However, when flow is turbulent, resistance becomes inversely proportional to the radius raised to the fifth power. Because of this, a small decrease in radius will dramatically increase resistance.[2,3] Compared to endotracheal tubes, a tracheostomy tube makes the elastic and resistive work of breathing easier. The shorter length of the tracheostomy tube, as well as its more rigid structure and placement in the subglottic region, makes it easier to facilitate effective bronchial hygiene.[3] By lessening the resistance that secretions create, intrinsic PEEP is reduced, thus decreasing the elastic work of breathing.

Pierson[4] clearly outlined the general principles of airflow with regard to artificial airways:

- The larger the inner diameter, the lower the resistance.
- The shorter the tube, the lower the resistance.
- Irregular walls of the tube (such as those produced by secretions) increase resistance.
- The sharper the curve of the tube, the greater the resistance.

All these factors contribute to the work of breathing and must be considered when fitting a tracheostomy tube. Major indications for placing a tracheostomy tube include prolonged mechanical ventilation with endotracheal intubation, upper airway obstruction, airway protection, and the facilitation of bronchial hygiene,[5] all of which make up the acronym VOPS (ventilation, obstruction, protection, secretions).

In hospitals, it is advisable to fit the tracheostomy patient with a tube with a standard 15-mm connector to enable the use of a mechanical resuscitation bag or ventilator in the event of an emergency. Some low-profile tubes eliminate the 15-mm connector for a more cosmetic appearance. However, many hospital-based practitioners are not familiar with the low-profile tracheostomy tube, nor that some can be converted to a standard inner cannula with a 15-mm connector, which could result in confusion during an emergency.

Clinical Scenario Cont'd.

The tracheostomy specialist returns two days later to change the tracheostomy tube for Patient A. The nurse reports that the patient has a large amount of thick secretions, so the tracheostomy specialist chooses a Shiley 6 CFS (cuffless, dual-cannula) tube. She places her finger over the tube to test the patient's ability to move air around the tube, knowing that airflow should be laminar around a smaller cuffless tube.

Choosing a Cuffed Versus Uncuffed Tube

The earliest tracheostomy tubes were cuffless. In the 1960s, tracheostomy tubes were constructed with small-volume cuffs. These cuffs were smaller than the airway, and pressures of 160 to 300 mm

Hg were required to fill the cuffs.[6] Larger volume cuffs that required lower inflation pressure were developed in the 1970s.

The first decision when choosing the type of tracheotomy tube is whether or not the patient requires a cuffed tube. Patients who require positive-pressure ventilation almost always require a cuffed tube. If the patient is ventilator-dependent, a tube with a low-pressure cuff would minimize pressure against the tracheal wall. However, the patient who is only partially dependent on positive-pressure ventilation could use a different tube (e.g., using nocturnal ventilation at night and a high-humidity tracheostomy collar during the day). In that case, a Bivona TTS tracheostomy tube could provide the added advantage of capping during the day. Any concerns about their high-pressure cuffs would be offset by intermittent inflation. Because the cuff lies completely against the shaft when deflated, creating no airflow obstruction, the Bivona TTS tube is the only cuffed tracheostomy tube that can be capped safely when the cuff is deflated. A properly fitted, fenestrated tube may also be capped, but this tube has a standard high-volume, low-pressure cuff.

Positive-Pressure Ventilation and Choice of Tube

Whenever positive-pressure ventilation is required, a cuffed tracheostomy tube is necessary to ensure the set tidal volume is delivered. If a cuffless tube is used with a ventilator-dependent patient, there will be a large leak of air around the tube because of the significant difference in delivered versus returned tidal volume. This difference can be problematic—not only in ventilator alarms sounding, but also in terms of respiratory distress, hypoxemia, and hemodynamic instability. Occasionally, however, some ventilator-dependent patients with cuffless tracheostomy tubes use what is called "leak speech" in order to phonate. (See chapter 6 for a detailed discussion about leak speech.) However, if these patients become unstable or critically ill, a cuffed tube is always advisable. In this circumstance, patients will need the benefit of receiving the entire tidal volume. Until a cuffed tracheostomy tube can be placed, ventilator settings should be adjusted by increasing flow and/or minute ventilation to compensate for the large deficit in returned tidal volumes.

The success of managing a ventilator-dependent patient with a tracheostomy revolves around several factors: volume delivered versus volume returned, adequate seal of the cuff within the airway, and resistance to gas delivered. When the volume returned is much less than the tidal volume delivered, ventilator alarms will sound with an alert indicator for a system leak. This leak could be in one of three main locations: the ventilator circuit, the seal of the cuff against the airway, or within the cuff itself. See chapter 5 for a comprehensive discussion about leaks.

CLINICAL SCENARIO CONT'D

Patient B has a Shiley 9 SCT tracheostomy tube and has been on full ventilator support for two weeks in the critical care unit, with high airway pressures. Cuff pressure has been increasing over the past few days, and the respiratory therapist reports copious thick secretions. This morning, cuff pressure was measured at 60 cm H_2O, with a continued leak around the cuff, so the tracheostomy specialist is called for help.

If it has been determined that there is sufficient air in the cuff and a leak remains, tracheomalacia is the presumed cause. Tracheomalacia is commonly caused by chronic overinflation of the cuff. This added pressure against the elastic tracheal tissue causes it to weaken and balloon out in the area of the cuff. Like overstretched elastic, the tracheal tissue appears to stretch in the area of increased pressure. This stretch is limited, however, and can result in tracheal erosion if the pressures are too great over a prolonged period of time. Tracheoscopy can be used to visualize the extent of the defect.

CLINICAL SCENARIO CONT'D.

Because of the history of increasing cuff pressures with a continuing cuff leak, the tracheostomy specialist presumes that tracheomalacia is present. Because of the report of high airway pressures and copious thick secretions, she is also concerned about accumulation of secretions within the single-cannula tube. She changes the tube to a Shiley 7 XLT tube because of its extended length and inner cannula. Airway pressures drop to normal and cuff pressure is now 24 cm H_2O.

The method to resolve a leak due to tracheomalacia is to place the cuff in a different location within the trachea. This is usually done by placing a tracheostomy tube with a slightly longer length so as to place the cuff inferior to the area of tracheomalacia (see **Figure 4.1**).

Figure 4.1 Tracheomalacia & repositioning

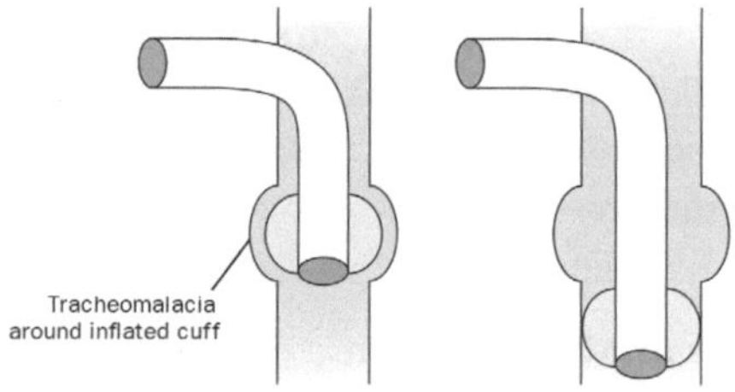

Tracheomalacia and repositioning the tracheostomy tube. On the left is an area of tracheomalacia around an inflated cuff. On the right, a longer tracheostomy tube has been inserted, allowing the cuff to be positioned below the level of tracheomalacia.

Airway Protection

Another important factor in determining the proper type of tracheostomy tube is airway protection. If the patient is able to protect his or her airway, then a cuffless tube usually offers the most benefits. However, without adequate intrinsic reflex airway protection, a cuffed tube must be chosen. Following this decision, other features can then be considered, such as phonation and single- versus dual-cannula tubes.

Airway protection is primarily influenced by intact swallow and adequate cough. The epiglottis closes over the trachea during swallowing in order to prevent food and fluid from entering the trachea. A study in normal adults by Mendell and Logemann[7] showed that the sequence of events in the pharyngeal swallow varied depending on the age of the patient and the volume and consistency of the bolus. The dominant sequence was hyoid and laryngeal elevation, followed by posterior tongue retraction and then laryngeal vestibular closure. On a larger bolus, laryngeal vestibule closure occurred before the tongue base movement—and it was thought this would add to airway protection. The sequence of events during the swallow was dependent on other factors such as age and comorbidities. Normal participants in their 60s and 70s had longer time differences between hyoid elevation and upper esophageal sphincter opening than younger subjects.[7,8]

A more recent study[9] studied swallow physiology in left versus right hemispheric strokes. Out of 46 subjects, the investigators concluded there were differences in swallow physiology, and patients with right strokes showed worse pharyngeal impairment. Lesion lateralization was found to be an important marker for severity of swallow impairment. Neurological injury or disease may greatly influence a patient's ability to swallow, so it is advisable to obtain a swallow evaluation from a speech pathologist whenever the patient's swallow is in question. A detailed discussion on the physiology of swallow is provided in chapter 1.

Strength of Cough

Strength of cough can be subjectively observed at the bedside, though a more objective measure is called vital capacity. Normal vital capacity is 50–70 ml/kg of body weight.[10] However, after days or weeks of oral intubation, the ability to cough can be compromised because the glottic mechanism is bypassed, and associated muscle weakness of critical illness. The lowest acceptable vital capacity that determines adequacy of cough is 15 ml/kg of body weight—or approximately 1 liter for most adults.[5] Another measure of cough strength is the peak cough flow, which should be at least 360 liters per minute;[11] lower than this indicates poor cough strength. The primary danger of poor cough strength is the inability to clear secretions, which can result in the retention of secretions, respiratory distress, and hypoxemia.

Usually, the best way to improve cough strength is vigorous exercise. In an unpublished case series by this author, a program of deep breathing and arm exercises was prescribed to tracheostomy patients who were able to independently move at least one of their upper extremities. Exercises were demonstrated to the patient, the primary nurse, and the family when available, and the patient was encouraged to do 10 (or more) repetitions per hour. All the patients who complied, even partially, demonstrated improvement in vital capacity after only two days—often by at least 100%, and in one case by 700%.

Incentive spirometry is ideal for tracheostomy patients who have the manual dexterity to use it. However, it can only be used for patients who are capped and breathing through their native airway, as it requires use of a mouthpiece.

Deep breathing *and* arm exercises can result in the enhanced early mobilization of secretions.

Swallowing

An intact swallow is essential for ensuring airway protection. The swallowing mechanism is disrupted by the prolonged presence of an endotracheal tube, and tracheostomy patients, particularly those with an inflated cuff, sometimes report discomfort with swallowing. Furthermore, the frequency of silent aspiration and reduced laryngeal elevation is increased with cuff inflation.[12]

Mental Status

Unresponsive patients usually present more of a challenge and often require a cuffed tracheostomy tube. However, unresponsive patients are sometimes able to protect their airway to a certain degree. Mental status alone is not a determining factor in fitting or downsizing a tracheostomy tube. If an unresponsive patient has an effective spontaneous cough and swallow, the patient can be considered for downsizing. The primary factors to be considered are swallow, cough, and secretions.

Choosing a Dual- Versus Single-Cannula Tracheostomy Tube

Another consideration is the choice between a dual- or single-cannula tube. The amount and thickness of secretions determines whether or not a dual-cannula tube is desirable. The primary advantage of a dual-cannula tube is that the inner cannula can be removed, inspected, and cleaned or replaced if necessary. Single-cannula tubes do not have this feature. Secretions accumulate and collect within the inner lumen of the tracheostomy tube, which results in a narrowing of the inner diameter of the tube and can contribute to increased resistance, work of breathing, or, worse, tube obstruction.

If other factors (such as the desire to speak, ventilator dependency, or altered anatomy) are considered, a single-cannula tracheostomy tube may be the better choice. Precautionary measures should be taken for patients who have large amounts of thick secretions, including offering optimal fluids to thin secretions and vigorous physical therapy to facilitate the mobility of secretions.

One bench study[13] found that pressures changed with increasing flow and the type of tube, as well as with the pattern affected by tube type. The single lumen reference tube created the lowest inspiratory and expiratory pressures when compared with all dual-lumen tubes tested. Placement of an inner cannula significantly increased resistance by factors of 0.3 to 4.0.

Secretions and Tube Obstruction

The amount and thickness of secretions are factors in the choice of tracheostomy tube. When the consistency of secretions is thin, it is easier for them to be coughed or suctioned out. Not all patients who have a large amount of secretions will require a cuffed tracheostomy tube. However, patients who cannot manage their secretions will require a cuffed tube. Thick secretions in a patient with a poor cough are the most worrisome because mucous plugs can readily develop. *Unresponsive patients who do not cough may be retaining secretions.* Patients with a poor cough reflex or who are unresponsive should be regularly stimulated. Frequent turning and increasing of the patient's range of motion will help mobilize secretions. Other bronchial hygiene maneuvers—such as percussion and vibration, postural drainage, and bronchodilators—may be necessary to mobilize secretions, but they are applied on an individual basis. All efforts to mobilize secretions should be followed by vigorous coughing or tracheal suctioning to remove secretions from the airway.

Suctioning

Suctioning a patient on a regular schedule is not recommended, but it is vital to prevent mucus plugging and ensure patency of the airway.[14] Patients with a weak or absent cough will require the most suctioning, regardless of the secretion consistency, because suctioning is one effective way to stimulate secretions. Passing a suction catheter will ensure patency of the tube, but there is no evidence to determine the optimal frequency of this maneuver. Patients with a strong cough will usually require less suctioning unless their secretions are very thick and they are unable to fully expectorate them.

The technique of suctioning has been described in several studies. Some authors suggest the suction catheter should not go past the tip of the tracheostomy tube to avoid causing unnecessary stimulation and possible damage to the tracheal wall. This shallow suctioning may be adequate in patients with a strong cough. However, the potential danger is to patients without a strong cough reflex. These patients are unable to effectively produce secretions and will require stimulation, often in the form of deep tracheal suctioning.

There are few studies on depth of suctioning, and most showed no preference of deep versus shallow suctioning. However, Irajpour[15] found that the use of deep suctioning required less passes of the suction catheter to clear the airway without a difference in heart rate, blood pressure, oxygen saturation, or arrhythmias.

The failure to provide effective stimulation and secretion mobilization in patients who are unresponsive can result in the inspissation of secretions, mucous plug formation, and obstruction of the tube—all of which have potentially serious consequences. See chapter 7 for further discussion of mobilization of secretions.

Choosing Optimal Tube Size

The choice of tracheostomy tube size goes hand in hand with determining the need for cuffed versus uncuffed and single- versus dual-cannula tubes. The appropriate size and type of tube for each patient are determined by the goal of the care plan, which takes the following factors into consideration: need for positive-pressure ventilation, phonation, amount and viscosity of secretions, hemodynamic stability, airway anatomy, and coexisting medical disorders. The initial step is to identify the inner diameter, outer diameter, and length of tube in situ and compare with the available choices. **Appendices A-C** list the inner and outer diameters and lengths by type and manufacturer. The information in the appendices facilitates the optimal choice of tube for each patient.

Appendix A: Tracheostomy tube measurements, adult

Appendix B: Laryngectomy tube measurements

Appendix C: Tracheostomy tube measurements, neonatal and pediatric.

If the patient is breathing exclusively through the tube, the largest inner diameter is recommended; if the patient is breathing at least partially around the tube, he or she could likely tolerate a tube with a much smaller outer diameter. The process of downsizing should enable the patient to breathe easier around the tube. **Figure 4.2** shows the difference in airflow through a larger versus a smaller tube. Refer to chapter 11 for a discussion about downsizing tracheostomy tubes.

Figure 4.2 Airflow larger vs. smaller tube

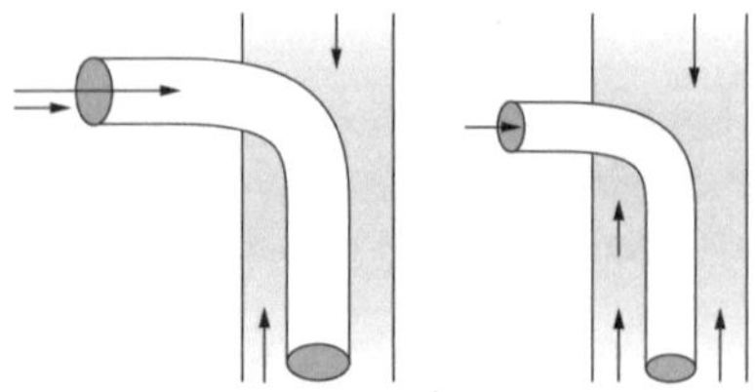

Airflow through a smaller tube compared with one that is larger. Note less resistance with breathing through a larger tube. As the tube gets smaller, resistance (hence, work of breathing) will increase.

Proper sizing will also ensure a low-pressure seal to the cuff. A tube that is too small will not adequately seal the airway and, thus, will create numerous problems (**Figure 4.3A**), including loss of airway pressures and overinflation of the cuff. This can lead to the development of ventilator-associated pneumonia.[6,16] A tube that is too large can damage the tracheal mucosa, leading to granulation tissue or stenosis of the trachea (**Figure 4.3B**). In this case, inflating the cuff will produce high cuff pressures. Thus, the ratio of size of cuff to size of trachea is an important factor for properly fitting a tracheostomy tube.[6]

Figure 4.3 Improperly sized tubes

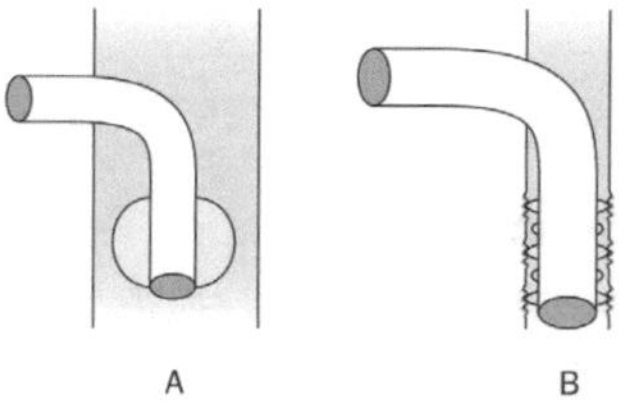

Improperly sized tubes. A) A tracheostomy tube that is too small, despite hyperinflation of the cuff. B) A tracheostomy tube that is too large; it leaves no room for the cuff and abuts the tracheal wall.

Choosing the Best Tube Construction

One consideration regarding the optimal tracheostomy tube is the tube's construction. For example, a patient with a tumor extrinsically compressing his or her airway might benefit from a tracheostomy tube with a more rigid shaft so the airway is not compromised. However, a patient with unusual airway anatomy might benefit from a more flexible tube. Generally speaking, tracheostomy tubes with less rigid construction tend to be more comfortable because they can conform to the morphology of the airway.

Polyvinyl chloride tubes can be either rigid or flexible. Silicone is known for its flexible properties, and secretions tend to adhere less to a silicone inner lumen. However, silicone does not prevent the accumulation of secretions. Changing a tracheostomy tube that is more flexible can be a challenge because it can change shape during insertion. Hence, the obturator is necessary to maintain the position of the tube during insertion. Once the tube is in place, the obturator is removed, and the tube is allowed to conform to airway anatomy.

Choosing Optimal Tube Length

When the tracheostomy tube is too short, it can easily slip out of the airway, exert excessive pressure on the anterior tracheal wall, create backward pressure against the posterior tracheal wall, and make suctioning difficult.[17] In fact, one study suggested that the standard tracheostomy tube should be longer with a redesigned angle. The basis for this European study was recurrent problems with too short tubes in critically ill patients. The study was conducted both in vitro and in vivo. Measurements from a variety of standard tracheostomy tubes were compared in vivo with measurements of the depth from the skin surface to the tracheal wall, as well as the angle of the tracheal stoma. Results suggested that tracheostomy tubes should be lengthened by 1 cm and the angle redesigned to 110–120 degrees in order to facilitate proper placement within the airway.[17] Since that study was published, there has been no corroborating work further suggesting a change in tube length or angle.

Longer tubes can be used in a variety of cases, including for patients with thick or obese necks or unusual anatomy. Ventilator-dependent patients with tracheomalacia will benefit from the placement of longer tubes where the cuff rests below the area of the tracheomalacia. By contrast, a longer tube can also act as a stent past an airway obstruction.

Matching Shape of Tube and Airway

The curvature of the tracheostomy tube will affect airway integrity and the work of breathing over time. A tube with too wide an angle can create erosion of the dorsal trachea where the shaft abrades the posterior wall. A tube with too narrow an angle can also create increased work of breathing[4] and potential erosion of the anterior wall. (**Figure 4.4**).

Figure 4.4 Wide angle vs. narrow, erosion

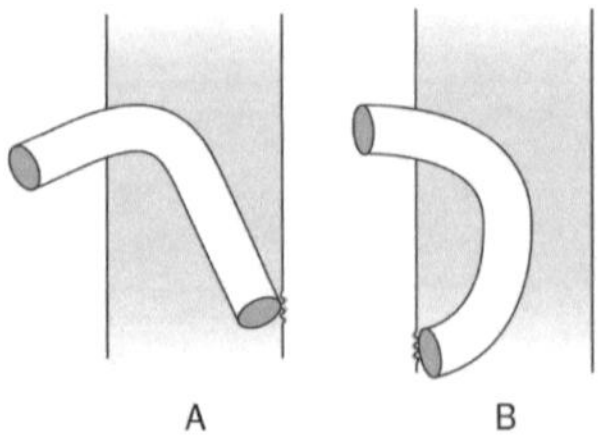

Tubes of different angles creating tracheal erosion. A) Poorly fitting wide-angle tube shows erosion of the posterior tracheal wall. B) Poorly fitting narrow-angled tube shows erosion of the anterior tracheal wall.

A patient with an irregular shape to his or her airway can develop increased airway resistance and work of breathing. For example, a neck mass can press against the airway, distorting its curvature and narrowing its diameter. In this example, it would be important to reinforce the airway to prevent narrowing and allow laminar airflow, thus optimizing the work of breathing.

Phonation and Tube Choice

There are numerous considerations involved in speech with tracheostomy patients. The details of phonation with a tracheostomy are discussed in chapter 6.

Tracheostomy Tube Changes

A tracheostomy tube change is not a benign procedure. The loss of the airway is a primary concern, especially in the early postoperative period. During the first postoperative week, the stomal tissue tract is not mature, and removal of the tube can result in the collapse of the tissue planes, making replacement within the airway difficult. Furthermore, attempts to replace the airway prematurely within the stoma can create a false passage if the tube is forced into the stoma and an initial caudal turn is applied. Continued efforts to insert the tube, inflate the cuff, and ventilate the patient will enlarge this false passage, compress the trachea, and potentially result in life-threatening pneumopericardium, pneumothorax, or widespread subcutaneous emphysema.[18] **Figure 4.5** shows the placement of a tracheostomy tube into a false passage within the pretracheal tissue. Thus, tube change or replacement should always be followed by confirmation of proper tube placement.

Figure 4.5 Premature caudal turn

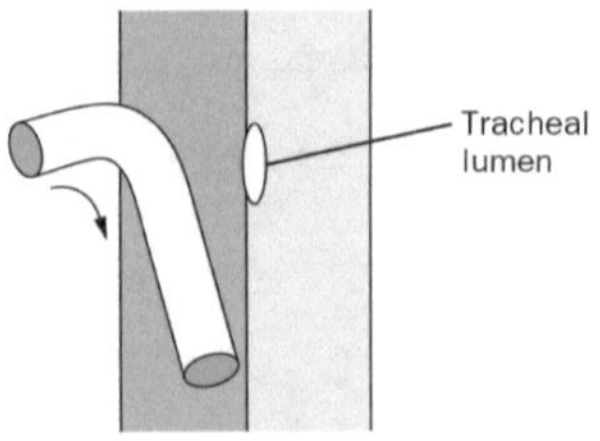

Premature caudal turn, placing tube in a false passage in the subcutaneous tissue anterior to the trachea.

Tabaee and colleagues[19] conducted a survey of chief residents of accredited otolaryngology programs to determine their practice patterns related to tracheostomy tube changes. Ninety-three percent of respondents indicated they used sutures to secure the tracheostomy tube. Seventeen percent reported they changed the tube before the fifth day, 55% changed the tube on the fifth postoperative day, and 28% changed the tube after the fifth day. The mean time interval between the tracheotomy procedure and the first tube change was 5.3 days, with a range of 3–7 days. Participants were asked if they were aware of any loss of airway or death as a result of the first tube change; 42% of respondents were aware of a loss of airway, and 15% were aware of a death. A higher percentage of respondents indicated there was a significantly higher incidence of loss of airway on the wards compared to the ICU, and the investigators suggested that tube changes might be delayed for patients on the wards in order to allow for a more mature stoma, but they could not conclude that tube changes on the wards are always problematic.

Factors that complicate a tracheostomy tube change include obesity, a short or edematous neck, anatomical anomalies, granulation tissue, copious tracheal secretions, and lack of patient cooperation due to pain, hypoxia, or neurological issues.[18] Before implementing the tracheostomy tube change procedure, it is advisable to determine what type of tube to place. This may be difficult to determine because a visual exam of the stoma and anterior airway without the tube in place affects the decision. In any case, it is wise to have at least one type of tracheostomy tube ready, and perhaps an alternate or two nearby.

Before beginning the procedure, it is important to gain the cooperation of the patient and/or his or her family by explaining the plan and the need for the tube change. A tube change may be fraught with anxiety for the patient and family. It is important to explain that the patient will feel a pulling sensation while the tube is being removed but that this is usually momentary. Patients should also be aware that coughing is common during the procedure. If the replacement tube has a smaller outer diameter, there is usually much less discomfort, especially with a cuffless tube. However, if the new tube has a larger outer diameter, it is usually more painful and traumatic. A small amount of limited bleeding should be expected after most tube changes.

One phenomenological study[20] determined that patients were quite anxious and experienced varying degrees of discomfort with the tube change despite the fact that many clinicians consider it a routine procedure. Patients who express anxiety may be offered premedication with a low dose of intravenous opioid or benzodiazepine. One can also premedicate the stoma—with 2% Xylocaine gel several minutes prior to the procedure—to lessen sensation at the site. Patients are less anxious when they know the entire procedure usually takes less than 1 minute.

Before the procedure, it is important to gather all the necessary supplies: tracheostomy tube and alternates, lubricating gel, new tracheostomy tube holder, precut tracheostomy dressing, a dampened cloth to cleanse the stoma of dried secretions and other debris, and a suture removal tray. Sometimes skin stay sutures are present under the neck flange but not otherwise readily visible. Lighting should be adequate, and suction and oxygen should be available. A variety of tracheostomy tube sizes and types should be available. In a critically ill patient, it is also advisable to have other equipment and supplies available, including pulse oximetry, capnography, tube exchangers, and tracheal dilators.[18]

If the patient is hemodynamically unstable, or if there is concern that the procedure may be difficult, preoxygenation with 100% oxygen for 10 minutes prior to the procedure will provide de-nitrogenation of the blood and maximize the patient's oxygen reserve. In these cases, it is also advisable to have an assistant at the bedside in case a difficult situation occurs.

A bedside tracheostomy tube change is done as a clean procedure unless there are extenuating circumstances requiring sterile conditions. After thorough hand washing, the tube itself is prepped. It is usually packaged with the inner cannula in place and the cuff deflated (one exception is the Bivona Fome-Cuf tracheostomy tube, and the procedure for that tube will be discussed separately). The inner cannula is removed from the outer cannula. The obturator is placed within the outer cannula, and the entire distal tip of the tube is well-lubricated. If the tracheostomy tube is a single-cannula tube, the obturator is placed inside it and prepped with lubricating gel. Xylocaine gel can also be used as a local anesthetic at this point. Mirza and Cameron[18] also recommended lidocaine spray into the stoma prior to the procedure to provide added local anesthesia within the trachea.

The patient is positioned with his or her neck fully exposed and lying flat unless otherwise indicated. If the patient is in a cervical collar, it must be removed, and in-line stabilization must be maintained at all times by an assistant. There is no evidence that specifies nil per os (NPO) guidelines prior to the procedure, so prudence should be a guide. If there is any concern, patients should be asked to refrain from food and fluids for a period of time prior to the procedure. Continuous tube feedings should be turned off prior to the procedure, primarily because of the risk of aspiration while in the supine position.

Deep subglottic suctioning should always be done prior to cuff deflation. Secretions collect above the cuff and can be a source of respiratory distress and potential pneumonia if not removed prior to deflation. A soft, flexible suction catheter should be used for deep oropharyngeal suctioning, as it will create less trauma and discomfort than a rigid suction catheter. The patient should be cautioned that the procedure is likely to cause gagging, but that it is vital to collect the pooled secretions prior to deflation of the cuff.

Even though most secretions are removed with this maneuver, some often remain above the cuff. The best way to prevent these remaining secretions from being aspirated is to actively engage the patient during this procedure. Ask the patient to take a deep breath and cough. The cuff can be quickly deflated following complete inhalation and the beginning of exhalation, when the patient begins to cough up the remaining secretions. An unresponsive or uncooperative patient should have this cuff deflation timed with exhalation, and a suction catheter should be used to remove the secretions.

Another approach is to use the manual resuscitation bag to provide an "inspiratory push" during cuff deflation to clear any remaining pooled secretions above the cuff.[21]

Cuff deflation may be timed to occur during exhalation, or it can be extended over a longer period of time. Rapid cuff deflation can sometimes promote patient discomfort due to coughing, which may be a reaction to airflow returning through the glottis,[21] so it may be helpful to give the patient a few moments to adjust to the sensation of breathing through the upper airway.

There are two primary methods of changing the tracheostomy tube: the classic method and the tube exchanger method, also known as the "railroad" method.[18] Both methods will be described here.

The Classic Method

The classic method involves the complete removal of the old tracheostomy tube before placing a new tube. Patient and operator positioning is important. The person changing the tube should stand on the same side of the bed as his dominant hand. In other words, if the operator is left-handed, he should stand on the patient's left when changing or manipulating the tracheostomy.

The tracheostomy tube holder should be loosened and the ties removed. After ensuring the cuff is deflated completely, the tracheostomy tube should be pulled out using a smooth, continuous motion. The cuff of the tube creates the most resistance and difficulty in replacement. Cuffless tubes offer less resistance and are easiest to remove and insert.

Examination of the Stoma

Tube replacement is an opportune time to assess the stoma and examine the free airway. The color of the stoma should be noted, along with the presence and color of any secretions. A moistened cloth can cleanse away encrusted secretions. The stoma and the definition of the edges should be noted. The stoma should be covered with a gauze pad to determine ease of ventilation, and the patient should be asked to phonate. The inability to breathe comfortably or phonate could be a sign of future difficulty with capping due to airway obstruction. The orientation of the internal tracheal lumen to the cutaneous stoma should be appraised. Horizontal, caudad, or, less commonly, cephalad orientations will determine the approach of the tube change.

The new lubricated tube is inserted by initially directing it into the stoma at a 90-degree angle and then turning caudad (**Figure 4.6**). An initial caudal approach or a premature caudal turn risks missing the tracheal lumen and creating a false passage within the tissues anterior to the trachea.

Figure 4.6 Proper approach for insertion, caudal turn

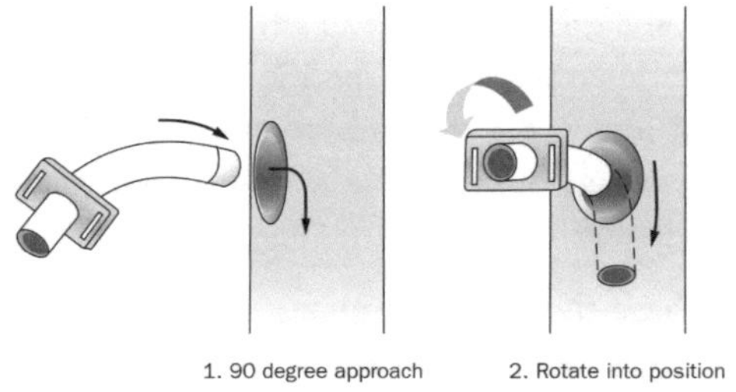

Proper 90-degree initial approach, followed by caudal turn.

Figure 4.7 shows the misalignment of the cutaneous stoma with the tracheal lumen, which can be recognized if the tracheal lumen is high and small in the 12-o'clock position when looking into the stoma. When inserting a tube into a cephalad orientation of the internal tracheal lumen, it is often necessary to begin with the tip of the tracheostomy tube pointed upward. During insertion, it is then possible to engage the internal tracheal lumen with the tip of the tube. Once engaged, one could then make the 180-degree caudal turn. However, a cephalad location of the internal tracheal lumen may not initially be evident. If the tube is not easily inserted on the first attempt, the clinician must reassess the stoma and consider if a cephalad approach is warranted. Indication for a cephalad approach can be confirmed by inserting the little finger in the stoma to palpate the location of the tracheal lumen.

Figure 4.7 Cephalad location of internal tracheal lumen

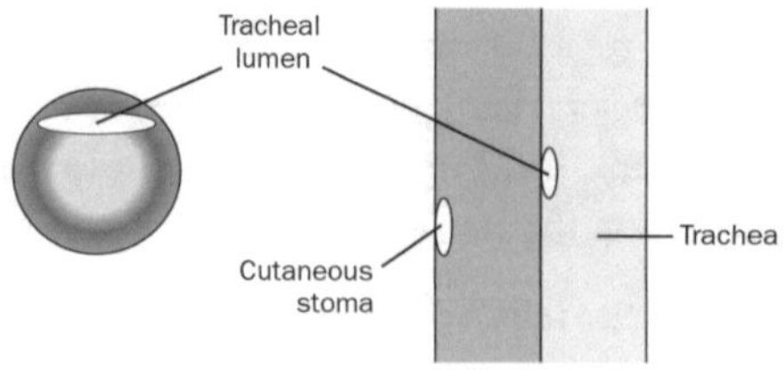

Cephalad location of internal tracheal lumen when the cutaneous stoma and tracheal lumen are not aligned. The tracheal lumen can sometimes be visualized through the cutaneous stoma high in a cephalad orientation.

After proper placement of the tube, the obturator is removed and replaced with the inner cannula. Proper placement should be confirmed by the presence of tracheal secretions, bilateral breath sounds, capnometry, and the ability to pass a suction catheter.

Patients who are hemodynamically unstable may require additional monitoring during the tube change, including electrocardiography, blood pressure, pulse oximetry, and capnography. In these patients, one must weigh the need for the tube change against the risk of hemodynamic embarrassment. Routine tracheostomy tube changes can and should be postponed until the patient is more stable.

The Tube Exchanger/Railroad Method

The tube exchanger technique is also known as the "railroad" method. If a tracheostomy tube must be changed during a period of hemodynamic instability or full mechanical ventilator support, caution is required. An additional assistant to manage the ventilator and the use of a tube exchanger can minimize the risk of loss of airway during the procedure.

Mimicking the Seldinger technique, the tube exchanger is used as a guidewire to maintain access to the airway as the old tube is removed and the new tube is inserted. Two types of tube exchangers are available: solid and hollow. An example of a solid tube exchanger is the Eschmann introducer ("bougie"). It has the advantage of maintaining its shape when placed at a specific angle, which can be especially helpful, if necessary, to find the tracheal lumen for an inadvertent decannulation. However, El-Orbany and Salem[22] suggested the Eschmann is not preferable as an airway exchange device because it does not allow for oxygenation or ventilation.

Several hollow tube exchangers are available and have the added advantage of using 15-mm connectors to which manual resuscitation bags can be applied for ventilation and supplemental oxygen. Other reports have described using suction catheters or nasogastric tubes as tube exchangers. However, these alternate tubes require modification before use.

Prior to initiating the tube exchanger method, the patient should be preoxygenated for several minutes. The inner cannula should be removed from both Tracheostomy Tubes: the one to be inserted and the one in situ. The tube exchanger will then be placed through the outer cannula of the tube in situ with at least 3 cm of the exchange catheter protruding past the distal end of the tube. The tube exchanger should be held in position by an assistant while the operator removes the old tracheostomy tube. Next, the exterior end of the tube exchanger should be placed through the distal end of the outer cannula of the tube to be inserted. The new tube can then be guided into position over the tube exchanger. The tube exchanger is then removed, the inner cannula replaced, and ventilation resumed. With a hollow tube exchanger, the 15-mm connector can be quickly applied for manual ventilation and oxygenation in case there is a delay or difficulty at any point during the procedure. The proper placement of the tube should be confirmed by any of the aforementioned measures.

PLACEMENT OF NONSTANDARD TRACHEOSTOMY TUBES

Foam Cuff Tracheostomy Tube

A foam cuff tube is different from the other tubes because its cuff remains inflated at all times unless actively deflated. To insert a foam cuff tracheostomy tube (e.g., Bivona Fome-Cuf), a 60-ml syringe fitted to a stopcock is used to deflate the large cuff. Complete deflation of the cuff is confirmed by observing the collapse of the pilot port. To prevent passive reinflation, the port is plugged with the attached stopper. The tip is lubricated with a water-based lubricant and inserted into place with its own obturator. Inserting a foam cuff tracheostomy tube generally takes more pressure exertion because the cuff is larger and bulkier. Once the foam cuff tube is in place, the pilot port should be unclamped and remain open to air, allowing the cuff to self-expand to fit the trachea. No additional air should be injected into this port.

The foam cuff tracheostomy tube should be power deflated at regular intervals in order to prevent moisture accumulation within the cuff. There is no recommended frequency for this power deflation, but failure to do so often results in the ventilator alarm indicating low returned volumes. Power deflation once every 8-12 hours is usually enough to prevent this accumulation of moisture. Before deflating any cuff, it is important to perform deep oropharyngeal suctioning to remove all secretions above the cuff.

Fenestrated Tracheostomy Tube

A fenestration provides an added flow of air up to the vocal cords to lessen resistance to airflow and facilitate phonation. Fenestrated tracheostomy tubes are available in cuffed and cuffless versions.

An in-vitro study by Hussey and Bishop[23] showed that fenestrated tracheostomy tubes provided significantly less resistance to airflow than non-fenestrated tubes of equal size. Their bench study on a tracheal model compared Shiley fenestrated tracheostomies in sizes 4, 6, 8, and 10 with the cuff deflated and the external opening occluded (simulating capping) while obtaining pressure measurements. They compared these airway pressure measurements to comparably-sized Shiley cuffless tubes where capping was also simulated. They found that in an average-sized trachea, all tube sizes greater than 4 substantially increased work of breathing, while the fenestration returned the pressure to acceptable levels. They reported that the fenestration reduced resistance by allowing airflow not only around the tube, but also through the lumen of the tube. Because of this substantial decrease in resistance, they recommended a fenestrated tracheostomy be used for all patients able to breathe through their native airway, except those with a size 4 tube. In theory, the fenestrated tracheostomy tube decreases resistance, but this depends on many factors, primarily the proper placement of the fenestration within the airway. **Figure 4.8** shows the proper placement of the fenestration within the airway.

Figure 4.8 Proper position of fenestration

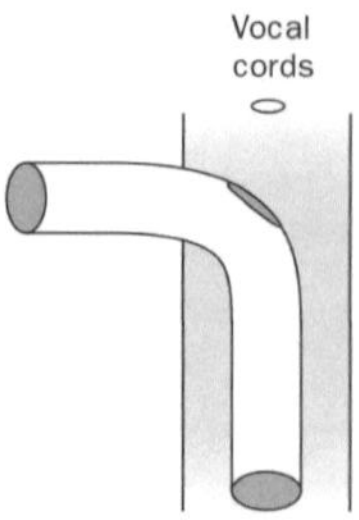

Proper placement of fenestration centrally within the airway. Note the fenestration is placed to avoid contact with anterior and posterior walls.

The position of the fenestration is affected by the curvature of the tube. The standard position of the fenestration on nearly all tracheostomy tubes is one-third of the way down the shaft from the neck flange, but this one-size-fits-all approach rarely produces a proper fit. The tracheas of most people are either too anterior or too posterior to ensure a proper fit with a standard fenestrated tube.

One of the most troubling problems with fenestrated tubes is the growth of granulation tissue within the fenestration, which was originally reported in tubes with one large fenestration. Since that time, fenestrated tubes with different designs have been developed. For example, the Shiley FEN and CFN tubes typically have one large oval fenestration, while the Shiley DCFN and DFEN as well as the Portex tubes have several elongated channels. Other tubes have a "sieved" fenestration. However, no matter what the design of the fenestration, *the risk of granulation tissue is greatest when the fenestration is not centered in the airway.* For this reason, many centers choose not to place fenestrated tracheostomy tubes. If a fenestrated tube remains the best option for phonation and ventilation, however, it is imperative to ensure a proper fit.

The procedure to fit a fenestration involves measuring the distance from the stoma to the anterior and posterior tracheal walls. Some modifications are no longer recommended practice, such as lengthening the established fenestration, as described by one group.[24] To measure the tracheal depth, one can use a probe, a cotton-tipped swab, or a bent pipe cleaner to mark the distance between the anterior and posterior walls. As shown in **Figure 4.9**, the "handle" of a cotton-tipped swab is placed at the anterior tracheal wall and a mark is made at the stomal opening. Then the applicator is placed further within the airway until it reaches the posterior wall. A second mark is made on the applicator at the stomal skin level. Alternatively, Boston Medical Products makes a handy measuring device called the Mongtomery Stomeasure.

Figure 4.9 Measuring tracheal depth

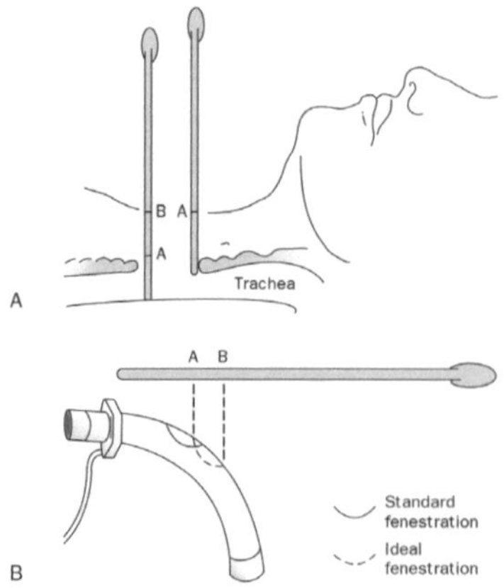

Fitting a fenestrated tracheostomy tube. The anterior and posterior tracheal walls are measured with a probe. These measurements are then compared to the fenestration on the tube. If the markings do not line up with the fenestration, a custom tube (ideal fenestration) should be ordered.

The two marks should be aligned with the intended fenestrated tube by placing the tip of the applicator on the neck flange of the tube to determine the ideal location of the fenestration. The fenestration should lie completely between the two marks to ensure proper fit. If the fenestration does not fit within these marks, a custom fenestration should be ordered, rather than cutting the shaft oneself. A cut tube may have irregular edges, which could result in inflammation or an even greater risk of granuloma. The Moore tracheostomy tube is the only one that can be modified, as small fenestration holes can be punched into the shaft with an awl that comes with the kit.

Great caution must be taken when removing a fenestrated tracheostomy tube. When granulation tissue has grown within the fenestration(s), manual removal is potentially dangerous. The mobility of a fenestrated tube should always be assessed by exerting gentle pressure to determine if it moves easily within the stoma. Shining a light within the tube itself will reveal a pinkish hue in the presence of granulation. In this case, an otolaryngologist should conduct a visual examination of the trachea. The forceful removal of a fenestrated tracheostomy tube can result in hemorrhage, leading to a surgical emergency.

Granulation tissue is not the only complication of a fenestrated tracheostomy tube. Subcutaneous emphysema has also been reported when the inner cannula is not properly aligned with the outer cannula and air escapes through the tissue planes. For this reason, a fenestrated tracheostomy tube should not be placed within an immature stoma.[25]

Another reported problem was resistance produced from a deflated cuff in a fenestrated tube. Criner, Make, and Celli[26] reported a case of a woman who experienced increased airway resistance and chronic airflow obstruction when using a fenestrated tracheostomy tube for nocturnal ventilation. The tube was confirmed to be in the correct position within the airway and the cuff was deflated, but her pressure measurements continued to be elevated. Upon decannulation and a return to mouth breathing, her minute ventilation and resultant exercise endurance dramatically increased. The investigators concluded that a deflated cuff on a fenestrated tracheostomy tube significantly increases airway resistance and can further limit ventilatory muscle performance in patients with compromised ventilatory reserve..

UPSIZING

Occasionally, there is a need to place a tracheostomy tube that is larger than the one in place. Typical conditions that require upsizing include a hemodynamically unstable patient who is exhibiting high airway pressures on the ventilator, or a patient who has been in the process of downsizing and breathing around the tube and is now presenting with respiratory distress. Either the tube itself or secretions within the tube can increase resistance and manifest as respiratory distress. For example, it is unreasonable to expect an average-sized adult to breathe through a size 4 cuffed tube; it is simply too small. If positive-pressure ventilation is applied to a small tube, the problem will manifest immediately as high airway pressures.

When possible, it is advisable to provide some analgesic premedication and/or benzodiazepine prior to upsizing a tracheostomy tube. Placing a larger tube often involves some degree of resistance and discomfort. In addition, lidocaine gel can serve a dual purpose as a local anesthetic and lubricant. Occasionally, it may be necessary to dilate the stoma in order to allow the placement of a larger tube. The cuff of the tracheostomy tube in situ can be used to dilate the opening of the stoma by maneuvering the tube in several positions and hyperinflating the cuff.

FITTING A TRACHEOSTOMY CANNULA OR STOMA STENT

A tracheostomy button or tracheostomy cannula is used as a stent to maintain patency of the stoma. However, the Olympic tracheostomy button is no longer manufactured. The tracheostomy cannula is usually intended for temporary use and is indicated in patients who may require repeated tracheostomies such as those who have spinal cord injuries or sleep apnea. It can also be used with patients who are undergoing rehabilitation while working toward decannulation, or in patients for whom a future surgery is planned.

When properly placed, the tracheostomy cannula fits solely within the stoma, eliminates resistance within the airway, and, when plugged, allows the patient to breathe entirely through his or her upper airway. However, if long-term access to the airway is required, such as for frequent suctioning, replacement of the cannula or stoma stent with a standard tracheostomy tube is recommended.

For a proper fit, the length of the stoma is measured as follows: the distance from the cutaneous stoma to the anterior tracheal wall. Two distances to the anterior tracheal wall should be measured, as they may be different, which includes the superior aspect of the stoma as well as the inferior aspect of the stoma.

When a tracheostomy cannula is properly placed, there is no obstruction within the airway. **Figure 4.10** illustrates a stoma stent that is properly placed.

Figure 4.10 Hood Stoma Stent in place

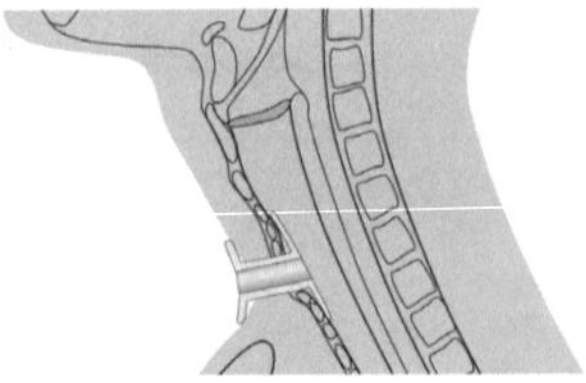

Stoma stent in place. Note that it creates no obstruction within the airway.

Hood Labs (Pembroke, Massachusetts)

SUMMARY

The process of sizing and fitting a tracheostomy tube requires planning and consideration of goals. The tube should be long enough for the patient's anatomy and large enough to provide adequate ventilation. There are several factors that must be considered when fitting and changing a tracheostomy tube. These include determining whether a cuff is necessary in addition to assessment of airway protection and secretions. Identifying goals is the first step toward a determination of the proper tube.

Key Points

- The first decision when fitting a tracheostomy tube is whether the patient requires a cuffed tube.
- A dual-cannula tube is optimal for a patient who has a large amount of thick secretions.
- A larger tube size is optimal for a patient breathing through the tube, whereas a smaller tube size is more appropriate for a patient breathing around the tube.
- The tracheostomy tube can be changed by using either the classic method or the tube exchanger method; the latter is used when the patient is hemodynamically unstable or there is concern about loss of access to the airway.
- Fenestrated tracheostomy tubes must be fitted carefully to prevent granulation growth in the aperture.

Review Questions

1. An ICU patient has required continuous mechanical ventilation for the past three weeks. However, for the last three days, he requires mechanical ventilation only at night. Today he tells you he wants to talk with his family. Which of the following tracheostomy tubes would allow him to be adequately ventilated at night and safely capped when off the ventilator?
    a. Bivona TTS
    b. Shiley SCT
    c. TRACOE Twist with air supply line
    d. Fahl Duravent

    ANSWER: A. Choice A is the only tube that provides a high-pressure cuff that can be inflated for ventilation and deflates tightly to the shaft of the tube, allowing laminar airflow around it. Choice B has a low-pressure cuff that cannot be safely capped. Choice C is a talking tracheostomy with a low-pressure cuff that cannot be safely capped. Choice D is a cuffless tube that cannot provide adequate ventilation.

2. A patient has a Shiley 8 cuffed tracheostomy tube on continuous mechanical ventilation. Cuff pressures are 60 cm H_2O, and the low-pressure alarm continues to sound, indicating a leak around the cuff. What is the likely diagnosis of the problem?
    a. Tube dislodgement
    b. Tracheomalacia
    c. Sepsis
    d. Ventilator-associated pneumonia

    ANSWER: B. The correct answer is B. A low-pressure alarm in the presence of elevated cuff pressure suggests tracheomalacia. Choice A is not correct because the high-pressure alarm would alert you if the tube were dislodged. Choices C and D are not related to the tracheostomy tube.

3. How would you properly treat the patient in the previous question?
    a. Change the tracheostomy tube to a longer one
    b. Mask ventilate and re-intubate
    c. Elevate the head of the bed 30 degrees
    d. Goal-directed therapy

    ANSWER: A. For a patient with tracheomalacia, the short-term treatment is to place a longer tube to bypass the area of tracheomalacia so that effective ventilation can be provided. All of the other choices are related to the distractors in the previous question.

4. When is the tube exchanger method recommended when changing a tracheostomy tube?
    a. During a period of desaturation
    b. During a period of sepsis
    c. During a period of hemodynamic instability
    d. During a period of ventilator-associated pneumonia

    ANSWER: C. The best answer is C because the tube exchanger method allows for oxygenation during the procedure, which may be necessary during periods of hemodynamic instability or full ventilatory support. In addition, the tube exchanger method minimizes the risk of loss of the airway.

5. Upsizing a tracheostomy tube is likely to be necessary in which of the following situations?
    a. A patient with a capped size 4 cuffless tube who is in respiratory distress
    b. A patient with a size 8 Portex Blueline Suctionaid who wishes to speak
    c. A patient with a size 8 talking tracheostomy who has been weaned from ventilator support
    d. A patient with a size 7 cuffed tube and a low-pressure alarm sounds in the presence of high cuff pressure.

    ANSWER: A. Choice A is the best answer because it is impossible to effectively ventilate a patient with a small cuffless tube. Choice B is incorrect because a tracheostomy tube change may be required to provide phonation, though a smaller tube would be desirable. Choice C is incorrect because a tube change may be helpful toward tracheostomy progression, though a smaller tube would be most helpful. Choice D is incorrect because this situation suggests tracheomalacia, in which a longer tube would be most helpful.

References

1. Fisher DF, Kondili D, Williams J, Hess DR, Bittner EA, Schmidt UH. Tracheostomy tube change before day 7 is associated with earlier use of speaking valve and earlier oral intake. *Respir Care.* 2013;58(2):257-263.
2. Beachey W. *Respiratory care anatomy and physiology.* St. Louis, MO: Mosby; 2007.
3. Epstein SK. Anatomy and physiology of tracheostomy. *Respir Care.* 2005;*50*(3):476-482.
4. Pierson DJ. Tracheostomy and weaning. *Respiratory Care.* 2005;*50*(4):526-533.
5. Shapiro BA, Harrison RA, Kacmarek RM, Cane RD. *Clinical application of respiratory care* (3rd ed.). Chicago: Yearbook Medical Publishers; 1985.
6. Rumbak MJ, Graves AE, Scott MP, Sporn GK, Walsh FW, Anderson WM, et al. Tracheostomy occlusion protocol predicts significant obstruction to air flow in patients requiring prolonged mechanical ventilation. *Crit Care Med.* 1997;*25*(3):413-417.
7. Mendell DA, Logemann JA. Temporal sequence of swallow events during the oropharyngeal swallow. *J Speech Lang Hear* Res. 2007;50(5):1256-1271.
8. Robbins J, Hamilton JW, Lof GL, Kempster GB. Oropharyngeal swallowing in normal adults of different ages. *Gastroenterology.* 1992;103:823-829.
9. Wilmskoetter J, Martin-Harris B, Pearson WG, Bonilha L, Elm JJ, Horn J, Bonilha HS. Differences in swallow physiology in patients with left and right hemispheric strokes. *Physiol Behavior.* 2018;194:155-152.
10. Douce FH. Pulmonary function testing. In R. L. Wilkins, J. K. Stoller, & C. L. Scanlan eds. *Egan's fundamentals of respiratory care.* 8th ed. St. Louis, MO: Mosby, 2003:391-425.
11. Bach JR. Mechanical insufflation-exsufflation comparison of peak expiratory flows with manually assisted and unassisted coughing. *Chest.* 1993;14:1553-1562.
12. Ding R, Logemann JA. Swallow physiology in patients with trach cuff inflated or deflated: A retrospective study. *Head and Neck.* 2005;27(9):809-813.
13. Pryor LN, Baldwin, CE Ward, EC, Cornwell PL, O'Connor SN, Chapman MJ, Bersten AD. Tracheostomy tube type and inner cannula selection impact pressure and resistance to air flow. *Respir Care,* 2016;61(5):607-614.
14. St. John RE, Malen JF. Contemporary issues in adult tracheostomy management. *Crit Care Nurs Clin North Amer.* 2004;16(3):413-430.
15. Irajpour A, Abbasinia M, Hoseini A, Kashefi P. Effects of shallow and deep endotracheal tube suctioning on cardiovascular indices in patients in intensive care units. *Ir J Nurs Midwif Res.* 2014;19(4):366-370.
16. Guyton D, Banner MJ, Kirby RR. High-volume, low-pressure cuffs: Are they always low? *Chest.* 1991;100:1076-1081.
17. Mallick A, Bodenham A, Elliot S, Oram J. An investigation into the length of standard tracheostomy tubes in critical care patients. *Anaesthesia.* 2008;63:302-306.
18. Mirza, S, Cameron DS. The tracheostomy tube change: A review of techniques. *Hosp Med.* 2001;62(3):158-163.
19. Tabaee A, Lando T, Rickert S, Stewart MG, Kuhel WI. Practice patterns, safety, and rationale for tracheostomy tube changes: A survey of otolaryngology training programs. *Otolaryngology.* 2007;117:573-576.
20. Donnelly F, Wiechula R. The lived experience of a tracheostomy tube change: A phenomenological study. *J Clin Nurs.* 2006;15:1115-1122.

21. Kazandjian MS, Dikeman KJ. Communication options for tracheostomy and ventilator-dependent patients. In E. N. Myers EN, Johnson JT. eds. *Tracheostomy: Airway management, communication, and swallowing.* San Diego, CA: Plural Publishing; 2008.
22. El-Orbany M, Salem MR. The Eschmann tracheal tube is not an airway exchange device. *Anesth Analg.* 2004;99(4):1269-1270.
23. Hussey JD, Bishop MJ. Pressures required to move gas through the native airway in the presence of a fenestrated vs. a nonfenestrated tracheostomy tube. *Chest.* 1996;110(2):494-497.
24. Cane RD, Woodward C, Shapiro BA. Customizing fenestrated Tracheostomy Tubes: A bedside technique. *Crit Care Med.* 1982;10(12):880-881.
25. Orme, RM, Welham, KL. Subcutaneous emphysema after percutaneous tracheostomy—time to dispense with fenestrated tubes? *Anaesthesia.* 2006;61:911-912.
26. Criner G, Make B, Celli B. Respiratory muscle dysfunction secondary to chronic tracheostomy. *Chest.* 1987;91(1):139-141.

5

Addressing Complex Tracheostomy Issues: Mechanical Ventilation, Altitude, Wounds, Cuff Leaks, and Airborne Infections

by Linda L. Morris

Objectives

- Compare the changes in aerodynamics through a tracheostomy and return to normal breathing
- Describe troubleshooting when a cuff leak is discovered
- Explain precautions used when caring for patients at altitude and during anesthesia
- Recommend precautions in patients with infectious airborne illness
- Identify causes and treatment of skin wounds.
- Discuss approach to management of defective tracheostomy tubes.

Introduction

Each patient with a tracheostomy is unique, with individual circumstances that direct assessment, planning, and management. When a critically ill patient on mechanical ventilation develops high airway pressures, one must assess whether there is increased resistance within the tracheostomy tube or whether lung compliance is decreased. The cough is the primary defense mechanism against retained secretions, and efforts to mobilize secretions are vital in tracheostomy patients. Leaks may develop within the cuff, around the cuff, or within the tube itself, and a plan for the management of cuff leaks is presented. A discussion is also included with regard to pistoning and the management of cuff changes that occur at altitude and with anesthesia. Lessons learned with the COVID-19 pandemic are presented regarding aerosol generation and tracheostomy precautions. Complex tracheostomy wounds can also be a challenging management issue. The chapter concludes with a discussion of tracheostomy as a lived experience and dealing with tubes with defects or missing parts.

The Critically Ill Patient on Mechanical Ventilation

Critically ill patients on mechanical ventilation present a challenge. There are numerous conditions that require intubation and consideration when on mechanical ventilation. These include acute respiratory failure, airway obstruction, and neurological conditions that deplete the patient's respiratory drive, adequate spontaneous endurance, or the ability to protect his or her airway. All these factors must be evaluated when planning for a long-term artificial airway. The majority of patients in ICUs receive tracheostomies because of prolonged mechanical ventilation and failure with the weaning process. The reasons for this difficulty in weaning vary according to the patient's underlying conditions. Like endotracheal intubation, the conditions that require a tracheostomy fall into four broad categories: difficulties with ventilation, airway obstruction, airway protection, and secretions (remember VOPS for a mnemonic).[1] Current practice in critical care reports a varied lifespan for the placement of an endotracheal tube in an adult that ranges from a few short days up to two weeks. A tracheotomy should be considered when the expected need for an artificial airway outlasts that time frame.

Time to Tracheotomy

When patients cannot be liberated from mechanical ventilation soon after intubation, the practitioner must determine whether to place a tracheostomy or whether efforts to wean ventilator support should continue. Tracheotomy is performed more frequently than in years past due to several factors, including increased use of percutaneous techniques, with several studies confirming their safety comparable with, if not preferable to, the open surgical technique.[2,3] Numerous studies have attempted to identify the optimal time to place a tracheostomy; however, no definitive recommendations have been developed. The difficulty lies in the interpretation of results because different studies use different populations, time frames, and outcome measures. Several authors have failed to show an improvement (i.e., decrease) in mortality rate with early tracheotomy,[4,5] while other studies have demonstrated a decreased mortality rate.[6,7] The definitions of early tracheotomy in these studies have included those done within 48 hours to one week of intubation.

Kluge and colleagues[8] used a questionnaire to survey physician directors of ICUs in Germany. They found that 67.2% of tracheostomies were performed during the second week of mechanical ventilation, while only 21.7% were performed within seven days.

Blot and others[9] recruited patients from 25 ICUs in France to show the benefit of early tracheostomy compared to prolonged intubation. They recruited patients on mechanical ventilation and randomized them into two groups: early tracheotomy within four days of intubation versus patients with prolonged intubation of at least 14 days. The projected sample size of the early tracheotomy group was calculated to be 470 patients; however the study was stopped early because there was no difference in the study's primary endpoint of mortality. They concluded that the sole benefit of the tracheostomy was greater comfort as self-reported by patients. One more recent meta-analysis showed a significant decrease in mortality, and duration of mechanical ventilation, ICU stay, and hospital stay when tracheotomy was performed between days three and seven of intubation and mechanical ventilation.[10]

Other studies have examined the benefit of tracheotomy on the discontinuation of mechanical ventilation. However, numerous factors affect the weaning process, including work of breathing, dead space, amount of respiratory secretions, sedation, and varied approaches of weaning protocols. One as yet unpublished study in a Midwestern academic medical center showed that 59% of ICU patients were liberated from mechanical ventilation within 0-5 days of tracheostomy placement.[11] Pierson[12] and Scales and Kahn[7] suggest that perhaps the benefit of tracheotomy on weaning can be appreciated in less dramatic ways, such as by decreasing complications from overexposure to mechanical ventilation, facilitating improved removal of secretions, and improved comfort leading to reduced sedation requirements.

Project IMPACT, a multi-institutional database adopted by the Society of Critical Care Medicine (SCCM), attempted to identify not only optimal time to tracheotomy but also to evaluate clinical and nonclinical factors on tracheostomy practice. With a database of nearly 44,000 patients, they found the median time to tracheotomy was nine days and that prolonged intubation led to increased duration of mechanical ventilation, increased ICU length of stay, and increased hospital length of stay.[13] A Cochrane review[14] concluded that their findings are "no more than suggestive" of the superiority of early over late tracheotomy because there was no high-quality information for selected populations. A more recent systematic review of 43 studies[15] found a significant difference in favor of early tracheotomy in adults, including reduced hospital-acquired pneumonia. In pediatric patients, they found a significant decrease in duration of mechanical ventilation, mortality, and ICU stay. Patients with tracheotomies performed within seven days had better outcomes than those performed within 14 or 21 days of intubation. Therefore, they recommended tracheotomy within seven days for both adults and pediatric patients.

The clear benefits of early tracheotomy lie within selected populations. McCredie and others[16] conducted a systematic review and meta-analysis, evaluating 10 trials in brain-injured patients. Early tracheotomy (less than 10 days after intubation) decreased long-term mortality, duration of mechanical ventilation, and ICU length of stay, but did not reduce short-term mortality. Kang and others[17] found significant benefits in early tracheotomy in trauma patients, including shorter duration of mechanical ventilation and ICU length of stay. Pizza and others[18] found a significant decrease in incidence of ventilator-associated pneumonia and days of mechanical ventilation with early tracheotomy in a pediatric ICU. Currently, the recommended critical care practice continues to be withholding sedation and initiating a weaning trial with spontaneous breathing on a daily basis. When the patient is unable to be liberated from mechanical ventilation after 7–10 days, a tracheotomy should be considered. See chapter 2 for further discussion on time to tracheotomy.

Airway Pressures and Work of Breathing

The tracheostomy patient on ventilator support presents unique challenges. It is important to minimize airway pressure and resistance and maximize the mobilization of secretions. A mechanical ventilator provides the power to insufflate the lungs, aerate the alveoli, and remove carbon dioxide. Numerous modes are used to adjust a graded work of breathing. Whenever a patient is mechanically ventilated, the clinician monitors the trend in compliance of the respiratory system (the balance between pressure and volume produced by the lungs, chest cavity, and respiratory circuit). Often the progression and selected mode of mechanical ventilation, whether volume-limited or pressure-limited, are driven by changes in lung compliance. Empirically, in a volume-limited ventilation mode, a preset tidal volume is delivered to the patient, and the pressure is dependent on compliance. With a pressure-limited ventilation mode, the ventilator delivers a flow of gas to the patient until a preset pressure is achieved, and the generated tidal volume is dependent on compliance. Of particular concern to the tracheostomy patient is the development of high airway pressures, and this concern is magnified as the tube caliber gets smaller or airway secretions accumulate.

Peak and Plateau Pressures

The peak pressure, or peak inspiratory pressure (P_{peak}), is the highest pressure generated in the system during inspiration. It is a dynamic pressure reflecting changes in compliance due to changes within the lung itself, secretions, obstruction, and other factors that affect driving pressure. When tidal volume is constant, an increased peak pressure can reflect reduced lung compliance or increased airway resistance.[19,20] Because peak pressure is measured during airflow, it consists of both lung and chest wall recoil plus the resistance created by the tracheostomy tube and the airway itself. Lung compliance is the change in volume (V) as a function of a change in pressure (P). The formula is as follows:[21]

$$Compliance = \Delta V \div \Delta P$$

Dynamic compliance varies per breath and is a function of the tidal volume (V_t), peak inspiratory pressure (P_{peak}), and PEEP. The formula for dynamic compliance is as follows:

$$Dynamic\ compliance = V_t \div (P_{peak} - PEEP)$$

The plateau pressure (P_{plat}) is measured in the absence of airflow and reflects static compliance. The absence of airflow is created by adding an inspiratory pause at the end of inspiration. The formula for static compliance is as follows:

$$Static\ compliance = V_t \div (P_{plat} - PEEP)$$

Factors that change compliance include level of PEEP, compliance of the chest wall and ventilator tubing, and all conditions that cause changes in the density and distensibility of lung tissue. Compliance can also be affected by tracheostomy tubes that are constructed of more distensible materials, such as silicone. Static compliance reflects the elastic recoil of the alveolar walls and thoracic cage against the volume of air in the lungs. It also reflects the recoil of the ventilator tubing on the volume of air in the circuit. It is difficult to measure accurately in spontaneously breathing patients because it cannot be measured when a patient is making active respiratory efforts. Decreased static compliance implies ventilation is less effective and can be caused by air trapping, pulmonary edema, pneumothorax, atelectasis, and other conditions that limit the compliance of the chest wall as well as the abdominal wall (pneumomediastinum and abdominal compartment syndrome).[19,20]

Because dynamic compliance consists of both compliance and resistance, it is actually a measure of elastance.[22] Lung problems can be differentiated from airway problems by monitoring changes between the peak and plateau pressure. If P_{peak} and P_{plat} are both increasing while volume stays constant, then lung compliance is decreasing.[19,20]

Assessing peak and plateau pressures is especially important in the mechanically ventilated patient with a tracheostomy. When peak or plateau pressures are high, the clinician must first ensure the patency and proper positioning of the tube. High peak pressure in the presence of normal plateau pressure indicates an airway problem such as obstruction due to secretions or a tracheostomy tube that is too small.

Work of Breathing

Work is required to overcome the forces that oppose lung inflation. High airway resistance contributes to work of breathing. The formula for work of breathing is calculated as follows:

Work of breathing (in joules) = (P × V) ÷ 10

The product of P and V is expressed as cm H_2O; however, mechanical work is usually not expressed in cm H_2O, but rather kg/m, or joules. To convert cm H_2O into joules, divide the product by 10.[23]

There are significant changes in aerodynamics associated with both tracheostomy and return to breathing through the native airway. Factors involved in the decision to place a tracheostomy tube are often complex, especially when attempting liberation from mechanical ventilation. It is often difficult to discern the causes for a failure to wean from mechanical ventilation, and it is even more of a mystery why many patients are able to wean shortly after the placement of a tracheostomy. Davis, Campbell, Johannigman, Valente, and Branson[24] explored this phenomenon by studying the effects of tracheostomy and work of breathing in a group of surgical patients who had failed two attempts at weaning from mechanical ventilation. Patients had an esophageal balloon inserted transnasally to monitor esophageal pressure 6 to 10 hours before tracheotomy. Esophageal pressures were taken as a surrogate for lung and chest wall pressure. Patients were disconnected from the ventilator and allowed to breathe with a continuous flow of gas at an oxygen concentration equal to that of the ventilator. After 10 minutes of stabilization, measurements were made of tidal volume, respiratory rate, airway pressure, flow, and esophageal pressure, and then work of breathing was calculated. Allowing for elimination of anesthetic gases, the same measurements were repeated 10 hours after tracheotomy. They found that all patients were successfully weaned to a high-humidity tracheostomy collar within 24 hours of tracheostomy placement. There was a statistically significant decrease in work of breathing and PEEP after tracheotomy, but the authors suggest these changes do not fully explain the facilitated weaning. The investigators proposed that facilitated weaning is promoted by the decreased length, rigid structure, and curvature of the tracheostomy tube, as well as its less tortuous path compared to an endotracheal tube.

Retained Secretions

Effective bronchial hygiene is of paramount importance to a patient with a tracheostomy. Normally, there is a continuous blanket of mucus covering the epithelial lining of the large airways. The forward motion of cilia propels this mucus lining toward the hilus of the lung, moving toward the larynx and the pharynx, where it is eventually swallowed. This mucus blanket moves at a rate of 1 to 2 cm per minute and can completely cleanse the entire lung in 20 minutes in a normal, healthy adult. Ciliary activity is diminished in conditions such as smoking, positive-pressure ventilation, high levels of inspired oxygen, dehydration, general anesthesia, and tracheal foreign bodies such as tracheostomy tubes.[1,25]

The cough is the primary defense mechanism against retained secretions. The purpose of the cough is to provide high-velocity airflow upon expiration. The cough mechanism consists of five components: deep breath, inspiratory pause, glottic closure, increased thoracic pressure, and glottic opening. Without adequate inspiration, a cough is ineffective. Vital capacity must be at least 15 ml/kg of ideal body weight to produce an adequate cough. Following deep inspiration, the breath-holding maneuver provides time for maximal distribution of air, followed by glottic closure. With the glottis closed, the primary mechanism for increasing intrathoracic pressure is to increase intra-abdominal pressure. This pushes the diaphragm upward and decreases the volume of the thoracic cavity. The primary muscles involved in increasing intra-abdominal pressure are the anterior abdominal wall muscles, which force the diaphragm up against the closed glottis. Suddenly, the glottis opens and allows high-velocity airflow from the lungs—as high as 300 liters per minute.[1,25]

Retained secretions can be caused by dehydration, pulmonary disease, artificial airways, generalized muscular weakness, central nervous system disorders causing bulbar malfunction, and limitation of the abdominal musculature as in spinal cord injury or abdominal surgery. Efforts to mobilize retained secretions should be directed to the cause(s), but the importance of the mobilization of secretions cannot be overstated. Specific measures to mobilize secretions are discussed further in chapter 7.

Cuff Leaks

One of the most common occurrences with a tracheostomy is a cuff leak. In order to provide proper management, the clinician must first determine whether the leak is coming from within the cuff, around the cuff, or within the inflation line or pilot balloon.

Leak Within the Cuff

The tight quality-control process of companies that produce airway appliances makes a defect within a tube cuff a rare occurrence. Nonetheless, cuff integrity should always be checked prior to the insertion of any tracheostomy tube. The simplest maneuver is to ensure the cuff sustains inflation against digital pressure. A second maneuver is to place an air-inflated cuff into a small basin of sterile water, where bubbling will indicate a leak within the cuff.

It is possible for a leak within a cuff to develop over time. Leaks in endotracheal tube cuffs are more common due to damage from the teeth and other airway appliances as tubes are introduced through the oropharynx. When the tracheostomy tube is in place, the easiest way to check for a leak within the cuff is to attach a syringe and deflate the cuff. If air can be continuously withdrawn, there is a leak in the cuff. Another easy way to check for a leak is to inflate the cuff with air and check for an adequate seal by ensuring integrity of delivered tidal volume on the ventilator and measured cuff pressure. If the cuff does not seem to hold air, damage to the pilot balloon valve, inflation line, or cuff should be suspected. The definitive treatment for any of these concerns is to change the tracheostomy tube.

Cuff leaks have also been reported following the percutaneous approach to tracheotomy, which presents a unique dilemma. With percutaneous placement, the tracheostomy tube is snug within the stoma. In fact, less bleeding has been reported with the percutaneous approach than with the surgical approach due to its tamponade effect within the stoma. Cuff leaks occurring after a percutaneous approach could be due to pressure applied during insertion through the stoma. For this reason, some practitioners prefer to delay the first tube change with a percutaneous tracheotomy until a more mature stoma has developed. Although the definitive treatment for a cuff leak is to change the tube, if a cuff leak is detected soon after the placement of a percutaneous tracheostomy, the advisable approach is to maintain constant close monitoring of the patient's gas exchange and hemodynamic status and later replace the tube in the presence of a specialized airway team, possibly in a controlled environment such as the operating room.

Leak Around the Cuff

Leaks around the cuff are much more common than leaks within the cuff and result from a less than adequate seal within the airway. Unless there is a risk for aspiration, a leak around the cuff is not usually a concern, nor is it even noticeable, in a patient free from mechanical ventilation. In fact, an imperceptible leak around the cuff might be an incidental advantage in minimizing pressure against the trachea. Patients with a cuff leak can often talk, indicating they are able to comfortably pass air not only through the tube but also to reach the vocal cords.

When the patient is ventilator dependent, however, a cuff leak can be quite exasperating for the nurse or respiratory care practitioner due to frequent ventilator alarms indicating low pressure. Naturally, a cuff leak in a mechanically ventilated patient who is hemodynamically unstable would require immediate exploration of the cause of the leak. There are numerous causes for a leak around the cuff, including the following:

- Cuff is not fully inflated to seal the airway.
- Cuff is inflated, but the tube is too small for the airway.
- Cuff is inflated, but air and secretions are leaking past the cuff.
- Leak is associated with changes in patient position.
- Patient is on mechanical ventilation with high airway pressures or high levels of PEEP.
- An area of tracheomalacia has developed.

Cuff Is Not Fully Inflated

In some cases, there is a very simple solution to a leak around the cuff. Sometimes all that is required is to put more air in the cuff. This can be assessed by palpating deeply on the pilot balloon. This maneuver is equivalent to adding air to the cuff because it pushes air from the pilot balloon into the cuff itself. The pilot balloon provides an indicator of cuff inflation but has no bearing on cuff pressure. It has been demonstrated that an estimation of cuff pressure with balloon palpation is often inaccurate.[26,27] However, palpation of the pilot balloon can provide information about the presence of air in the cuff. A flat pilot balloon indicates there is no air in the cuff, whereas a tense pilot balloon indicates there is a large volume of air in the cuff relative to the diameter of the trachea. If the leak disappears with deep palpation of the pilot balloon, then more air should be added to the cuff. However, cuff inflation should not always be an automatic response to a leak. For a cuff that repeatedly loses air, the clinician should explore further to determine the cause of the leak.

Cuff Is Inflated, but the Tube Is Too Small for the Airway

The pilot balloon should first be palpated for the presence of air when investigating a cuff leak in an inflated cuff. If the pilot balloon is tense, the cuff is probably overinflated, and can be confirmed with manometry. Frequently, the cuff may be overinflated in an attempt to create an adequate seal. However, an overinflated cuff with a continued leak is indicative of a tracheostomy tube that is too small to create an adequate seal within the airway (see Figure 5.1). Besides palpation, the manufacturer's recommendations regarding inflation volumes should be reviewed. For example, Shiley provides leak test inflation volumes for its cuffed tracheostomy tubes that list the maximum volume to be added to the cuff to seal the airway. For the Shiley LPC and FEN tracheostomy tubes, the leak test inflation volumes are 11, 14, 17, and 20 ml for the size 4, 6, 8, and 10 tubes, respectively. When these volumes are exceeded, the cuff can be considered overinflated. An optimal treatment in this case is to place a larger tracheostomy tube. (See discussion on upsizing in chapter 4.)

Figure 5.1 Tube too small with hyperinflation

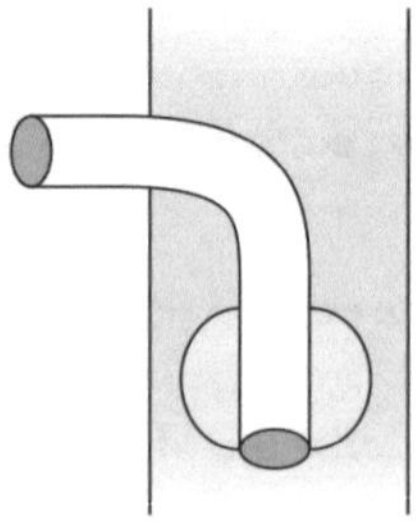

Tracheostomy tube that is too small for the airway despite hyperinflation of the cuff.

Cuff Is Inflated, but Air and Secretions Are Leaking Past the Cuff

Up to 150 ml of oropharyngeal secretions can be removed per day from ICU patients, while it has been reported that over 50 ml of secretions per hour have been removed from patients in the prone position.[28]

Longitudinal channels can occur in high-volume, low-pressure cuffs, and these folds appear upon inflation of the cuff because the diameter must be greater than that of the trachea for intracuff pressure to equal tracheal wall pressure. Winklmaier, Wüst, Schiller, and Wallner[29] studied leakage around the cuffs of three different Tracheostomy Tubes: Rüsch Ultra-Tracheoflex, TRACOE Vario, and Portex Blue Line Ultra. They injected 6 ml of water or artificial saliva into a tracheostomized pig model and measured the volumes that leaked past the inflated cuff after 5, 10, and 15 minutes. They studied these conditions with and without artificial ventilation. They found that when water runs into the subglottic space, it disappears almost completely down the longitudinal channels. The increased viscosity of saliva reduced this leakage significantly compared to water.

The investigators found that the Portex Blue Line Ultra was the most effective of the tubes studied in preventing leakage of fluid and that leakage was higher without artificial ventilation. An interesting observation was that cuff pressure in all three tubes dropped significantly after 15 minutes. All tubes were initially measured at 25 cm H_2O; after 15 minutes, the pressure dropped to an average of 18.76 cm H_2O in the TRACOE tube, 19.54 in the Rüsch tube, and 19.07 in the Portex tube. The researchers concluded that leakage of fluid was associated with the thickness of the cuff membrane, and they projected that ultrathin polyurethane might be the cuff material of the future.

Miller and others[30] compared the use of conventional endotracheal tubes with a polyurethane cuff endotracheal tube. They found that the rates of ventilator-associated pneumonia dropped significantly from 5.3 per 1,000 ventilator days to 2.8 per 1,000 ventilator days. Young and colleagues[28] performed similar testing in a model lung and trachea and found that leakage occurred down the longitudinal folds in all cuffs tested. They found that the application of lubricant around the cuff helped protect it from leakage, and the use of PEEP and CPAP also protected against leakage.

The leakage of secretions around the cuff may not be clinically evident. The normal response to the leakage of secretions around the cuff is continued coughing, but sedation blunts this response. Normal glottic function is impaired with prolonged intubation. Silent aspiration is common in certain patients who have been orotracheally intubated for mechanical ventilation and in those with neurologic deficits.

Leak Is Associated With Changes in Patient Position

In some cases, the leak is present when the patient is in a certain position but disappears when the patient's position is changed. Tracheostomy and endotracheal tubes can move within the airway when the patient's head is moved in different positions, which, secondarily, alters the position of the cuff within the airway. Simple repositioning will often eliminate the leak. Frequently, leaks result not only from head movement and repositioning of the cuff within the airway but also from external forces on the tube. The presence of added weight on the tracheostomy tube from filters, in-line suctioning systems, or unsupported circuit tubing will cause traction or torque on the tracheostomy tube. If this is the case, the added weight should be removed, and the ventilator tubing should be adequately supported. If the leak remains after these maneuvers, the tracheostomy tube should be changed to a longer tube for improved placement in the airway.

Patient Is on High Levels of PEEP

When the level of PEEP is high, it is sometimes difficult to maintain an adequate seal because air pushed through the tube can also push against the cuff. With higher levels of PEEP (usually greater than 10 cm H_2O), the tracheostomy tube can often be displaced outward. The movement of the tube in the airway with the respiratory cycle is called pistoning, which will be discussed in more detail later. A patient on high levels of PEEP should be closely monitored not only for hemodynamic stability and evidence of barotrauma, but also for proper tube placement.

An Area of Tracheomalacia Has Developed

If the tube is of adequate size for the patient's airway and the leak remains following full inflation of the cuff, one can assume tracheomalacia has developed. Tracheomalacia can be definitively diagnosed by endoscopy. Chronic overinflation of the tracheostomy tube cuff can create an area of tracheal ischemia, which later becomes a localized softening of the tracheal tissue known as tracheomalacia (see **Figure 5.2**). Upon direct visualization, a floppy area moves freely with breathing; depending on the location of the defect, it can result in a severe narrowing of the trachea. Extrathoracic tracheomalacia (above the chest cavity) can cause collapse during spontaneous inspiration, while intrathoracic tracheomalacia (within the chest cavity) can collapse the airway on exhalation.[31] While on mechanical ventilation, the short-term correction of the leak associated with tracheomalacia is to place a longer tracheostomy tube to position the cuff in a more distal location within the trachea. However, surgical resection of the trachea is the long-term solution to this problem. See chapter 10 for more discussion about tracheomalacia.

Figure 5.2 Tracheomalacia & repositioning

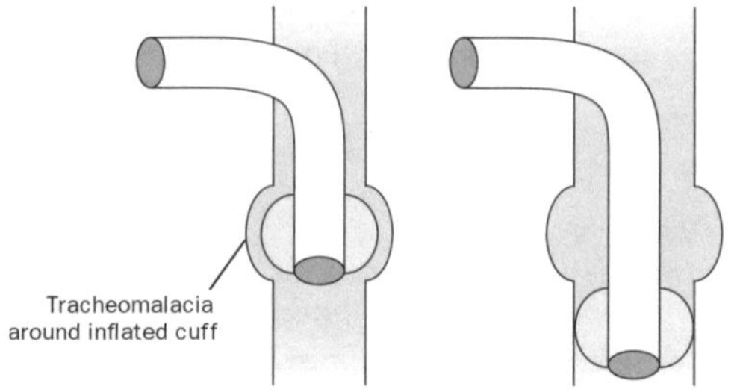

Tracheomalacia and repositioning the tracheostomy tube. On the left is an area of tracheomalacia around an inflated cuff. On the right, a longer tracheostomy tube has been inserted, allowing the cuff to be positioned below the level of tracheomalacia.

Though it is not clinically feasible to continually place progressively longer tracheostomy tubes, one can alternate placing a longer and shorter tube. Another alternative is to use an adjustable-neck flange tracheostomy tube, though it is not recommended for long-term use.

Leak Within the Tube

Rarely, a leak can occur within the tracheostomy tube itself and can result from several factors: a poor fit of the inner cannula into the outer cannula, imperfect connections, or damage during placement. A leak caused by poor fit occurs when there is a size difference between the inner cannula and the outer cannula. When a smaller inner cannula is placed into a larger outer cannula, air will leak between them. Similarly, a leak can be caused when a properly sized inner cannula is not locked into place and air escapes around it. Rarely, a leak can be caused as a result of a manufacturing defect, such as a non-fitting connection between the inner cannula and the outer cannula. More often, a leak within a tube occurs as a result of damage to the tube during insertion, such as during percutaneous insertion, where a higher degree of force is necessary to insert the tube. Any suspected defects in a tube must be reported promptly to the manufacturer and, in some cases, to the Food and Drug Administration (FDA).

Managing cuff leaks can be challenging; therefore, it is important to evaluate them following a systematic method. **Figure 5.3** shows an algorithm for detecting the cause of a cuff leak.

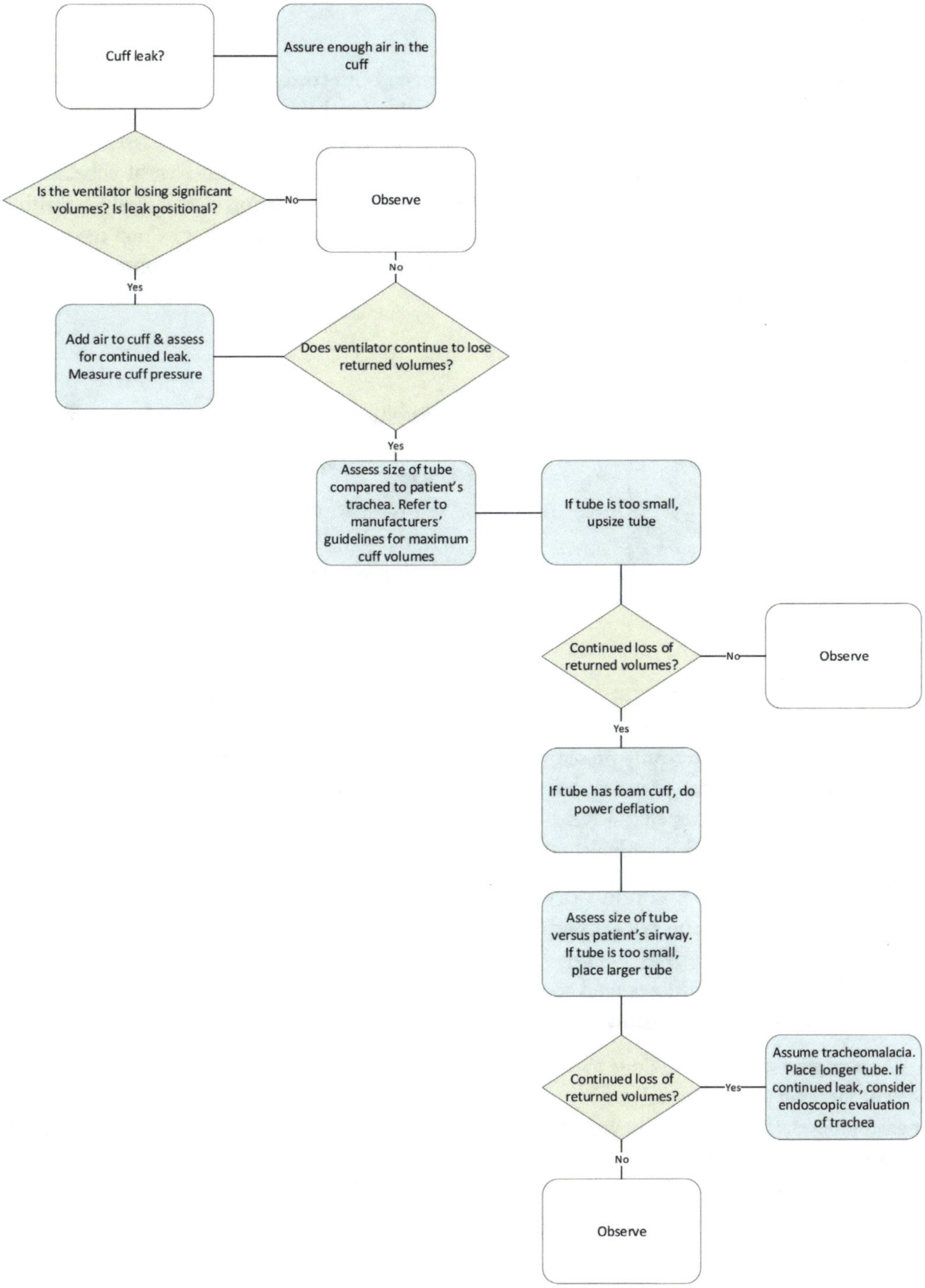

Figure 5.3 Cuff Leak Algorithm

PISTONING

During positive-pressure ventilation, a tube with an inflated cuff tends to move up and down within the airway as the ventilator cycles while the cuff remains fixed in place. Pistoning describes the movement of the tracheostomy tube inside the trachea with the fully inflated cuff fixed in place (see **Figure 5.4**). Pistoning is more apparent with the larger cuff of the endotracheal tube, but it frequently occurs with the tracheostomy tube as well. Over time, this action creates weakness within the integrity of the cuff and adds pressure against the tracheal mucosa as it drags along the walls of the trachea. Even though it is suggested that teardrop-shaped cuffs may prevent this pistoning action, there are no studies to support this claim.

Figure 5.4 Pistoning

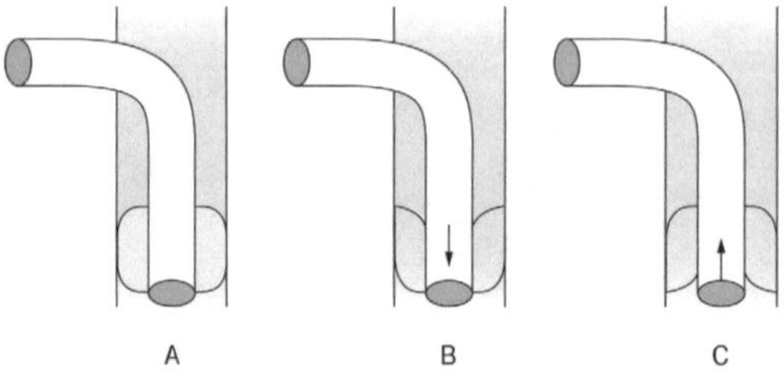

Pistoning of tracheostomy tube against the tracheal wall. Note the cuff stays fixed in place. A) Tube at rest. B) Downward movement of tube with positive-pressure ventilation. C) Upward movement of tube with positive-pressure ventilation.

CUFF CHANGES AT ALTITUDE

The patient with a tracheostomy presents significant complications when traveling by air. During ascent to altitude, ambient pressure decreases. As altitude increases, pressure within the cuff also increases. Boyle's law states that a fixed volume of gas will expand as pressure decreases,[32] so as barometric pressure decreases with altitude, tracheal tube cuffs will expand.

Air-filled cuffs expand with increasing altitude at a rate of 30 mbar/1,000 feet (one millibar equals 0.0145038 psi). The critical perfusion pressure of the tracheal mucosa is exceeded at an altitude of 1,820 feet, so it is important to control for cuff volume expansion in aeromedical transport.[33] Commercial airlines tend to pressurize cabins to 6,000 to 8,000 feet. Helicopters are unpressurized and fly at approximately 5,000 feet.[32]

Several studies have been done to demonstrate the deleterious effect of pressure on tracheal tube cuffs. Stoner and Cooke[34] conducted an early study of endotracheal tube cuffs in anesthetized dogs. At ground level, the cuff pressure was 45 torr in a Portex tube and 78 torr in a Rüsch tube (one torr equals 1.33322 millibars). However, at 8,000 feet, the pressures measured 64 torr in the Portex tube and 130 torr in the Rüsch tube. Upon decompression to 35,000 feet, pressures in the cuffs exceeded 135 and 230 torr, respectively. Interestingly, at compression back to ground level, both cuffs were 60% and 45% of their original pressures, respectively.

Henning and colleagues[32] measured the cuff pressures of 10 patients during aeromedical flights in helicopters and fixed-wing aircraft. All patients began the flight with a cuff pressure of 22 cm H_2O at ground level, and pressure was measured again at 3,000 feet (one centimeter of water pressure equals 0.735559 torr). The investigators found that all pressures had significantly increased, ranging from 40 to 51 cm H_2O.

Normally, it is possible to determine adequate cuff inflation by using either the minimal occlusive volume or the minimal leak technique. (See chapter 7 for a description of methods to minimize pressure in the cuff.) In air transport, however, the noise level is too high to use these methods effectively. Current evidence in the aeromedical transport literature supports the use of cuff inflation with saline, an alternate balloon to vent air from the cuff, or deflation of the cuff at altitude.[33]

Yoneda, Watanabe, Hayashida, Kanno, and Sato[35] described a method to vent air from the cuff by using a separate balloon attached directly to the cuff of an endotracheal tube. They chose balloons of different sizes and connected them to the endotracheal tube with a roller clamp and three-way stopcock. With no pressure-controlling device, they found the tracheal pressure rose 20.8 cm H_2O per 1,000 feet and reached 228.7 cm H_2O at 10,000 feet. Following decompression, tracheal pressure rose from 21.2 cm H_20 at 8,000 feet to 259.0 cm H_2O at 22,000 feet. With the pressure-control device, however, they found no significant increases in cuff pressure. Upon ascent, the pressure with the controlling device was 20.9 cm H_2O at ground level and 20.3 cm H_2O at 10,000 feet. Upon descent, pressure was 19.8 cm H_2O and 20.7 cm H_2O at ground level.

Rather than using a venting device, Mann and colleagues[33] described a formula for the removal of air from the cuff at altitude. They recommended an air-filled cuff should have 0.3 ml of air removed per 1,000 feet during ascent to control for rising pressure. During descent, the cuff should be inflated at the same rate. Smith and McArdle[36] recommended air be removed after reaching altitudes as low as 2,000 feet.

Kaye[37] suggested that the use of saline in the cuffs of tracheal tubes is an easier and more effective method for controlling gas expansion and contraction during air transport. Smith and McArdle[36] found that replacing air with saline resulted in much smaller increases in cuff pressure. The study by Henning and colleagues[32] reported that even with saline in the cuff, there still may be a rise in pressure with altitude, and the pressures even at ground level may be variable. The use of an automatic device to continuously monitor and adjust cuff pressure might be an ideal solution for air transport with cuffed tracheostomy tubes.

Cuff Changes With Anesthesia

It is common knowledge among anesthesiologists that nitrous oxide increases cuff pressure because of easy diffusion into the cuff. This increased cuff pressure manifests as postoperative complaints of sore throat, with severity dependent on the length of the operative procedure. Numerous methods have been employed during nitrous oxide administration to prevent these high cuff pressures. These include high-volume, low-pressure endotracheal tube cuffs; balloon-limiting pressure; inflation of the cuff with a mixture of nitrous oxide and oxygen or saline; a gas barrier cuff; an ultrathin endotracheal tube; and continuous monitoring of cuff pressure.[38]

Karasawa, Hamachi, Takamatsu, and Oshima[39] tested the time required to achieve a stable cuff pressure during 67% nitrous oxide anesthesia. Air-filled cuffs of a standard endotracheal tube were aspirated every 30 minutes for the first three or four hours, and cuff pressures were monitored for an additional three hours. Intracuff concentrations of nitrous oxide increased during the repeated cuff deflation and continued to increase during the additional three-hour monitoring period, from 39.8 cm H_2O to 44.3 cm H_2O. When the cuff was deflated periodically over a four-hour period, it was possible to maintain a stable cuff pressure, implying that cuff pressures continue to increase even after the completion of nitrous oxide anesthesia.

Dullenkopf and investigators[40] tested cuff compliance and pressure during nitrous oxide exposure with a new polyurethane material compared with standard polyvinyl chloride cuffs. They found that the ultrathin polyurethane cuff demonstrated a higher permeability for nitrous oxide and led to a rapid increase in cuff pressure when exposed to nitrous oxide.

Postaci and colleagues[41] compared intracuff pressures during high-flow and low-flow nitrous oxide anesthesia. Cuff pressures were measured continuously with a pressure manometer, and inspired oxygen and nitrous oxide levels were noted every 10 minutes. The time required to reach maximum cuff pressure was significantly shorter in the low-flow anesthesia group.

Navarro and others[42] studied endotracheal cuffs filled with air versus alkalinized lidocaine. In their sample of 50 patients, endotracheal cuff pressures were recorded at 30, 60, 90, and 120 minutes after starting and after ending nitrous oxide anesthesia. Patients were randomly assigned to one of two groups: one group was given a cuff inflated with air to attain a pressure of 20 cm H_2O, while the other used a cuff filled with 2% lidocaine plus 8.4% sodium bicarbonate to attain the same pressure. Pressures in the lidocaine cuffs were significantly lower than those filled with air, and postoperative complaints of sore throat also decreased.

Sato and investigators[43] measured changes in intracuff pressure using an endotracheal tube with the Portex Soft-Seal Cuff. Patients were randomly selected to use a standard endotracheal tube or the Soft-Seal tube. Cuffs were inflated with air and intracuff pressure was measured during 67% nitrous oxide anesthesia. The investigators noted that cuff pressure gradually increased in both groups, but the mean pressure of the Soft-Seal cuffs was significantly lower than the standard tube. The incidence of postoperative sore throat was not significantly different between the two groups.

Combes and others[44] randomly assigned patients to two groups—those with cuffs filled with air and those with cuffs filled with saline during nitrous oxide anesthesia—at 20–30 cm H_2O pressure. In their study of 50 patients, they found that cuff pressure gradually increased during anesthesia in cuffs filled with air but remained stable in those filled with saline. In addition, the incidence of sore throat was greater in patients whose cuffs were filled with air. At the time of extubation, tracheal lesions were seen in all patients with air-filled cuffs, compared to 32% of patients with saline-filled cuffs.

Tracheostomy in Infectious Airborne Illness

Experience with the COVID-19 pandemic has provided clinicians of the world a new opportunity for learning and collaboration in studying virulence and mortality, methods of transmission, and the importance of patient safety. In addition, it has underscored the need for staff protection; even the term PPE (personal protective equipment) has become a part of common vocabulary to those outside of healthcare.

Tracheotomy, by its very nature, is one of the highest aerosol-generating procedures, and any infectious airborne illness magnifies the risk to the healthcare team members. As such, the risks and benefits of the procedure should be examined for each individual case.[45]

The standard of care for tracheostomy placement is within 14 days of intubation and mechanical ventilation, but in the case of COVID-19, some papers have recommended waiting at least 14 days to decrease viral load. However, there is evidence that viral loads are detectable up to three weeks after the onset of symptoms, with the longest documented case lasting 37 days.[46] Takhar and investigators[47] reported that a significant proportion of their COVID-19 positive patients were weaned from mechanical ventilation and successfully extubated between days five and 10. Further, they also suggested that tracheotomy may be considered futile if performed too early.

Givi and investigators[45] recommended that a percutaneous tracheotomy can be considered if it can be accomplished with minimal to no bronchoscopic guidance. However, Tay and investigators[48] recommended against percutaneous tracheotomy because of the increased aerosolization caused by bronchoscopy and serial dilations. Takhar's group[47] provided recommendations to minimize aerosolization with percutaneous tracheotomies, including:

1. Avoid the use of a bronchoscope for guidance. Percutaneous ultrasound is an alternative method of guidance that avoids aerosol generation.
2. Instead of bronchoscopy, use a catheter mount with a sealed port for bronchoscopy to minimize aerosol generation.
3. Perform the procedure under deep sedation and full neuromuscular blockade.
4. Overinflate the cuff of the endotracheal tube (ETT) during the procedure to ensure there is no leak throughout the procedure.
5. Pause ventilation and clamp the ETT at end expiration to reduce aerosol generation during the following critical steps:
    a. While changing the catheter mount
    b. During repositioning of the ETT cuff to the level of the vocal cords
    c. During removal of the large Rhino dilator
6. Cover the tracheal puncture site with a swab throughout the procedure to minimize aerosol spread.
7. Use a single-stage 'Rhino' dilator to avoid multiple entries into the airway.

Tube Choice

There are no clear recommendations for tube choice in infectious airborne illness, although a dual-cannula tube may be the best choice to manage a large amount of thick secretions. Givi and colleagues[45] recommended a smaller than normal tube because it will create a reduced surgical stoma. However, to facilitate bronchial hygiene, Takhar and investigators[47] proposed using a larger diameter tube (8.0-9.0 mm for adults).

Transportation of Patients

In order to minimize risk of transmission of the viral infection during necessary transport throughout the hospital, masking of the patient is required. For patients with cuffed tubes, cuff inflation is recommended to minimize aerosolization. In certain situations, Lambe (2020)[49] recommended using two masks: one covering the patient's mouth and nose, and the other covering the tracheostomy tube:

a. When traveling outside the room
b. When oxygen flow is higher than 6 liters
c. When staff enter the room
d. When oxygen is not delivered in a closed system (if mechanical ventilation is not in use)

Methods to Minimize Aerosol Generation

Several authors have recommended other methods to decrease droplet and aerosol spread while providing tracheostomy care.

1. Use an HME with a filter on an open tracheostomy to "close the system."[50]
2. Use disposable inner cannulas rather than cleaning and reusing them.[50]
3. Use in-line suction systems with HME and filter.[48, 50, 51]
4. Use T-piece with in-line suction, humidification, and filter.[50]
5. Keep cuff pressure greater than 20 cm H_2O to minimize aerosol generation.[52]
6. Avoid cool or heated aerosol systems.[52]
7. Remember cuff deflation is an aerosol-generating procedure, so cuff inflation is recommended at all times. Use caution when deflating cuff.[53]
8. Apply a mask to patients when the cuff is deflated.[53]
9. All communication interventions are considered aerosol-generating.[53]
   a. Above the cuff ventilation, talking tracheostomy
   b. One-way speaking valve
   c. Leak speech
10. Delay videofluoroscopic swallowing study (VFSS) or fiberoptic endoscopic evaluation of swallowing (FEES).[54]
11. Avoid ventilator disconnections.[54]
12. Careful consideration during other aerosol-generating procedures.[55]
    a. Open suctioning
    b. Manual ventilation: If bag-mask ventilation is needed, place a filter between the bag valve and the mask/tracheostomy tube.[51] We recommend use of a HEPA (high-efficiency particulate air) filter.
    c. Flexible tracheoscopy
    d. Tracheostomy tube changes

THE COMPLEX TRACHEOSTOMY WOUND

Patients with complex stomal wounds require extra attention. Occasionally, traction against the stoma will create a widened area of erosion or maceration of tissue. These wounds can become inflamed or infected and turn into cellulitis. Some of the more common problems involved with these lesions and their prevention is described in this section.

Stomal Erosion

Erosion of the stoma is caused by either outward or inward traction. Outward traction is excessive outward pressure on the tracheostomy tube resulting from poorly supported ventilator tubing with devices added to the circuit (such as HMEs, in-line closed suction systems, or filters). This added traction introduces the risk of inadvertent tube dislodgement, which often results from internal erosion of the stoma. The erosion can be so severe that it widens the stoma enough for the entire shaft and cuff to be visible. The only way to prevent this type of erosion is to eliminate excess weight and traction forces. Methods to prevent this internal erosion include the following practices:

- Support the ventilator circuit with support arms, or strategically cushion it with a well-placed towel roll.
- Survey the security of the tracheostomy ties/holder frequently.
- Minimize traction/torque whenever the patient is moved. Whenever turning a patient, always turn him or her first toward the ventilator, then away from the ventilator, and avoid traction throughout the turn.
- Remove the in-line suction system when feasible.
- Replace the HME with a heated humidity unit when feasible.

Inward forces can cause stomal erosion by pressing the neck flange into the tissues of the neck. The effect can be magnified when a twisting force is applied at the pivot points of a rigid neck flange. The only way to prevent this type of stomal erosion is to remove these traction forces by eliminating all mechanisms that cause it and by ensuring proper patient positioning. Other preventive steps include supporting the ventilator circuit, using a tracheostomy dressing to cushion the neck flange against the skin, preventing neck flexion when possible, removing excess weight from the circuit, and, if necessary, changing the tracheostomy tube to one with a soft and flexible neck flange.

Inflammation/Cellulitis

Most inflammation of the stoma is caused by moisture. The prolonged contact of secretions with the skin creates irritation and inflammation of the skin—not unlike diaper rash—and can lead to the maceration of tissue and the development of cellulitis. These complications can be prevented by keeping the stoma dry, particularly in patients who produce copious amounts of secretions. If frequent changes of the gauze dressing are not enough to keep the stoma dry, then absorbent dressings may be required. Two examples of absorbent dressings are Lyofoam and Mepilex, which come in a precut form for use as a drain sponge.

Infected, erosive wounds present a greater challenge. Systemic antibiotics may be indicated if the patient exhibits signs of systemic infection, including fever, elevated white blood cell count, tachycardia, etc. In most cases, adequate local treatment is effective in preventing systemic infection. Hotter and Warfield[56] described an approach to care for deep, erosive, infected wounds. They used a product called Mesalt, a thin cloth ribbon impregnated with 15% sodium chloride. The wound was gently packed with the ribbon to absorb excess secretions and bacteria and was changed every two to three hours. The researchers hypothesized that the hypertonicity of the product provided an osmotic effect within the wound bed to increase oxygen delivery and decrease edema. For deeply erosive wounds, they also used DuoDERM as a platform to support the neck flange from digging into the skin. DuoDERM is a hydrocolloid wafer that forms a gel when it comes in contact with moisture or exudate. The authors suggested that DuoDERM can be left in place for up to 10 days; the manufacturer recommends only up to seven days. **Figure 5.5** shows a complex tracheostomy wound using DuoDERM as a platform for stomal erosion.

Figure 5.5 Stomal Erosion

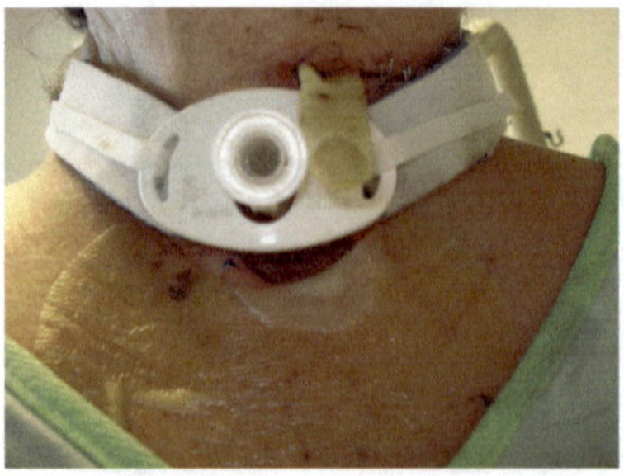

A complex tracheostomy wound. Note hydrocolloid dressing is used as a platform.

Silver-impregnated pads have been shown to be effective on infected wounds. Direct contact with silver disrupts the bacterial cell membrane and results in a significant bactericidal effect. Aquacel Ag is one such silver-infused product, and it can be used for infected and draining wounds. It turns to a hydrocolloid gel that absorbs secretions and can be left in place for up to seven days.

Tracheostomy as a Lived Experience

The experiences of patients and caregivers have not been well reported in the literature, but there have been a few notable studies which provide insight to clinicians. Sherlock, Wilson, and Exley[57] reported the results of their semi-structured interviews with eight patients still in the hospital. Though their sample size was admittedly small, their results gave quite a powerful message to clinicians. The study shed light on the limited amount and quality of information provided to patients while in the hospital. The researchers found that clinicians were provided little information about the tracheostomy procedure and their overall condition. Patients' responses fell into several categories, including physical sensations, feelings related to the tube, eating and drinking, suctioning, and communication. All the patients described the bulkiness of the tube as restricting their freedom of movement. They also reported their fears associated with the tube. One patient reported, "For a couple of days, I was really scared of moving my head, 'cos [sic] there was something new stuck in my neck." All patients who had commenced oral intake commented on the difficulty they experienced with swallowing. One patient reported, "I was uncomfortable with it because every time you tried to swallow you could feel this lump there."

All the patients understood the necessity of suctioning for removal of secretions, but they also described their fear of and discomfort with the procedure. One patient described his experience: "The worst part was when it needed to be cleaned with suction… I would panic because I couldn't breathe. I had no control over what was happening." Another patient reported, "Every time they put it [the suction catheter] down, you coughed violently. You felt as if you were going to explode and then sort of relief because they'd taken all the mucus away…It's a most uncomfortable process."

Every patient expressed frustration at his or her inability to communicate effectively. One patient stated, "That's terrible. The fact that you can't communicate. You can open, close your mouth and know what you're saying, knowing that nobody else can hear what it is that you are trying to say, so we got a board in the end and I used to have to write messages."

Patients reported they received little, if any, information about the tracheostomy and its implications. One patient responded, "They come and have a few words with you and then go on their way and not have time to sit and explain...It would have been nice to have had more [information]." Three patients reported being given information but still awoke feeling shocked that the tracheostomy tube was in place. "They tell you what's going to happen. They're going to put this tube in your throat to help you breathe, but with me it wasn't until I actually realized I'd got it there that I thought, 'What's this thing?"[57]

Segaran[58] studied the experience of eating with a tracheostomy during critical illness. The responses of the subjects fell into several categories, including regaining control, self-determination, sensory impact, and apprehensions. Patients were interviewed either while still in the ICU or within seven days of leaving the ICU. Unstructured interviews were used, and the patients' responses were analyzed using a phenomenological approach. Patients started to develop goals in an effort to regain control over their situation. One subject reported the need to start "shedding attachments" and that his "number one goal was to get the tracheostomy out." Eating and drinking were key priorities, but many became frustrated at their inability to meet those goals. Subjects reported the difficulty they had with eating with a tracheostomy: "Eating with a tracheostomy was very cumbersome. That was frustrating, as I couldn't eat properly, really. Well, not what I really wanted, like coke or fish and chips." Subjects also described eating as a difficult procedure that added to their frustration. When finally allowed to eat or drink, patients reported their fears about eating and drinking for the first time with a tracheostomy, especially after having been cautioned about the risks of aspiration. They also identified a restriction in their throat that they could always feel. Patients who had been decannulated reported the impact it had on their sense of taste and smell. One patient reported: "When I had the trache [sic] in, nothing tasted or smelt [sic] as it should. But I think it's getting better now the trache is out. I'm definitely starting to smell things again now."[58]

Rwakonda[59] studied quality of life in 10 tracheostomy patients on home mechanical ventilation for at least six months. They reported that their quality of life improved when they were on home mechanical ventilation compared to the hospital and felt empowered that they had control in their daily lives when they had competent caregivers and family members. She found several themes that emerged in the data: autonomy, significance of the ventilator for well-being, feeling tied-up, creating meaning, tipping point, reminiscence, building trust and confidence, adjusting to technology, family support and relationships, and meaning of life.

Gilony and colleagues[60] studied body image and quality of life in patients with tracheostomy and found that quality of life scores were diminished in patients with a tracheostomy when compared with non-cannulated patients. To study body image, they used the Body Cathexis Scale, focusing questions on the neck and general health. They found that the scores of cannulated and decannulated patients were significantly lower than those who never had a tracheostomy tube. Scores of decannulated patients were significantly higher than those who remained cannulated, indicating improved body image perception after decannulation.[60]

Morris and colleagues[61] used a different approach to study body image in patients with a tracheostomy. They used the qualitative approach of naturalistic inquiry to ask patients their responses to four open-ended questions about body image. They found four major themes in the responses of patients: patient feelings, patient perception of others' feelings, interaction with others, and social activity. The majority of patients (67%) were concerned with what others thought about their tracheostomy, but most were not embarrassed or emotionally uncomfortable (58%), did not avoid social situations (67%), and did not think they made others uncomfortable (58%). Some of their comments included:

- "Sometimes I gaze into the dark hole during trach changes and I almost feel sick. I have tried to accept my trach but I hate that I can't swim anymore and miss how my throat used to look and I hate how it hurts so often and how it gets infected. I am grateful that having it saves my life, but there's a definite cost."
- "...the stares used to bother me at first, but not so much anymore."
- "My first trip to a restaurant, I sat next to people who loudly requested that they be moved, my 'thing' disturbed them, as did the gauze I wore under the flange."
- Only when an ER doctor pointed out that I should not be able to speak with a trach. She was clueless and did that in front of a large group of my peers."[61]

Nakarada-Kordic and others[62] conducted an important systematic review of the literature on patient and caregiver experiences with a tracheostomy. They reviewed 17 adult studies and included only experiences from the patient/family perspectives, excluding children and laryngectomy patients. Five main themes emerged in the studies they reviewed: care, support, and management of the tracheostomy, speech and communication, well-being and quality of life, disfigurement and body image, and stigma and social withdrawal.

One study[63] described how the tracheostomy brought about new problems such as disability for work. None of the participants returned to work after the tracheostomy, noting the employers' reluctance to rehire them due to legal concerns.

Defective Tracheostomy Tubes

Manufacturing defects are relatively rare in airway devices, but they do occur. Fused parts may become disconnected or detached; pieces may be missing or not fit properly. It is better to discover a problem before the device is placed into a patient, but often defects are not discovered until the tube has been in place for some time. In any case, it is wise to always save the packaging for a device. The package identifies the batch number (and sometimes the serial number) so the problem can be more easily traced. Ideally, this identifying information should be recorded in the medical record when the device is placed in the patient. One company (TRACOE) provides a wallet-sized identification card for their tracheostomy tubes that includes the serial number, model number, size, and length along with the company's contact information.

When a defect is identified, the manufacturer must be contacted immediately and notified of the problem. Manufacturers usually have a system in place for the return shipping of equipment for a safety inspection. Ideally, all parts of the tracheostomy tube should be returned with the package it came in. In many cases, these defects must also be reported promptly to the Food and Drug Administration (FDA). This is required if an adverse event occurred because of the defective device.

The FDA maintains the Manufacturer and User Facility Device Experience (MAUDE) database.[64] This database houses reports submitted to the FDA from healthcare professionals, patients, and consumers. It is updated monthly and is limited to adverse event reports in the preceding 10 years. Manufacturers are required to submit reports to the FDA when they become aware of information that suggests one of their devices may have malfunctioned, causing or contributing to a death or serious injury. The information provided in this database can be surprising to clinicians with regard to the potential for tracheostomy tube malfunctions.

Tracheostomy tubes can also become damaged during the tracheotomy procedure itself, especially during percutaneous insertion. A tracheostomy tube inserted percutaneously creates a much tighter fit than one inserted with a standard surgical approach. Because of this tight fit, excessive pressure must sometimes be used to insert the tube. The neck flange may be weakened during insertion and may not become noticeable until hours or days later. This situation presents a unique dilemma. Ordinarily, a damaged tube must be replaced immediately. However, the replacement of any tracheostomy tube in the early postoperative period is fraught with the risk of loss of airway access. It is usually preferable that measures be taken to stabilize the tube until a more mature stoma can develop; if this is not possible, the tube should be replaced in a controlled environment using a well-developed plan.

Missing Parts

Tracheostomy tubes are packaged as a set, with all the pieces fitting together. All the parts within a set are designed to be used together. With few exceptions, these parts are not interchangeable with other tubes. For example, a missing inner cannula should not be replaced with an inner cannula from a different set; the entire tube should be changed. Frequently, lengths will be different between two identical tubes of the same size. The inner cannula may be longer than the outer cannula and may create erosion of the tracheal wall as it protrudes from the end of the outer cannula. In addition, disposable inner cannulas may not be used with non-disposable outer cannulas because of the different locking mechanisms.

Summary

There are many special considerations for a patient with a tracheostomy. Airway pressures must be closely monitored for patients who are ventilator dependent. The retention of secretions is a particular concern with a tracheostomy, and increased airway pressure is an early sign of secretion accumulation within the tracheostomy tube. Cuff leaks are a particular concern in the mechanically ventilated patient and can be managed with a methodical approach. Care should be taken to minimize pressure against the stoma, as both inward and outward traction forces can cause erosion of the stoma. This erosive action can be prevented by eliminating excessive weight from the ventilator tubing and by strategically placing a towel roll to support it. Altitude and nitrous oxide anesthesia cause large increases in cuff pressure, so paying careful attention to optimal cuff pressure and volume will prevent complications. Though rare, manufacturing defects do occur in tracheostomy tubes, and damage may be caused to the tube during the insertion procedure. With careful assessment and a methodical approach, the experienced practitioner can expertly manage all of these challenges, including managing tracheostomies in highly infectious settings.

Key Points

- For the patient on mechanical ventilation, high peak pressure in the presence of normal plateau pressure indicates an airway problem, including an obstruction due to secretions or a tracheostomy tube that is too small.
- Cuff leaks can occur within the cuff, around the cuff, or within the tube itself. A systematic approach should be used to determine the cause of a cuff leak.
- Stomal erosion commonly occurs from traction caused by the ventilator circuit against the tracheostomy tube.
- Cuff pressures dramatically increase at altitude and with administration of nitrous oxide anesthesia. Close attention to cuff pressure is warranted in these situations.
- Encounters with patients who have viral/bacterial respiratory infections require meticulous attention to containment of aerosol as well as patient-healthcare worker-patient contact. A practiced methodology serves as an important checklist for procedures and transporting these patients.
- To minimize apprehension and fear, patients need continued guidance and information about how to manage specific functions such as tube care, feeding, and phonation.

REVIEW QUESTIONS

1. Patient A is critically ill on mechanical ventilation. If peak pressures are high and plateau pressures are normal, what does this indicate?
    a. Decreasing lung compliance
    b. Increasing lung compliance
    c. Possible tube obstruction
    d. Decreasing work of breathing

    ANSWER: C. Choice C is correct because it indicates resistance to dynamic airflow in the presence of tube obstruction. Choices A and B are incorrect because, in the presence of normal lung volumes, lung compliance would be decreased when both peak and plateau pressures are increasing. Choice D is a distractor and incorrect.

2. Over the previous 8 hours, you notice the cuff of the tracheostomy tube has required the addition of air on three separate occasions. What is the most likely explanation?
    a. Decreasing tidal volumes on the ventilator
    b. Increasing compliance of the lungs
    c. Tracheomalacia
    d. Damage to the cuff or pilot balloon

    ANSWER: D. Damage to the cuff or pilot balloon is the most likely situation to require repeated addition of air to the cuff. Choice A is possible but would not cause repeated cuff leak. Choice B is a distractor. Tracheomalacia is a consideration because it often initially presents as a cuff leak, though the leak develops over a longer period of time. A cuff that seems to lose air over a relatively short period of time should be suspicious of damage to the cuff or pilot balloon. In that case, the tube should be changed.

3. Aerosol generation during tracheostomy care can be minimized by which of the following?
    a. Use in-line (closed) suctioning system
    b. Keep the cuff deflated or use cuffless tube
    c. Use leak speech for phonation
    d. Use heated aerosol tracheostomy collar to loosen thick secretions

    ANSWER: A. A closed suctioning system is the only choice that lessens aerosol generation. All of the other choices promote aerosol generation.

4. If you are transporting a tracheostomy patient by airplane, which of the following is the recommended method to manage cuff pressure?
    a. Inflate cuff with 0.5 ml of air for every 1,000 feet of ascent
    b. Deflate cuff 0.3 ml for every 1,000 feet of ascent
    c. Inflate cuff 0.3 ml for every 1,000 feet of descent
    d. Inflate cuff with saline

    ANSWER: D. Choice A is incorrect because cuff pressure increases with ascent, and inflating the cuff worsens the problem. Choices B and C are based on the study from Mann and colleagues[33] and could be used. However, choice D is more reliable and the recommended method.

5. Methods to prevent skin issues with a tracheostomy include all of the following EXCEPT:
    a. Prevent traction against the tracheostomy tube
    b. Administer preventative antibiotic
    c. Keep the stoma clean and dry
    d. Use absorbent dressings if gauze dressings cannot keep the stoma dry

ANSWER: B. The correct choice is B. All of the other choices are recommended methods to prevent skin issues.

REFERENCES

1. Shapiro BA, Harrison RA, Kacmarek RM, Cane RD. *Clinical Application of Respiratory Care.* 3rd ed. Chicago: Yearbook Medical Publishers; 1985.
2. Oliver ER, Gist A, Gillespie MB. Percutaneous versus surgical tracheotomy: An updated meta-analysis. *Laryngoscope.* 2007;117:1570-1575.
3. Fernandez-Bussy S, Mahajan B, Folch E, Caviedes I, Guerrero J, Majid A. Tracheostomy tube placement: Early and late complications. *Journal of Bronchology Interventional Pulmonol.* 2015;22(4):357-364.
4. Marsh HM, Gillespie DJ, Baumgartner AE. Timing of tracheostomy in the critically ill patient. *Chest.* 1989;96(1):190-193.
5. Arabi YM, Alhashemi JA, Tamim HM, Esteban A, Haddad SH, Dawood A, et al. The impact of time to tracheostomy on mechanical ventilation duration, length of stay, and mortality in intensive care unit patients. *J Crit Care.* 2009;24(3):435-440.
6. Rumbak MJ, Newton M, Truncale T, Schwartz SW, Adams JW, Hazard PB. A prospective, randomized study comparing early percutaneous dilational tracheotomy to prolonged translaryngeal intubation (delayed tracheotomy) in critically ill medical patients. *Crit Care Med.* 2004;*32*(8):1689-1694.
7. Scales DC, Kahn JM. Tracheostomy timing, enrollment and power in ICU clinical trials. *Intens Care Med.* 2008;34(10):1743-1745.
8. Kluge S, Baumann HJ, Maier C, Klose H, Meyer A, Nierhaus A, et al. Tracheostomy in the intensive care unit: A nationwide survey. *Anesth Analg.* 2008;107(5):1639-1643.
9. Blot F, Similowski T, Trouillet JL, Chardon P, Korach JM, Costa MA, et al. Early tracheotomy versus prolonged endotracheal intubation in unselected severely ill ICU patients. *Intens Care Med.* 2008;34:1779-1787.
10. Shan L, Hao P, Xu F, Chen Y. Benefits of early tracheotomy: A meta-analysis based on 6 observational studies. *Respir Care,* 2013;58(11):1856-1862.
11. Morris LL. Tracheostomy database, Northwestern University, 2020.
12. Pierson DJ. Tracheostomy and weaning. *Respir Care.* 2005;50(4) 526-533.
13. Freeman BD, Borecki IB, Coopersmith CM, Buchman TG. Relationship between tracheostomy timing and duration of mechanical ventilation in critically ill patients. *Criti Care Med.* 2005 33(11):2513-2520.
14. Andriolo BN, Andriolo, RB, Saconato, H, Atallah AN, Valente I. Early versus late tracheostomy for critically ill patients. *Cochrane Database Syst Rev.* 2015;1: CD007271.
15. Adly A, Youssef TA, El-Begermy MM, Younis HM. Timing of tracheostomy in patients with prolonged endotracheal intubation: A systematic review. *Eur Arch Otorhinolaryngol.* 2018;275(3):679-690.
16. McCredie VA, Alali AS, Scales DC, Adhikari NK, Rubenfeld GD, Cuthbertson BH, Nathens AB. Effect of early versus late tracheostomy or prolonged intubation in critically ill patients with acute brain injury: A systematic review and meta-analysis. *Neurocrit Care.* 2017;26(1):14-25.
17. Kang BH, Cho J, Lee JC, Jung K. Early versus late tracheostomy in trauma patients: A propensity-matched cohort study of 5 years' data at a single institution in Korea. *World J Surg.* 2018;42(6):1742-1747.
18. Pizza A, Picconi E, Piastra M, Genovese O, Biasucci DG, Conti G. Early versus late tracheostomy in pediatric intensive care unit: Does it matter? A 6-year experience. *Minerva Anestesiol.* 2017;83(8):836-843.

19. Pilbeam SP. Basic patient assessment and methods to improve ventilation. In Pilbeam SP. ed., *Mechanical ventilation: Physiological and Clinical Applications*. St. Louis, MO: Mosby; 1998:244-261.
20. Esan A, Khusid F, Raoof S. Ventilator technology and management. In Oropello JM, Pastores SM, Kvetan V. eds. *Critical Care*. New York, NY: McGraw-Hill; 2017.
21. Gomella LG, Haist SA. Critical care. In Gomella LG, Haist SA *Clinician's Pocket Reference: The Scut Monkey*. 11th ed. Columbus, OH: McGraw-Hill; 2006.
22. Bone RC. Monitoring ventilatory mechanics during respiratory failure. *Respir Care*. 1983;28(5):1287.
23. Beachey W. Mechanics of ventilation. In W. Beachey, *Respiratory care anatomy and physiology* (2nd ed.). St. Louis, MO: Mosby; 2007.
24. Davis K, Campbell RS, Johannigman JA, Valente JF, Branson RD. Changes in respiratory mechanics after tracheostomy. *Arch Surg*. 1999;134:59-62.
25. Levitsky MG. Nonrespiratory functions of the lung. In Levitsky MG. ed. *Pulmonary Physiology*. New York, NY: McGraw-Hill; 2018.
26. Fernandez R, Blanch L, Mancebo J, Bonsoms N, Artigas A. Endotracheal tube cuff pressure assessment: Pitfalls of finger estimation and need for objective measurement. *Crit Care Med*. 1990;18(12):1423-1426.
27. Hoffman RJ, Parwani V, Hahn I. Experienced emergency medicine physicians cannot safely inflate or estimate endotracheal tube cuff pressure using standard techniques. *Amer J Emerg Med*. 2006;24:139-143.
28. Young PJ, Rollinson M, Downward G, Henderson S. Leakage of fluid past the tracheal tube cuff in a benchtop model. *Brit J Anaesth*. 1997;78:557-562.
29. Winklmaier U, Wüst K, Schiller S, Wallner F. Leakage of fluid in different types of tracheal tubes. *Dysphagia*. 2006;21(4):237-242.
30. Miller, MA, Arndt, JL, Konkle, MA, Chenoweth, CE, Iwashyna, TJ, Flaherty, KR, Hyzy, RC. A polyurethane cuffed endotracheal tube is associated with decreased rates of ventilator-associated pneumonia. *J Crit Care*. 2011;26(3):280-286.
31. Zur KB, Schilero GJ. Pulmonary physiology and mechanical ventilation. In Van de Water TR, Staecker H, eds. *Otolaryngology: Basic Science and Clinical Review*. New York: Thieme; 2006.
32. Henning J, Sharley P, Young R. Pressures within air-filled tracheal cuffs at altitude— An in vivo study. *Anaesth*. 2004;59(3):252-254.
33. Mann C, Parkinson N, Bleetman A. Endotracheal tube and laryngeal mask airway cuff volume changes with altitude: A rule of thumb for aeromedical transport. *Emerg Med J*. 2007;24:165-167.
34. Stoner DL, Cooke JP. Intratracheal cuffs and aeromedical evacuation. *Anesthesiol*. 1974;41(3):302-306.
35. Yoneda I, Watanabe K, Hayashida S, Kanno M, Sato T. A simple method to control tracheal cuff pressure in anaesthesia and in air evacuation. *Anaesth*. 1999;54:975-980.
36. Smith RP, McArdle BH. Pressure in the cuffs of tracheal tubes at altitude. *Anaesth*. 2002;57(4):374-378.
37. Kaye P. Effects of altitude on endotracheal tube cuff pressure. *Emerg Med J*. 2007;24:605-607.
38. Tu HN, Saidi N, Lieutaud T, Bensaid S, Venival V, Duvaldestin P. Nitrous oxide increases endotracheal cuff pressure and the incidence of tracheal lesions in anesthetized patients. *Anesth Analg*. 1999;89:187-190.

39. Karasawa F, Hamachi T, Takamatsu I, Oshima T. Time required to achieve a stable cuff pressure by repeated aspiration of the cuff during anesthesia with nitrous oxide. *Eur J Anaesth*. 2003;20(6):470-474.
40. Dullenkopf A, Gerber AC, Weiss M. Nitrous oxide diffusion into tracheal tube cuffs: Comparison of five different tracheal tube cuffs. *Acta Anaesthesiol Scand*. 2004;48(9):1180-1184.
41. Postaci A, Karabeyoglu I, Erk G, Ayerden T, Sastim H, Barcin S, et al. A comparison of intra cuff pressures in high-flow and low-flow nitrous oxide anesthesia. *Saudi Medical J*. 2008;29(12):1719-1722.
42. Navarro LHC, Braz JRC, Nakamura G, Lima RME, Silva FDPE, Modolo NSP. Effectiveness and safety of endotracheal tube cuffs filled with air versus filled with alkalinized lidocaine: A randomized clinical trial. *Sao Paolo Med J*. 2007;125(6):322-328.
43. Sato K, Tanaka M, Nishikawa T. Changes in intracuff pressure of endotracheal tubes permeable or resistant to nitrous oxide and incidence of postoperative sore throat. *Masui Jap J Anesthesiol*. 2004;53(7):767-771.
44. Combes X, Schauvliege F, Peyrouset O, Motamed C, Kirov K, Dhonneur G, et al. Intracuff pressure and tracheal morbidity. *Anesthesiol*. 2001;95(5):1120-1124.
45. Givi B, Schiff BA, Chinn, SB, Clayburgh D, Iyer NG, Jalisi S, Moore, MG, Nathan, CA, Orloff LA, O'Neill JP, Parker N, ZSender C, Morris LGT, Davies L. Safety recommendations for evaluation and surgery of the nead and neck during the COVID-19 pandemic. *JAMA Otolaryngol Head Neck Surg*. 2020;146(6):579-584. doi:10.1001/jamaoto.2020.0780.
46. Zhou F, Yu T, Du R, Fan G, Liu Y, Liu Z, Xiang J, Wang Y, Song B, Gu X, Guan L, Wei Y, Li H, Wu X, Xu J, Tu S, Zhang Y, Chen H, Cao B. Clinical course and risk factors for mortality of adult inpatients with COVID-19 in Wuhan, China: A retrospective cohort study. *Lancet*. 395:1054-1062. https://doi.org/10.1016/S0140-6736(20)30566-3.
47. Takhar A, Walker A, Tricklebank S, Wyncoll D, Hart N, Jacob T, Arora A, Skilbeck C, Simo R, Surda P. (2020). Recommendation of a practical guideline for safe tracheostomy during the COVID-19 pandemic. *Eur Arch Oto Rhino Laryngol*. 2020;277:2173-2184. [https://doi.org/10.1007/s00405-020-05993-x].
48. Tay JK, Khoo ML-C, Loh WS. (2020). Surgical considerations for tracheostomy during the COVID-19 pandemic. Lessons learned from the severe acute respiratory syndrome outbreak. *JAMA Otolaryngol Head Neck Surg*. 2020;146(6):515-518. doi:10.1001/jamaoto.2020.0764.
49. Lambe, L. (2020). Putting safety first during the COVID-19 pandemic: Practical strategies for healthcare workers and patients with a tracheostomy. Global Tracheostomy Collaborative webinar, April 10, 2020. https://www.gotostage.com/channel/c4d2288975ce453daf8d9e09860c8da4/recording/5684b06d845b4dd58ee404534687749b/watch?source=CHANNEL.
50. DeRose, T. Putting safety first during the COVID-19 pandemic: Practical strategies for healthcare workers and patients with a tracheostomy. Global Tracheostomy Collaborative webinar, April 10, 2020. https://www.gotostage.com/channel/c4d2288975ce453daf8d9e09860c8da4/recording/5684b06d845b4dd58ee404534687749b/watch?source=CHANNEL.
51. Ferioli M, Cisternino C, Leo V, Pisani L, Palange P, Nava S. (2020). Protecting healthcare workers from SARS-CoV-2 infection: Practical indications. *Eur Respir Rev*. 29:200068. [https://doi.org/10.1183/16000617.0068-2020].
52. Walsh B. Putting safety first during the COVID-19 pandemic: Practical strategies for healthcare workers and patients with a tracheostomy. Global Tracheostomy Collaborative webinar, April 10, 2020.

https://www.gotostage.com/channel/c4d2288975ce453daf8d9e09860c8da4/recording/5684b06d845b4dd58ee404534687749b/watch?source=CHANNEL.

53. Zaga C. Putting safety first during the COVID-19 pandemic: Practical strategies for healthcare workers and patients with a tracheostomy. Global Tracheostomy Collaborative webinar, April 10, 2020. https://www.gotostage.com/channel/c4d2288975ce453daf8d9e09860c8da4/recording/5684b06d845b4dd58ee404534687749b/watch?source=CHANNEL.
54. Cameron T. (2020). Putting safety first during the COVID-19 pandemic: Practical strategies for healthcare workers and patients with a tracheostomy. Global Tracheostomy Collaborative webinar, April 10, 2020. https://www.gotostage.com/channel/c4d2288975ce453daf8d9e09860c8da4/recording/5684b06d845b4dd58ee404534687749b/watch?source=CHANNEL.
55. Watters K. Putting safety first during the COVID-19 pandemic: Practical strategies for healthcare workers and patients with a tracheostomy. Global Tracheostomy Collaborative webinar, April 10, 2020. https://www.gotostage.com/channel/c4d2288975ce453daf8d9e09860c8da4/recording/5684b06d845b4dd58ee404534687749b/watch?source=CHANNEL.
56. Hotter AN, Warfield K. Technique for promoting healing of complex tracheostomy wounds. *Otolaryngol Head Neck Surg.* 1997;11(6):693-695.
57. Sherlock ZV, Wilson JA, Exley C. Tracheostomy in the acute setting: Patient experience and information needs. *J Crit Care.* 2009;24(4):501-507.
58. Segaran E. Returning to normal: The role of eating in recovery from a critical illness. *Brit J Neurosci Nurs.* 2006;2(3):141-148.
59. Rwakonda M. Lived experiences of individuals quality of life on prolonged home mechanical ventilation. (Doctoral dissertation). Retrieved from ProQuest Dissertations and Theses database. (UMI No. 10684192), 2017.
60. Gilony D, Gilboa D, Blumstein T, Murad H, Talmi YP, Kronenberg G, Wolf M. Effects of tracheostomy and well-being and body image perceptions. *Otolaryngol Head Neck Surg.* 2005;133:366-371.
61. Morris LL, Lupei M, Afifi MS. Body image perception after tracheostomy. *ORL Head Neck Nurs.* 2017;35(4):13-18.
62. Nakarada-Kordic I, Patterson N, Wrapson J, Reay SD. A systematic review of patient and caregiver experiences with a tracheostomy. Patient Centered Outcomes Res. 2018;11(2):175-191.
63. Laakso K, Markstrom A., Idvall M. Havstam C, Hartelius L. Communication experience of individuals treated with home mechanical ventilation. *Int J Lang Communic Dis.* 2011;46(6):686-699.
64. MAUDE, Manufacturer and User Facility Device Experience. https://www.accessdata.fda.gov/scripts/cdrh/cfdocs/cfmaude/search.cfm. Accessed April 29, 2020.

6

Phonation with a Tracheostomy

by Linda L. Morris

Objectives

- List principles of voice restoration for patients with tracheostomies
- Discuss methods to restore phonation with and without assisted ventilation
- Differentiate use of speaking valves compared to capping
- Illustrate airflows necessary for phonation with different tracheostomy tubes

Introduction

Phonation is the creation of sound, while articulation is the creation of words. Sound is created as air passes through the vocal cords. Speech is the effective blending of both phonation and articulation. The ability to communicate is vital for effective overall medical care, psychological function, and social interaction. Speech allows patients to express needs, communicate with caregivers, use the telephone, and maintain personal relationships.[1] The inability to speak greatly restricts patients' abilities to participate meaningfully in their health care plan.[2] The inability to speak is often fraught with frustration for patients and caregivers alike.[3] Patients who cannot speak may feel an additional loss of control and powerlessness, which can often lead to depression and other behavioral concerns. One small pilot study of five critically ill patients found that pain and speech were the two most important factors contributing to their quality of life in the intensive care unit.[4] Freeman-Sanderson and colleagues[5] found that quality of life scores improved in ICU patients when their voice was restored.

General Principles of Voice Restoration

The tracheostomy tube redirects air, and normal speech is interrupted as air bypasses the vocal cords. A tracheostomy results in a loss of subglottic air pressure, which creates many other sequelae in addition to the loss of speech. An unoccluded tracheostomy tube interferes with effective swallowing, coughing, and defecation,[6] as well as taste and smell.

The restoration of patients' voices is often a surprising and emotional moment for them and their loved ones. Many times, patients haven't heard their own voices for weeks or months, and the opportunity to vocalize again is a surprise. They frequently don't remember that they can use their voices and will often begin with a whisper. Hearing their own voices speak even a few words can provide great comfort and restore a sense of well-being.

There are several mechanisms to restore speech. All of them require some manipulation of the tracheostomy tube or ventilator circuit, and almost all require cuff deflation.

There also are several factors that must be considered when planning for phonation with a tracheostomy. The first consideration is whether or not the patient requires cuff inflation. Most often, patients require cuff inflation because of the need for positive-pressure ventilation, airway protection, or both. Not all patients who require positive-pressure ventilation also require cuff inflation. The most challenging patient is the one who requires cuff inflation for both airway protection and continuous positive-pressure mechanical ventilation. For these reasons, it is necessary to have a clear understanding of the patient's medical status and treatment plan before attempting to restore speech.

Risk of Aspiration

There are several possible explanations for the risk of aspiration with a tracheostomy tube. The first is decreased elevation and anterior rotation of the larynx because the trachea is anchored to the strap muscles with the inflated cuff. It is also thought that esophageal compression causes the cuff to impinge against the esophageal wall. There is also an attenuation of the reflex of the vocal cords because airflow is redirected away from the upper airway. In addition, there is a reduction in subglottal air pressure.[7]

Leder and Ross[8] examined 20 consecutive patients using a swallow study before and after tracheotomy. They found no causal relationship between tracheostomy and aspiration. All these patients had the same aspiration status before and after the test. The authors concluded that a number of these patients had multiple risk factors other than the presence of the tracheostomy tube that would predispose them to aspirate.

Several studies by speech language pathologists have shown that, contrary to common belief, an inflated cuff actually increases the risk of aspiration by anchoring the trachea to the anterior part of the neck, reducing movement of the larynx, and obstructing the esophagus.[9-13] Amathieu and colleagues[13] found that the swallowing reflex was progressively more difficult to elicit as cuff pressure increased.

REQUIREMENTS FOR SUCCESSFUL PHONATION

Patients must be cognitively intact and attempt to communicate before phonation is initiated. Patients who are able to respond to questions appropriately may be ready to be evaluated for phonation. If a patient is not making some attempt to speak, he or she is probably not ready to do so. In order to achieve adequate voice quality, a patient must be able to generate a tracheal pressure of at least 2 cm H_2O. Normal tracheal pressure is 5–10 cm H_2O during speech, and airflow through the upper airway during speech is 3–18 liters per minute.[14,15,16]

Current methods to restore speech can be divided into three major groups: methods for patients who do not require mechanical ventilation, methods for those who require intermittent mechanical ventilation, and methods for those who require continuous positive-pressure ventilation.

As long as the vocal cords are intact, it is usually relatively easy to restore speech for patients who do not require positive-pressure ventilation. Most often, all that is required is cuff deflation or a cuffless tube and capping or finger occlusion. Let us first discuss the more straightforward approaches to phonation, followed by the more complicated approaches. It may also be helpful to refer to **Figure 6.1** Phonation Algorithm.

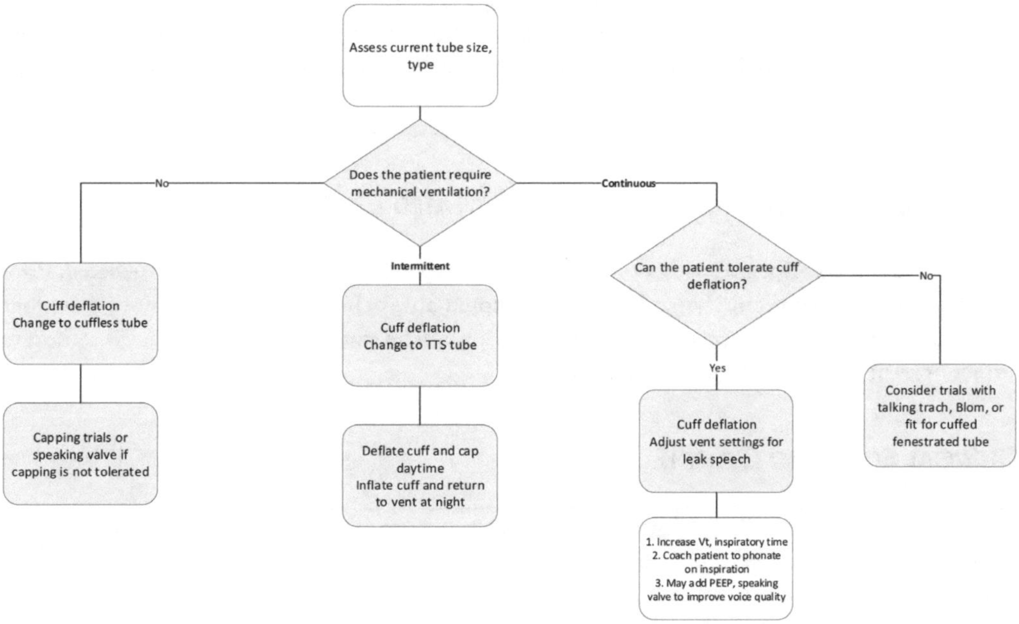

Figure 6.1 Phonation Algorithm

PATIENTS WHO DO NOT REQUIRE MECHANICAL VENTILATION

First, phonation should not be attempted in a patient who is not cognitively aware and making an effort to speak. **Table 6.1** summarizes several methods that will allow speech for patients who do not require mechanical ventilation.

Table 6.1. Methods of Phonation for Patients Who Do Not Require Mechanical Ventilation

Method of Phonation	Special Considerations
Digital occlusion	Requires cuffless or cuffed tube with cuff fully deflated
Capping	Requires cuffless tube or TTS tube
Cuffless fenestrated tube	Requires capping with removal of the standard inner cannula or with fenestrated inner cannula
Speaking valve	Patient must be able to tolerate cuff deflation, preferably cuffless tube; requires sufficient air to pass around outside of the tube
Speak EZ tracheal cannula	Tracheal cannula with built-in speaking valve; low profile, does not require tracheostomy ties; fits only within the stoma

Clinical Scenario

The tracheostomy specialist was contacted to evaluate a patient who had just been liberated from mechanical ventilation. She evaluates the patient and deflates the cuff. The patient appears to tolerate cuff deflation, so she instructs the team to assess the patient for signs of respiratory distress over the next day.

Digital Occlusion (Cuffless Tube or Deflated Cuff)

Digital occlusion is performed with a cuffless tracheostomy tube or with the cuff fully deflated. Prior to cuff deflation, deep oropharyngeal suctioning should always be performed to remove secretions accumulated above the cuff. In addition, cuff deflation can be timed to coincide with exhalation to further prevent secretions from being aspirated.

Clinical Scenario Cont'd.

Since there were no episodes of distress, the tracheostomy specialist returns the following day and changes the tube to a Shiley 6 CFS cuffless tube. She provides digital occlusion over the tube, and the patient is able to breathe comfortably, so the specialist applies a cap to the tracheostomy tube. The patient is able to breathe comfortably and phonate with strong voice quality. The patient is pleased at her ability to communicate her needs with her family and the medical team.

Digital occlusion should never be attempted with the cuff inflated, and ideally, should be done with a cuffless tube. After cuff deflation, the gloved finger of a caregiver or patient is placed over the opening of the tube. This maneuver redirects air to the upper airway and allows it to pass through the vocal cords, thus producing sound. If the tracheostomy tube is too large, resistance to airflow around the tube will prevent comfortable breathing as well as phonation. If the tracheostomy tube is too small, the patient's voice will be breathy, as most of the air will escape through the stoma rather than through the vocal cords.

The biggest safety advantage of digital occlusion is that the patient must be alert and coordinated enough to perform it. Patients who are not alert can quickly develop respiratory distress and be unable to summon help. This problem is magnified when the tracheostomy tube is capped. In order for these patients to speak, an assistant must be present in the patient's room. Patients who are cognitively alert but unable to use their upper extremities may experience frustration with the digital occlusion method if they have a lot to say.

Capping, Corking, and Plugging (Cuffless Tube)

Capping is the process of blocking the opening of the tracheostomy tube with a cap, a cork, or a plug. The nuances of these devices are reviewed in chapter 3, but they are all designed to prevent air from entering and exiting through the tracheostomy tube itself. As a result, some or all of the airflow is redirected around the tube and up to the vocal cords.

Not all patients should be capped. Capping should not be attempted in those who cannot tolerate cuff deflation and who are at risk for aspiration. With the exception of properly fitted fenestrated tubes, *capping should never be applied on a standard cuffed (low-pressure, high-volume) tracheostomy tube, even if the cuff is completely deflated.* If the cuff is deflated and the tube is capped, the patient is forced to breathe around the tracheostomy tube *and* the deflated cuff. The bulk of the deflated cuff adds a great deal of resistance, and it may be difficult or impossible for the patient to ventilate adequately. Additionally, the patient may be unable to effectively clear secretions around the tube and cuff. The patient may complain that when coughing, the secretions seem to "get stuck" in his or her neck. A classic example is a patient with a cuffed tracheostomy tube who had been capped at an outside hospital. She complained that, as much as she tried, she was never able to cough out her secretions. Once her tube was changed to a cuffless version, she immediately coughed out several large mucous plugs and expressed immediate relief from her symptoms. **Figure 6.2** shows the airflow around a capped tracheostomy tube. Note that both inspiration and expiration are around the tube, and that the outer diameter of the tube must be small enough to allow the easy passage of air around it.

Figure 6.2 Airflow around cuffless, capped

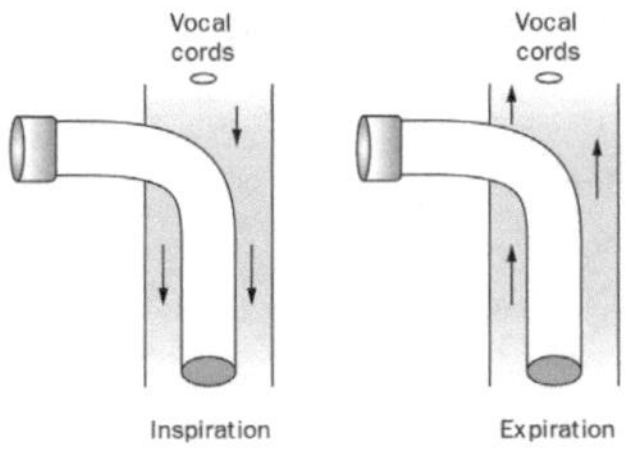

Airflow with cuffless tracheostomy tube, capped. Note both inspiration and expiration are around the outside of the tube.

The Bivona TTS tracheostomy tube is the only exception to the general clinical rule of not capping a cuffed tube. In this case, the TTS cuff functions exactly like cuffless tracheostomy tubes because its cuff essentially disappears when deflated (**Figure 3.32**). The deflated cuff on this tube assumes the shape of the tube around the shaft, creating no additional resistance when moving air around the outside of the tube. (Refer to **Figure 12.5** for an illustration of the inflation and deflation characteristics of high-volume, low-pressure versus low-volume, high-pressure cuffs.)

When capping a tracheostomy tube, it is important to monitor the patient's ability to breathe comfortably around the tube. Often, simply changing the tube to a cuffless version of the same size provides sufficient space to move air. However, if the patient is unable to breathe comfortably, either there is still not enough room to move air around the tube, or there is an obstruction within the airway. In this case, the tube should be downsized. If efforts to phonate are still unsuccessful, use of a speaking valve can be attempted (discussed later in this chapter). However, the patient's airway should be examined for the cause of the obstruction. Chapters 11 and 12 provide a broader discussion of the issues associated with downsizing tracheostomy tubes.

The act of capping a tracheostomy tube not only restores phonation, but it also restores subglottal pressure and improves taste, smell, swallow, cough, and the Valsalva maneuver. Additionally, the quantity of tracheal secretions tends to diminish after the tracheostomy tube has been capped.

CUFFLESS FENESTRATED TRACHEOSTOMY TUBE

Another option for phonation is the use of a fenestrated tracheostomy tube. The fenestrated tube provides an opening on the dorsal aspect of the shaft that should align centrally within the airway. When properly fitted, it provides an additional boost of air up to the vocal cords. (See chapter 4 for a discussion of how to properly fit a fenestrated tracheostomy tube.)

Great care must be taken when using a fenestrated tracheostomy tube. These tubes can have single or dual cannulas. The dual-cannula fenestrated tube usually has both a fenestrated and non-fenestrated inner cannula; the outer cannula is always fenestrated. The fenestrated inner cannula is used when phonation is desired. In this case, air passes around and through the tracheostomy tube. **Figure 6.3** shows airflow through a cuffless fenestrated tracheostomy tube. Note that the resistance of the tube is decreased because air also moves through the fenestration upon inspiration and expiration. When a fenestrated tracheostomy tube is capped, quality of voice improves because all the exhaled air passes through the upper airway as shown in **Figure 6.4**.

Figure 6.3 Airflow with cuffless fenestrated trach

Airflow with cuffless fenestrated tracheostomy tube, uncapped. Note airflow around and through fenestrated tube.

Figure 6.4 Airflow cuffess, fenestrated, capped

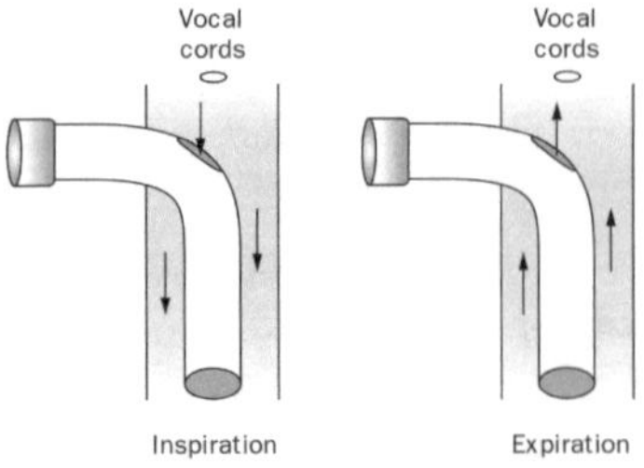

Airflow with cuffless fenestrated tracheostomy tube, capped. Note inspiration and expiration around and through the tube.

When the non-fenestrated inner cannula is used, the fenestration mechanism is lost because air cannot reach the vocal cords. However, the non-fenestrated inner cannula should be used when the patient requires suctioning so that the suction catheter does not get lodged within the fenestration.

To use the fenestrated tracheostomy tube for phonation, one can either keep the fenestrated inner cannula in place, or remove it, so that only the fenestrated outer cannula remains. One of two occlusion methods can be used: digital occlusion or capping. When the fenestrated inner cannula is in place, digital occlusion should initially be used to ensure the patient is able to breathe comfortably. Capping can take place with a regular cap (inner cannula in place; **Figure 3.90**) or decannulation plug (inner cannula removed; **Figures 3.93 and 3.94**). When the cuffless fenestrated tracheostomy tube is occluded, the patient breathes around *and through* the tracheostomy tube. The additional airflow through the fenestration minimizes the obstruction of the tube itself within the airway. The decision about whether or not to cap the fenestrated tracheostomy tube depends on the patient's mental status. Digital occlusion should be reserved for initial and limited vocalization trials in the patient with slightly less than optimal cognitive and respiratory reserve.

When phonation is achieved without the fenestrated inner cannula in place, the inner diameter of the tube is larger, imposing less resistance to airflow and providing easier breathing. Often, 1 or 2 mm enhance the patient's ease of breathing. The inner cannula should only be removed in patients with minimal secretions.

With the fenestrated inner cannula removed, some tracheostomy models cannot be capped in the standard way. For example, the inner cannulas of the Shiley, TRACOE Twist, Blom, and several models of the Fahl tracheostomy tubes provide a 15-mm connector, so a standard cap cannot be applied when the inner cannula is removed. A decannulation plug is made for this purpose. After the removal of the inner cannula, the decannulation plug is attached directly to the hub of the outer cannula to allow continuous occlusion of the opening so that airflow is directed through the fenestration and to the upper and lower airway.

SPEAKING VALVES (CUFFLESS TUBE OR CUFF DEFLATED)

Speaking valves are one-way valves that allow air into the tracheostomy tube but prevent it from being exhaled through the valve. Instead, exhaled air is redirected around the tracheostomy tube and through the upper airway. Ideally, a cuffless tube is used with a speaking valve to minimize untoward events. If using a cuffed tube, a TTS cuff is ideal, but it is essential that the cuff be completely deflated and that air can move easily around the tube. The deflated cuff of a standard low-pressure, high volume tube creates an obstruction itself, so the ability of air to move around it should be tested before a speaking valve is applied. This can be done by digitally occluding the tube and asking the patient to take a few breaths (simulating capping). If the patient is unable to breathe comfortably with this maneuver, the clinician can simulate a speaking valve by allowing the patient to inspire through the tube and occluding it during exhalation. If it is still uncomfortable for the patient to breathe with this maneuver, the clinician should consider downsizing the tracheostomy tube or evaluate the patient for upper airway obstruction.

In order to safely use a speaking valve, the patient should be awake, alert, attempting to communicate, able to tolerate cuff deflation, and medically stable. If the patient is at risk for aspiration, a speaking valve should not be used.[16] **Figure 6.5** shows airflow with a speaking valve and a cuffless tracheostomy tube. Air is inspired through the tube, and the valve closes upon expiration, forcing air through the upper airway. There are several different types of valves available, and they all have slightly different characteristics (**Table 6.2**).

Figure 6.5 Airflow with cuffless tube and speaking valve

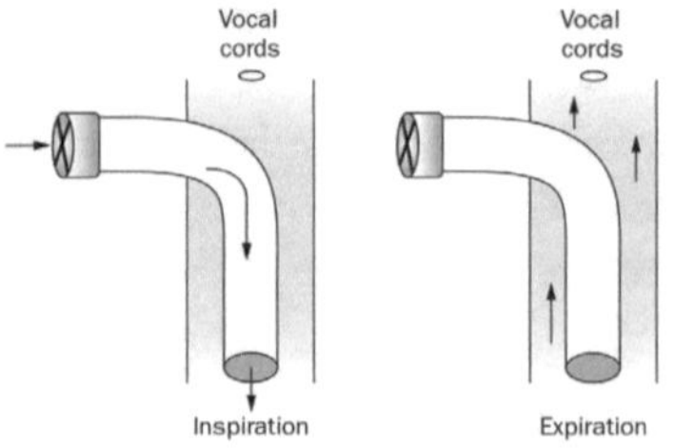

Airflow with cuffless tracheostomy tube and speaking valve. Note inspiration is through the tube, but expiration is around the tube.

Table 6.2. Types of Speaking Valves

Valve	Design	Unique Features
Montgomery Ventrach	Bias open flap valve	For ventilator-dependent patients
Passy Muir	Bias closed flap valve	Several models are available: PMV 005 (white), 2000 (clear); the following can be used within a ventilator circuit: 007 (aqua), and 2001 (purple), with adapter
Shiley Phonate	Bias closed flap valve	Silicone diaphragm with hinged cap; one model has oxygen port
Montgomery speaking valve	Bias closed flap valve	Cough-release feature Removable cover for suctioning
Eliachar speaking valve	Flap valve	For use with Hood stoma stent
TRACOE Phon Assist	Flap valve	Oxygen supply port Adjustable airflow mechanism With twist of housing, patients can "dial-up" desired level of airflow
Shikani	Ball valve	For use with either plastic or metal tubes Less inspiratory effort than others tested
Tucker	Flap valve	Fenestrated flap on inner cannula that opens on inhalation and closes on exhalation
Speak EZ	Flap valve	Tracheal cannula with built-in speaking valve

Early piston-type valves included the Toremalm valve, a flap valve by Emery, an adaptation of a Jackson tube by Cowan, and a two-way valve that could be rotated to allow inspiration only or both inspiration and expiration. When this two-way valve was used for inspiration only, it could also be used as a speaking valve.[17-19] It is unclear whether any of these older valves are still in clinical use.

In 1993, Fornataro-Clerici and Zajac[20] completed a study on the commercially available valves at that time, including those made by Kistner, Montgomery, Olympic, and Passy-Muir. They evaluated each valve's individual aerodynamic characteristics. The internal diaphragm of one-way valves is either in the open position (bias open) or closed position at rest (bias closed). This initial position of the diaphragm may have implications for work of breathing. The Kistner valve, which is no longer manufactured, was bias closed and attached to a metal tracheostomy tube. The Montgomery valve is bias open and has a unique "cough release" feature. This eliminates the possibility of the valve being blown off the tube. When the patient coughs, the diaphragm partially dislodges from the housing and must be pushed back into place. The Olympic valve is also a bias open valve. It is T-shaped and can be used for oxygen delivery. It also has a removable cover that permits suctioning without removal of the valve. The Passy-Muir valve is bias closed in design, which means the valve stays closed except when inspiratory effort is used to open the valve. None of these early valves were designed for use with a patient on a mechanical ventilator.

These valves were tested in a laboratory for their aerodynamic properties at four different flow rates. Resistance was calculated with each valve alone or with the valve attached to a tracheostomy tube. The results showed that the Kistner valve created significantly more resistance at all flow levels than the other valves available at that time. Since then, several new valves have been developed, and others have been redesigned. Zajac, Fornataro-Clerici, and Roop[21] updated their previous study with six valves on the market in 1999—the Montgomery speaking valve, the Olympic Trach Talk, the Shiley Phonate Speaking valve, the Montgomery Ventrach and the Passy-Muir PMV™ 007 (aqua) and PMV™ 2001 (purple), as seen in **Figure 6.6**.

Figure 6.6 Passy-Muir Valves

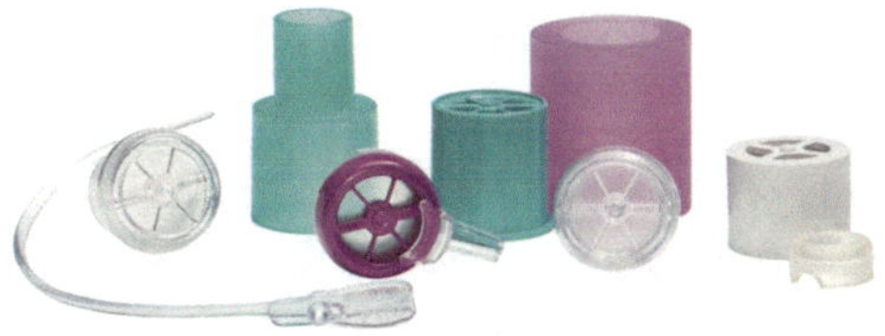

Passy Muir valves from left to right, PMV 2000 (clear), PMV 2001 (purple), PMV 007 (aqua), PMV 2000 (clear), PMV 005 (white)

Image courtesy of Passy-Muir, Inc., Irvine, CA

The new Montgomery speaking valve has a bias-closed diaphragm—a change in design from its previous configuration. It was designed for use with the Montgomery cannula and comes in compatible sizes. The Shiley Phonate speaking valve (**Figure 6.7**) is bias-closed with a silicone diaphragm. It has a hinged cap that makes the diaphragm available for cleaning. One model has a port to attach to an oxygen source. However, this model was not included in the study. The Montgomery Ventrach has a bias-open silicone diaphragm and can be used with ventilator-dependent patients. The Passy-Muir PMV™ 005 (white), PMV™ 007 (aqua), PMV™ 2000 (clear), and PMV™ 2001 (purple) can also be used for ventilator-dependent patients. The PMV™ 007 can be used within the ventilator circuit, but the others require an adapter. All the Passy-Muir valves are bias closed.[21] The PMV™ 2020, a modified version of the PMV™ 2000, was designed for use with metal tracheostomy tubes without 15-mm adapters (Passy-Muir product information, www.passy-muir.com/valves).

Figure 6.7 Shiley Phonate speaking valve with oxygen port

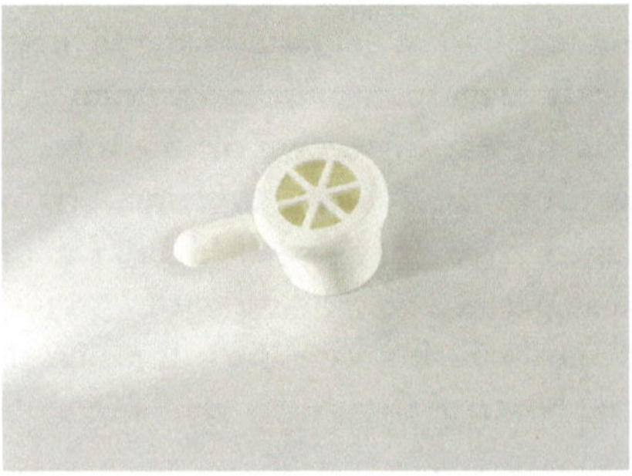

Each of these valves was tested using different flow rates. The flow rates in the 1999 study were higher than in the earlier work because they were associated with patients on mechanical ventilation. Except for minor differences, all the valves exhibited similar low resistance—even those with a bias-closed design. There were some differences in manufacturing specifications between the 1993 and 1999 studies. The researchers measured the thickness of the PMV™ 007 and found a thinner diaphragm than in the earlier study. This could explain the finding of reduced resistance, but they were unable to confirm a design change with the company.[21]

These six valves were also tested in vivo with the use of a mouthpiece; patients repeated the sound */pa/,* and the researchers tested for leakage of air through the valve. They found that both the Olympic Trach Talk and the Montgomery Ventrach showed significant air loss during expiration when the valves should have been closed.[21]

The Eliachar speaking valve (**Figure 6.8**) is made of silicone and is designed for use with the Hood stoma stent. It has a low-profile appearance and flap design that provide low resistance. The Hood speaking valve and the TRACOE Phon Assist (**Figure 6.9**) are both flap valves. The Phon Assist has an oxygen supply port, but its most unique feature is an adjustable airflow mechanism that patients can use to dial up their desired level of airflow.

Figure 6.8 Eliachar speaking valve

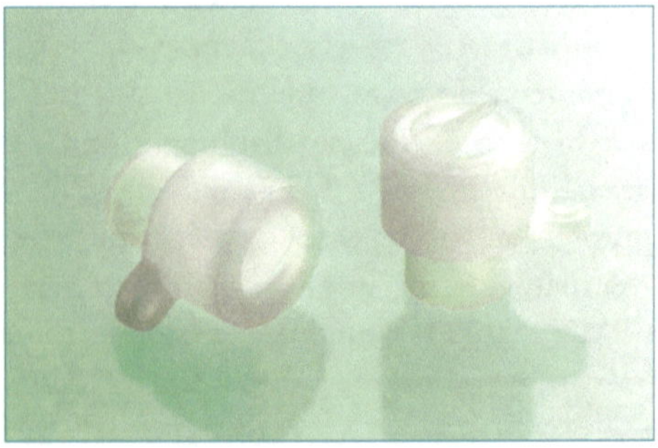

Hood Labs, (Pembroke, Massachusetts)

Figure 6.9 TRACOE speaking valve

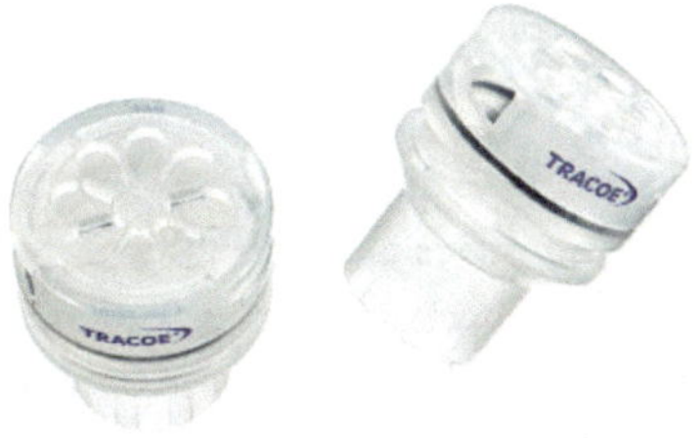

TRACOE Phon Assist

Courtesy of TRACOE medical GmbH, Germany. All rights reserved

The Speak-EZ tracheal cannula (**Figure 6.10**) is a unique stoma maintenance device with a built-in flap valve on the proximal end. It is made of soft silicone and may be an option for patients who wish to speak, but who cannot tolerate capping because of obstruction or resistance to airflow.

Figure 6.10 Speak-EZ

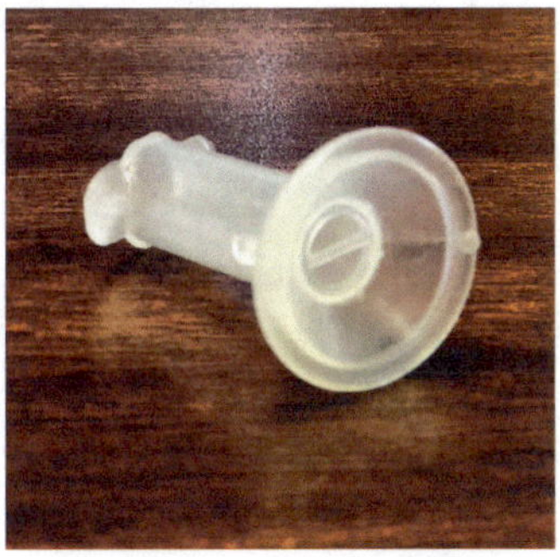

Speak-EZ tracheal cannula

Photo courtesy of Technical Products Inc of Georgia, Lawrenceville, Georgia (www.tpi-ga.com).

The Shikani valve uses a different mechanism than the other diaphragm valves—a unidirectional flow ball valve. It has lower resistance, a lower profile, and is more easily hidden under clothing than the other valves.[22] Originally called the Hopkins valve, the Shikani valve has been adapted for use with plastic as well as metal tracheostomy tubes. In the resting state, the ball lies on the wall of the air chamber (A). Upon inspiration, the ball moves toward the opening of the cannula, allowing air to enter the cannula (B). Airflow pushes the ball back, but it is prevented from entering the cannula by a wire stop. On expiration (C), the ball seals the port, forcing air into the upper airway. Because of this design, less pressure is required for valve closure, which is almost instantaneous. This is especially important in patients with very low tidal volumes and vital capacities. The valve is more compact than the other valves and can be used in the standard versions of all commercially available tracheostomy tubes. The valve can also replace the inner cannulas of these tubes and provide lower resistance.[22]

One study compared the Shikani ball valve (named Hopkins at the time of the study) with the Passy-Muir valve and found less inspiratory resistance and easier cleaning with the ball valve.[19]

The Tucker valve uses a different mechanism. The Tucker tracheostomy tube is composed of metal with a fenestrated flap on the inner cannula that opens upon inhalation and closes upon exhalation. This action forces air up through the upper airway.[19] Airflow during inspiration rotates the flap to an open position and then to a closed position during expiration.[23]

The Clinical Use of Speaking Valves

With the exception of the Tucker valve and the Speak-EZ, speaking valves are externally placed on the 15-mm or low-profile connector of a cuffless or deflated-cuff tracheostomy tube. Patients and their caregivers require education to effectively use the valve and to alleviate any anxiety about shortness of breath. They also need to know how to remove the valve in the event of acute dyspnea. Patients should not be left unsupervised with the valve in place until their ability to tolerate it has been established.[19]

Initially, a schedule for using the speaking valve should be structured to target continuous wearing during daytime hours. The manufacturer recommends that the Passy-Muir valve not be used while sleeping. However, two studies have confirmed its safety during sleep. Gross and colleagues[24] established the overnight usefulness in seriously ill tracheostomy patients without any untoward effects such as apnea, desaturation, respiratory distress, or cardiac arrhythmias. Accordingly, they recommended testing these valves for longer night duration.[24] Barrazza and others[25] studied nine children overnight and found no major events and no significant variations between the baseline night (without the valve) and the study night (with the valve). They recommended that the speaking valve might be safely used during sleep in children.

Studies have shown that speaking valves provide more benefits than merely verbal communication. Lichtman and colleagues[26] studied the potential secondary benefits of speaking valves. They found that patients had significantly fewer secretions with speaking valves than without. Other reported benefits included more effective swallowing, more effective coughing, a restoration of intrinsic PEEP, an enhanced Valsalva maneuver, and the prevention of aspiration.

Several studies have specifically examined the effect of speaking valves on aspiration. Dettelbach, Gross, Mahlmann, and Eibling[27] studied 11 patients with tracheostomies and clinical evidence of aspiration. They found that aspiration was reduced or eliminated in all patients when a speaking valve was in place. Suiter and others[7] studied swallow physiology as well as the incidence of aspiration with tracheostomized non-ventilator-dependent patients under three different conditions: cuff inflated, cuff deflated/cuffless tube, and with a Passy-Muir speaking valve. They found that cuff deflation significantly improved swallowing ability by increasing both pharyngeal transit duration as well as duration of hyoid excursion. In addition, they found that cuff status had no effect on aspiration. However, there was significantly less incidence of aspiration with the speaking valve when compared to the cuff-inflation and cuff-deflation conditions. Eight out of 10 patients who aspirated thin liquids with cuff inflation or deflation were able to safely take liquids with the valve in place. The authors concluded that the speaking valve might restore the subglottal air pressure lost with the use of a tracheostomy tube and that patients who are unable to tolerate thin liquids may be able to ingest them safely with the valve in place.

Elpern and co-investigators[28] also studied the effect of the Passy-Muir valve on aspiration and obtained different results. In their study of 15 patients with tracheostomies and evidence of aspiration, seven patients aspirated thin liquids, five patients aspirated only when the valve was not used, and two patients aspirated with and without the valve. They found that aspiration was less frequent with the valve in place and concluded that a speaking valve can reduce, but not eliminate, aspiration in patients with a tracheostomy.

Manzano and colleagues[29] found that the use of a speaking valve decreased the amount of secretions, improved the ability to cough, reduced the need for tracheal suctioning, and improved the sense of smell in patients. Although they did not specifically study patient mood, they also found that patients appeared to be happier and interacted better with their families and nursing staff.

One more recent study[30] compared the ball valve (Shikani) to the Passy-Muir and Shiley valves on olfaction, speech, and oxygenation. They found that the ball valve was significantly superior to the others in terms of olfaction, voice or pitch tests, speech naturalness, and several other speech parameters. Results showed no difference in oxygen saturation among the three valves. Eight of the 10 patients tested preferred the ball valve, and two preferred the Passy-Muir valve. Six subjects reported that the most important characteristic of a speaking valve is its low profile, and four reported that ease of breathing was the most important characteristic.

Prigent and colleagues[31] studied the effect of a speaking valve on the interaction of breathing and swallowing. They found that synchronization of breathing and swallowing were not influenced by use of the speaking valve. Thus, they recommended that a speaking valve should be routinely offered during periods off mechanical ventilation to facilitate expiration through the upper airway after swallowing and to decrease the risk of laryngeal penetration of solids or fluids leading to aspiration.

Contraindications for Speaking Valves

While speaking valves provide many benefits in addition to speech, not all patients can tolerate them. Patients with poor pulmonary reserves can develop hypercarbia. Because some degree of air trapping can occur with speaking valves, patients with severe lung disease may not be able to fully exhale.[6] The contraindications for the use of a speaking valve are listed as follows:

- Inability to tolerate cuff deflation (risk of aspiration)
- Hemodynamic instability
- Severe pulmonary disease
- Total laryngectomy
- Vocal cord paralysis

Patients Who Require Intermittent Positive-Pressure Ventilation

It is clear that patients who require continuous positive-pressure ventilation need a cuffed tube. However, patients who use intermittent ventilation require cuff inflation only during that time. Intermittent positive-pressure ventilation is applied to patients during weaning from mechanical ventilation, for nocturnal ventilation, and for bronchial hygiene. As patients are weaned from continuous mechanical ventilation, they spend increasing amounts of time free from the ventilator, at which time the cuff can be deflated. During the weaning process, altering the tracheostomy tube can accommodate the patient's changing goals. **Table 6.3** summarizes methods of phonation for patients who require intermittent mechanical ventilation.

Table 6.3. Methods of Phonation for Patients Who Require Intermittent Mechanical Ventilation

Method of Phonation	Special Considerations
Digital occlusion	• Can be done on cuffed tube with cuff down only
Capping trials when not on ventilator	• Tight to shaft (TTS) tube is the ideal choice for a patient who requires intermittent cuff inflation
Leak speech	• Requires cuff deflation • Procedure involves increasing tidal volume and adjusting to comfortable ventilation and optimal voice quality • Procedure increases inspiratory time • The addition of PEEP may improve voice quality and increase duration of speech time • Ventilator alarms must be adjusted because exhaled volume is lost through the upper airway
Leak speech with speaking valve	• Requires cuff deflation • Procedure involves increasing tidal volume and adjusting to comfortable ventilation and optimal voice quality • Procedure increases inspiratory time • The addition of PEEP may improve voice quality and increase duration of speech time • Ventilator alarms must be adjusted because exhaled volume is lost through the upper airway • The addition of a speaking valve may improve swallowing and decrease secretions • HME is ineffective with the valve
Fenestrated cuffed tracheostomy tube	• Cuff can remain inflated • Requires proper fit of fenestration • Requires adjustment of ventilator settings and alarms because exhaled volume is lost through the upper airway • Subcutaneous emphysema can occur if using a fenestrated tube through an immature stoma
Speaking tracheostomy tube	• Cuff can remain inflated • Involves adjusting gas flow of 2-10 liters per minute for optimal voice quality • Requires patient or caregiver assistance to occlude port for phonation • Subcutaneous emphysema can occur if using a speaking tracheostomy tube in an immature stoma
Blom tracheostomy tube	• Cuff can remain inflated • Upon inhalation, air is delivered to the lungs through the flap valve. Upon exhalation, air passes through the bubble valve and fenestration • The exhaled volume reservoir helps prevent ventilator alarms from sounding due to lost returned volume through the upper airway

When patients do not require continuous cuff inflation, it is usually relatively easy to restore phonation when they are free from ventilator support. This can be done by simply deflating the cuff and occluding the tube to allow air up to the vocal cords, while assessing for the adequate movement of air around the deflated cuff. However, cuffed tubes should never be capped. Thus, these patients will require a different type of tracheostomy tube.

The Bivona TTS tube can be the ideal choice to accommodate a patient who requires intermittent cuff inflation. In contrast to standard low-pressure, high-volume cuffs, these tubes have low-volume, high-pressure cuffs. When inflated, they can exert high pressures against the tracheal wall, so careful attention to minimizing cuff pressure should guide practice. The significant advantage of this type of tube is its deflation characteristics, which allow it to lie flush against the shaft of the tube when deflated, creating no obstruction to airflow around the tube (**Figure 6.11**). When deflated, the TTS tube functions as a cuffless tube, and is the only cuffed tube currently on the market that can be capped safely.

Figure 6.11 Inflation & Deflation Characteristics

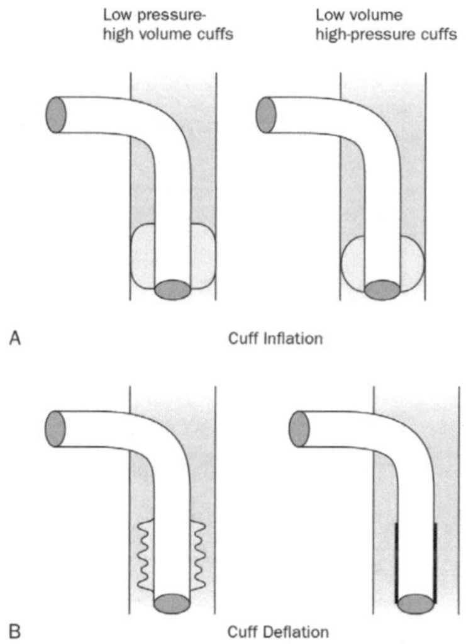

Inflation and deflation characteristics of high-volume, low-pressure cuffs compared to low-volume, high-pressure cuffs. (A) During cuff inflation, high-volume, low-pressure cuffs distribute pressure over larger surface area. With low-volume, high-pressure cuffs, pressure is concentrated into a very small surface area. (B) During cuff deflation, the folds of the deflated high-volume, low-pressure cuff occupy a large surface area and create resistance to airflow around the outside of the tracheostomy tube. In contrast, the deflated low-volume, high-pressure cuff lies snugly along the shaft of the tube, creating no resistance to airflow around the outside of the tube.

A TTS tube can be capped while the patient is free from the ventilator, and the cuff can be inflated when returning to the ventilator. This technique often speeds up the weaning process and frequently marks the beginning of freedom from the ventilator.

When inflating the cuff of the TTS tube, the clinician must take care to ensure minimal pressure in the cuff. Because of the inflation characteristics of the high-pressure cuff, direct cuff pressure measurement will result in a high reading; thus, the minimal leak technique is recommended. In order to distribute pressure evenly and prevent a loss of cuff volume from the diffusion of gas, the cuff should be inflated with sterile water (not saline).

A TTS tube is also ideal for patients who require intermittent cuff inflation because of bronchial hygiene or administration of inhaled medications. The cuff can be inflated during these maneuvers and deflated after completion.

In addition to concerns with the high-pressure cuff, the primary disadvantage of the TTS tube is that it is a single-cannula tube. Patients who have large volumes of thick secretions may be at particular risk for tube obstruction because these tubes lack an inner cannula. In this case, measures should be taken to ensure optimal mobilization of secretions, or it may be necessary to change to a tube with an inner cannula.

PATIENTS WHO REQUIRE CONTINUOUS MECHANICAL VENTILATION

Unless there are extenuating circumstances, phonation should not be attempted in patients who are hemodynamically unstable and on mechanical ventilation. In most cases, it is best to wait until patients are more stable and can tolerate cuff deflation because most options for phonation require cuff deflation or tube change. **Table 6.4** summarizes phonation options for those patients who require continuous mechanical ventilation.[32]

Table 6.4. Methods of Phonation for Those who Require Continuous Mechanical Ventilation

Technique	Pro	Con	Special Considerations
Leak speech	Allows speech despite the need for continuous mechanical ventilation.	Patient must be coached to speak on inspiration. Requires patience and practice.	Used only in patients who can tolerate cuff deflation. Ventilator settings are adjusted to compensate for air loss.
Talking tracheostomy tube	Used for patients who cannot tolerate cuff deflation.	Depends on manual occlusion of the port by patient or caregiver. Airflow line can become clogged. Discomfort and drying of mucous membranes with higher air flows.	Extra air port above the cuff. Remove pooled secretions above the cuff to improve voice and maintain patent airway. Increase airflow to allow phonation. May also connect to suction to allow phonation with retrograde airflow.
Cuffed fenestrated tracheostomy tube	Allows air to travel through fenestration and above the cuff, decreasing resistance caused by the tube itself.	Risk for aspiration. Fenestration must fit precisely in the center of the airway, or granulation may result.	Volumes may need to be adjusted to accommodate the exhaled volume lost through the upper airway. Fit requires evaluation by a tracheostomy specialist.
Blom tracheostomy tube system	Fenestration is located just above the cuff to minimize risk of granulation.	Requires additional training for proper use of the tube.	System uses a speech cannula with two valves: flap valve and bubble valve. Exhaled volume reservoir can minimize low exhaled volume alarms.

There is competition between airflow requirements for speech and gas exchange in the ventilator-dependent tracheostomy patient.[33] Normally, people speak during expiration using air that has already been used for gas exchange. Competition occurs when patients "steal" air from alveolar ventilation during the inhalation phase, producing sound by diverting air around the tracheostomy tube and up to the larynx. Speech during inhalation produces relative hypoventilation.

Shea and others[33] asked five patients with long-term tracheostomies to perform two speaking tasks. The patients read a standard text and spoke extemporaneously while the investigators measured speech ventilation volumes. All the subjects had either a fenestrated tracheostomy tube or a deflated cuff. They performed both tasks under normal conditions with 100% oxygen and under experimentally induced hypercapnic conditions using a mixture of carbon dioxide and oxygen. Normal individuals at rest will hyperventilate during speaking. The investigators noted an average loss of 14% of alveolar ventilation when speaking. During induced hypercapnia, which caused shortness of breath, all the subjects could still speak adequately. Two patients adapted to hypercapnia by reducing the amount of air used for speaking. One patient increased the airflow used per syllable during hypercapnic speech, which is a maladaptive strategy. The investigators concluded that there is complete antagonism between the airflow requirements for speaking and gas exchange during the ventilator's inspiratory phase. In their experiment, the behavioral drive to speak was modified but never fully suppressed by increasing respiratory drive.

Leak Speech (Cuff Deflated)

Clinical Scenario Cont'd.

> Patient C has been on continuous mechanical ventilation in the critical care unit after a devastating injury and currently has a Shiley 8 LPC tracheostomy tube in place. After several weeks in the ICU, she is now alert most of the time, but is unable to effectively communicate her needs. After a great deal of frustration on the part of both the patient and the care team, the tracheostomy specialist is contacted for assistance.

Leak speech involves creating a leak in the seal between the cuff and the trachea so some air can be diverted up to the vocal cords. The ventilator provides the power behind the voice, and ventilator settings are adjusted to accommodate the leak. Leak speech is possible only when the patient uses a deflated cuff, a cuffless tube, or a fenestrated tracheostomy tube.[34] In addition, leak speech is possible only when airflow is sufficient to generate adequate subglottal pressure. This pressure is usually limited to the inspiratory cycle and the beginning of the expiratory cycle. For this reason, leak speech is characterized by bursts of short phrases and long pauses.[1,3,4,5]

Clinical Scenario Cont'd.

> The tracheostomy specialist understands that the patient still requires full ventilator support. She calls the respiratory therapist and the speech pathologist to evaluate the patient together. They discuss the need for the cuff and are not sure whether the patient can tolerate cuff deflation. After deep subglottic suctioning, the cuff is deflated. The specialist cautions the patient that she may hear and feel a large air leak and ventilator alarms, but this is normal. A large leak is heard around the tube, and returned volumes fall.

Leak speech is beneficial because it improves patient quality of life by restoring communication, and the required cuff deflation reduces pressure against the trachea. However, it also involves trial and error until the optimal settings are achieved. Optimal leak speech requires ventilator adjustments to produce the best voice quality without discomfort or shortness of breath.

Clinical Scenario Cont'd.

The tracheostomy specialist instructs the respiratory therapist to increase tidal volumes by 50% and increase inspiratory time. Meanwhile, she coaches the patient to use her voice whenever the ventilator delivers a breath. Vital signs are monitored and ventilator settings are frequently adjusted during this initial trial for optimal speech and patient comfort. The speech pathologist instructs the patient to tighten the back of her throat to lessen air loss. The patient is able to make herself understood after several tries, although voice quality is weak.

Inspiratory speech is something of a paradox because normal speech commences during expiration. Competition of tidal volume use between speech and ventilation varies with glottic resistance, which can be consciously controlled by the patient. When the glottis is narrowed, more tidal volume is delivered to the lungs; when there is little laryngeal resistance, less tidal volume is delivered to the lungs.[19]

Typically, the first step toward leak speech is to assess the size of the tracheostomy tube with the cuff deflated. One must ensure the patient can move enough air comfortably around the deflated cuff. If the patient is unable to move enough air, it may be necessary to downsize the tracheostomy tube. Following cuff deflation, the tidal volume should be increased up to 50% more than for resting ventilation, and the inspiratory time can also be increased to permit comfortable and longer speech. During initial trials, the patient will require some coaching to speak on inspiration when the ventilator breath is delivered. Inspiratory speech often requires some practice because it is the opposite of normal speech.

Some patients report anxiety or discomfort with leak speech because of the flow of air through the upper airway; this is especially common in those who have not experienced this sensation for a long time. Anxiety is often resolved by coaching the patient to time their voicing with inspiration. It may also help to instruct patients to push down, hold their breath, or tighten their throat. Patients can be taught to widen or narrow their glottic aperture in order to increase or decrease the volume delivered to the lungs.[19]

If patients become breathless during a leak speech trial, tidal volume or inspiratory flow rate can be increased. Another strategy is to add PEEP. The addition of PEEP has several advantages, including lengthening the duration of tracheal pressure into the exhalation phase for voicing. Adding PEEP can allow patients to speak through 80% of the respiratory cycle.[1,16,33-36] The addition of 4–15 cm H_2O of PEEP can extend speech duration, produce higher quality speech, and allow more syllables per ventilator cycle. Patients using leak speech with PEEP have been observed to speak through the entire ventilator cycle without any pauses for breathing.[16]

Garguilo and colleagues[37] studied the effectiveness of patient-controlled delivery of PEEP to improve voice quality and ensure optimal respiratory comfort. They found that text reading time, phonation flow, use of the respiratory cycle for phonation and speech comfort significantly improved with increasing PEEP. They recommended that patient-controlled PEEP could be added to home ventilators to improve speech and patient autonomy.

Clinical Scenario Cont'd.

The patient has tolerated several short sessions of leak speech without changes in vital signs. Because the patient has reported episodes of shortness of breath, a speaking valve is added, and her voice becomes stronger.

Leak Speech with a Speaking Valve

Leak speech can also be used with a speaking valve rather than PEEP. Only three speaking valves are approved by the FDA for use with ventilator-dependent patients—the Montgomery Ventrach and Passy-Muir models PMV™ 005 and PMV™ 007.[34]

Speaking valves allow the ventilator to deliver a breath through the tracheostomy tube while the exhaled air is redirected around the tube—and so, it is essential that the cuff be completely deflated. Manzano and others[29] used the Passy-Muir valve in their series of ventilator-dependent patients to determine its usefulness, advantages, and disadvantages during mechanical ventilation. Because cuff deflation is vital to the use of the speaking valve, they recommended that a cuffless tracheostomy tube be used while the valve is in place. The presence of a deflated cuff makes aspiration possible, and because of this, it is necessary to closely monitor tidal volume, peak inspiratory pressure, thoracic movements, the elimination of secretions, and continuous airflow through the mouth and nose. **Figure 6.12** shows the placement of the valve within the ventilator circuit.

Figure 6.12 Placement of speaking valve in circuit of ventilator

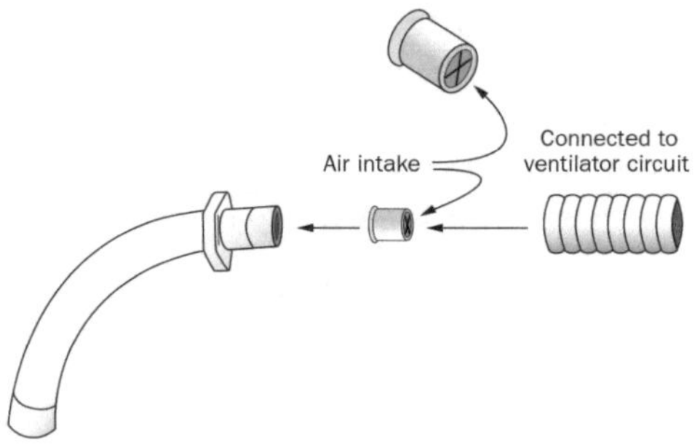

Proper placement of speaking valve within ventilator circuit. Valve is positioned between the tracheostomy tube and ventilator circuit to allow intake of air into the tube.

The speaking valve can be applied one of two ways. For patients with a closed suction system, the valve should be applied to the side port to allow the suction catheter to pass easily into the tracheostomy tube.[16] For patients who are not using a closed suction system, the valve can be applied directly between the ventilator circuit and the 15-mm connector. An HME is not functional with a speaking valve because no exhaled gas will pass through it when it is in place. Some patients report discomfort when initially using a speaking valve due to drying of the pharyngeal membranes or decreased tone from weakness and lack of airflow through the upper airway. This effect can be mitigated by slow cuff deflation over several minutes.[16]

In a study of 15 ventilator-dependent patients, Passy and colleagues[38] found that all the subjects using the Passy-Muir valve showed marked improvement in speech intelligibility, speech flow, elimination of speech hesitancy, and speech time. MacBean and colleagues[33] studied the use of leak speech in two patients with cervical spinal cord injuries. They found that the use of PEEP in addition to a speaking valve provided the best quality speech.

Figure 6.13 shows airflow when a speaking valve is used with a ventilator. With a speaking valve, air will be redirected through the upper airway upon exhalation and not returned to the ventilator. Therefore, the exhaled tidal volume alarm must be adjusted accordingly. In addition, the tidal volume and high-pressure alarms must be carefully monitored to avoid excessive air trapping.[6]

Figure 6.13 Airflow with valve and ventilator circuit

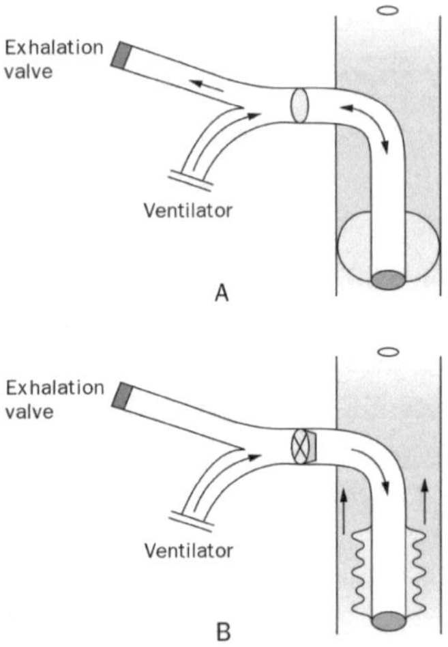

Airflow with valve and ventilator circuit. A) Normal ventilator circuit. Note inflation of the cuff with inflow of air from the ventilator, and exhaled air through exhalation valve. B) Ventilator circuit with speaking valve. Note deflation of the cuff, with all exhaled air passing through the upper airway and bypassing the ventilator.

Most ventilators will not easily tolerate a speaking valve.[16] The Respironics Esprit and the Respironics V200 ventilators have speaking modes in which the exhalation valve is closed, allowing gas flow past the vocal cords. In speaking modes, exhaled gas pressure is measured to evaluate whether the tube has become disconnected or obstructed. However, these ventilators are no longer manufactured. A new model of Trilogy ventilator is currently being developed with a speaking valve mode.

Cuffed Fenestrated Tracheostomy Tube (Cuff Inflated))

Patients who are ventilator dependent will usually require a cuffed tracheostomy tube. In order for these patients to phonate, one option is a cuffed fenestrated tracheostomy tube. The proper fit of the fenestration within the airway is vital for the proper functioning of the tube as well as preventing complications such as granulation tissue. See chapter 4 for a discussion of the proper fitting of a fenestrated tracheostomy tube.

Figure 6.14 shows airflow through fenestrated tracheostomy tubes. View A shows inspiration and expiration through a cuffless fenestrated tracheostomy tube. Air moves through the upper airway and through the tube. In View B, when the cuff is inflated on a cuffed fenestrated tube, inspiration and expiration occur primarily through the tube. However, a small amount of air moves through the upper airway. In View C, the cuff is deflated on a cuffed fenestrated tube. Inspiration is primarily through the tube, but a small amount of air is also inspired though the upper airway. On exhalation, air must pass around the deflated cuff and through the fenestration to reach the upper airway.

Figure 6.14 Airflow in 3 types of fenestrated trachs

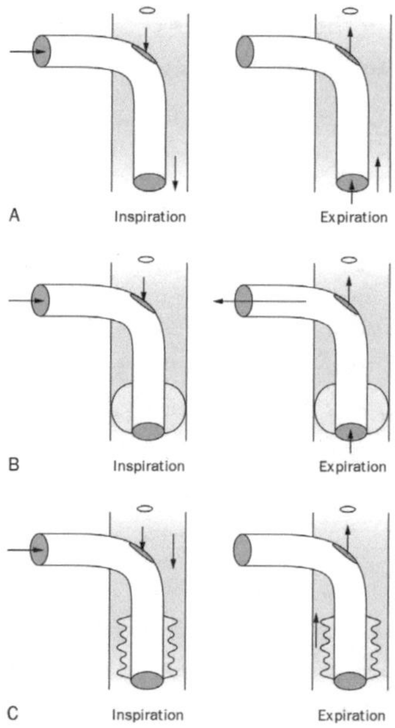

Airflow of fenestrated tracheostomy tubes on inspiration and expiration.

A) Cuffless fenestrated tracheostomy tube. Note inspiration around and through tube and expiration around and through the tube, with boost of air up to the vocal cords.

B) Cuffed fenestrated tracheostomy tube with cuff inflated. Note inspiration and expiration through (but not around) the tube. A small amount of air is directed to the vocal cords on expiration.

C) Cuffed fenestrated tracheostomy tube with cuff deflated. Note inspiration is through the tube and around the deflated cuff. A small amount of air is directed to the vocal cords on expiration.

Several authors have reported cases of subcutaneous emphysema with the use of fenestrated tracheostomy tubes.[39,40] Orme and Welham[40] reported a case of massive subcutaneous emphysema shortly after the percutaneous placement of a fenestrated tracheostomy tube. Later, these clinicians were directed to the manufacturer's instructions, which stated that a fenestrated tube should not be used in the early postoperative period, and that the position of the fenestration should be checked once placed. Prior to the maturation of the stoma, air can become displaced into the pre-tracheal tissues with the use of a fenestrated tube.

Talking Tracheostomy Tube (Cuff Inflated)

A talking tracheostomy is a tube that allows a ventilator-dependent patient to speak; unlike other methods, it does not require cuff deflation. Now known as above the cuff vocalization (ACV), the talking tracheostomy tube was designed for the ventilator-dependent patient who is at high risk for aspiration or cannot otherwise tolerate cuff deflation. An additional air supply line provides an extra source of air independent of ventilation. This supply line carries air from a regulated compressed source and terminates with an opening just above the cuff. When connected to a source of compressed air or oxygen, occlusion of the air control port allows gas flow to be directed to the vocal cords. **Figure 6.15** shows airflow with a talking tracheostomy tube.

Figure 6.15 Talking Trach

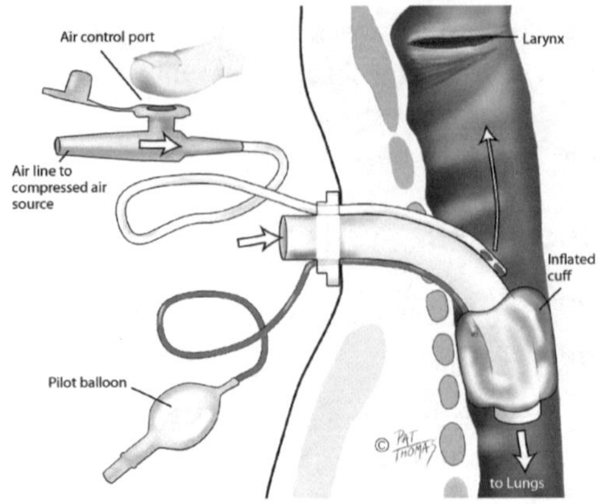

Airflow with talking tracheostomy tube. Note that a talking tracheostomy tube has a separate air supply line that terminates above the cuff. Phonation can be produced by manually occluding the air control port, directing air to the vocal cords.

© *Pat Thomas, CMI 2013*

For optimal use of the talking tracheostomy, airflow must be adjusted. Starting at 4 liters per minute, the flow can be increased up to 12–15 liters per minute until optimum voice quality is reached. However, high flow rates could be associated with a greater risk of airway injury.[16] At these high flow rates, humidification is important to prevent drying of laryngeal tissues.[6] Because of the continuous independent flow of air, talking tracheostomy tubes allow speech throughout the entire respiratory cycle.[23]

Tippet and Vogelman[19] suggested that the adjustment of airflow is a delicate balance between patient comfort and clarity of speech. A flow rate between 2–15 liters per minute is compatible with speech. A rate of 5 liters per minute is necessary to produce a whisper, and 8–10 liters per minute is necessary for speech with normal volume. Flow rates above 10 liters per minute have been reported to be uncomfortable and may necessitate warming and humidifying the airflow to make it more comfortable and reduce the drying effect. McGrath and colleagues[41] reported that laryngeal airflow used with above the cuff ventilation revived vocal fold vibration producing voice, and it also appeared to improve glottic closure reflexes.

In another study, McGrath and colleagues[42] investigated the use of retrograde gas flow via the suction port and its effect on phonation. They studied 10 patients with a Blue Line Ultra Suctionaid tracheostomy tube, using retrograde gas flow via the suction port. They found that eight of 10 patients achieved audible voice using this method.

Talking tracheostomy tubes have some disadvantages. Speaking is dependent on a caregiver and a source of compressed gas. The air supply line frequently becomes clogged with secretions and prevents airflow above the cuff. In this case, it is acceptable to flush the air supply line with 5 ml of sterile water.[43] A source of suction should be provided to remove the secretions from above the cuff. The accumulation of secretions is a persistent complication of speaking tracheostomy tubes, and deep subglottic suctioning above the cuff may be necessary before beginning speaking trials.[19]

The production of speech with talking tracheostomy tubes requires some trial and error in order to produce optimal voice quality. Patients need time to adjust to the new sensation of airflow and practice occlusion of the airflow port. Theoretically, patients can speak throughout the entire respiratory cycle with this tube, but Leder and Tranquina[44] reported that some patients have difficulty speaking through inspiration because it feels unnatural. They recommended that tube occlusion be timed for the expiratory phase of the ventilator.

Some difficulty has been reported with positioning the tube so its openings are unobstructed. Positioning is also an issue because of the weight of the ventilator circuit, which can pull the tube down and away from the stoma, resulting in an air leak. The weight of the ventilator circuit can also cause the rotation of the tube and the blockage of air vents coming into contact with the tracheal wall.[19] A malpositioned tube leaks air around the stoma and makes loud gurgling sounds. In addition, voice quality with this type of tracheostomy tube may not reach more than a whisper.[16,43] For these reasons, the use of talking tracheostomy tubes with rehabilitation patients may be limited.[23]

The speaking tracheostomy tube has also been used to provide continuous suction above the cuff in patients at risk for aspiration from a large amount of oropharyngeal secretions. When connected to suction, the removal of up to 600 ml of secretions per day has been reported.[43]

A waiting period of 3-5 days is recommended after the initial tracheotomy procedure before using a talking tracheostomy tube. The waiting period allows the tract to heal and prevents air leaks through the fresh tissue planes, which could lead to subcutaneous or mediastinal emphysema.[19]

Nomori[45] developed a prototype talking tracheostomy tube with a different mechanism. The tube has slits along the sides of the shaft with an elastic cuff and inflates and deflates in synchrony with respirations. In the initial trial with 16 patients, all patients except one were able to vocalize. One of the most notable factors from this initial clinical trial is that there were no complications from this tracheostomy tube. It never became occluded with secretions, and no cuff problems developed. Unfortunately, however, the tube has not been approved for use.

Blom Tracheostomy Tube System

The Blom tracheostomy tube system has a unique design and comes in four sizes: 4, 6, 8, and 10. The fenestrated aperture on the outer cannula is located only 1 mm above the cuff. This unique placement is intended to prevent contact with the tracheal mucosa when the cuff is inflated. It has a subglottic suctioning port to reduce the incidence of ventilator-associated pneumonia when connected to continuous suction.

In addition to a standard inner cannula and a subglottic suctioning cannula, the Blom tracheostomy tube system (**Figure 6.16**) also has two additional cannulas that can provide speech. The speech cannula is designed to allow speech to those patients who require a fully inflated cuff, while the low-profile cannula is designed for use with patients who can tolerate cuff deflation. The speech cannula is soft and floppy, fits within the outer cannula, and has two unique valves—a flap valve and a bubble valve—that function at different parts of the respiratory cycle.

Figure 6.16 Blom Tracheostomy Tube System

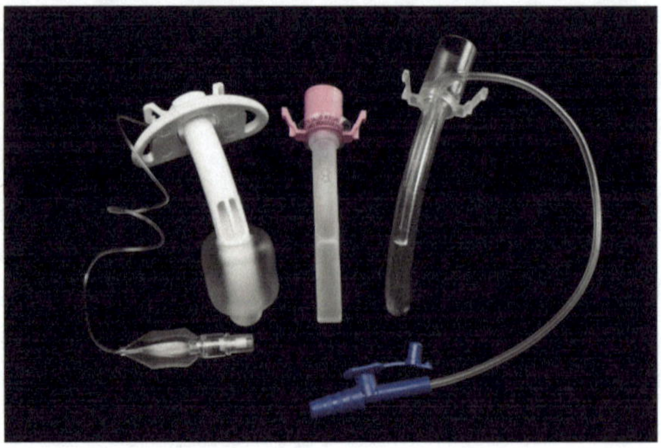

Blom tracheostomy tube system. Note fenestration of outer cannula just above the cuff, speech cannula, and inner cannula with subglottic suction port.

Reprinted with permission of Dr. Eric Blom

Figure 6.17 shows the airflow with the Blom tracheostomy tube system. The flap valve, located at the tip of the speech cannula, opens during inhalation, allowing air to flow through the tube and into the trachea. At the same time, the bubble valve, located along the dorsal aspect of the speech cannula, expands into the fenestration and seals it, preventing air from escaping into the upper airway. On exhalation, the flap valve closes and the bubble valve collapses, exposing the fenestration and directing the airflow through it and up to the vocal cords. Another unique feature of this tracheostomy tube is the exhaled volume reservoir, which prevents the ventilator from recognizing false low-volume readings as air is redirected through the upper airway rather than through the ventilator. This feature is likely to be appealing to practitioners who manage ventilators, because, to date, there are no described methods to prevent low-volume alarms as exhaled air is diverted from the expiratory limb of the ventilator. The manufacturer recommends that use of laser or electrosurgery electrodes should be avoided with this tube to prevent the release of toxic gases and fire in an oxygen-rich environment.

Figure 6.17 Airflow with Blom Trach

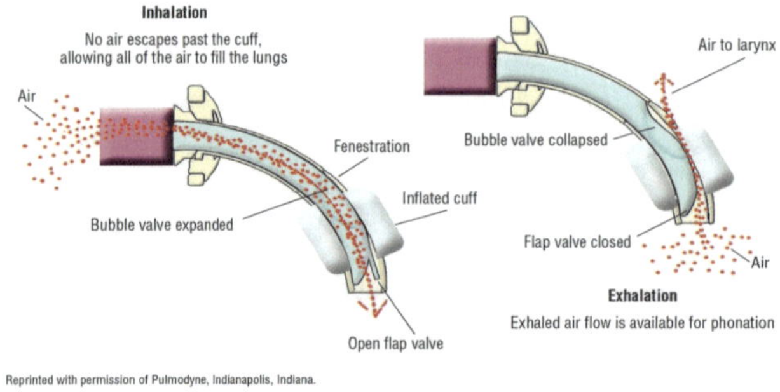

Reprinted with permission of Dr. Eric Blom

Airflow with Blom tracheostomy tube on inspiration and expiration. As air is inspired through the tube, the flap valve (located at the distal tip of the tube) opens. The flexible bubble valve (located on the dorsal shaft of the tube) also expands, covering the fenestration in the outer canula. On exhalation, the flap valve closes, allowing airflow around it and collapsing the bubble valve to allow air through the fenestration and to the vocal cords.

Adam and investigators[46] compared the Blom low profile and the Passy-Muir speaking valves on 30 tracheostomized patients who had never used a speaking valve before. They found no significant differences between these valves on oxygen saturation, respiratory rate, heart rate, speech tasks, voice intensity, and functional verbal communication.

Summary

The many options available to restore phonation make it difficult at times to determine the best method for a particular patient. The best method is often the simplest, but numerous factors must be considered. The first factor in determining the optimal choice for phonation is if the patient requires mechanical ventilation. The second factor is whether the patient can tolerate cuff deflation. When continuous mechanical ventilation is not required, a cuffless tube with capping trials works well for the majority of patients. For patients who require intermittent mechanical ventilation, a TTS tube with capping trials allows the flexibility of a cuff and provides minimal resistance to airflow. Patients on continuous mechanical ventilation who can tolerate cuff deflation can be managed with leak speech. Those patients who are on continuous mechanical ventilation and require cuff inflation usually provide the greatest challenge. Available options are talking tracheostomy tubes and the Blom tracheostomy tube system. Fenestrated tracheostomy tubes are rarely used and must be fit individually to ensure the central placement of the fenestration within the airway.

Health professionals must recognize the importance of a patient's voice to his or her well-being and for effective communication with the health care team. The restoration of a patient's voice is often an emotional moment and can represent the beginning of a return to normal for the patient. It requires patience and an individual, methodical approach to determine the best strategy for each individual patient.

Key Points

- Speaking valves are ideally used with a cuffless tracheostomy tube but may be used with a completely deflated cuff, as long as the patient's ability to breathe comfortably has been thoroughly assessed.
- For patients who do not require continuous mechanical ventilation, a cuffless tube with capping trials allows phonation for the majority of patients.
- For patients who require intermittent mechanical ventilation, a TTS tube with capping trials allows the flexibility of a cuff and offers minimal resistance to airflow when deflated.
- Ventilator-dependent patients who can tolerate cuff deflation can be managed with leak speech, but those who are on continuous mechanical ventilation and who require cuff inflation usually provide the greatest challenge.

REVIEW QUESTIONS

1. An alert patient with good cognitive function has a Shiley 6 cuffless tube and can tolerate digital occlusion. Which method of phonation is likely to be most appropriate for this patient?
    a. Change to a cuffed fenestrated tube with a speaking valve
    b. Capping, with oxygen delivered by nasal cannula, if needed
    c. Change to a talking tracheostomy tube
    d. Speaking valve, with oxygen delivered by nasal cannula, if needed

    ANSWER: B. Choice B is the most appropriate answer. Choices A and C are incorrect because there is no need to change to a cuffed tube because the patient can already tolerate a cuffless tube. Choice D is incorrect because there is no need to use a speaking valve if the patient can tolerate capping. In addition, oxygen should be given by tracheostomy collar when using a speaking valve.

2. Which of the following is NOT an example of a speaking valve?
    a. Shikani
    b. Speak EZ
    c. Jackson Trach Talk
    d. TRACOE Phon Assist

    ANSWER: C. All of the choices are speaking valves, except Choice C. However, technically, the Speak EZ is a tracheal cannula with a built-in speaking valve.

3. A patient is on continuous mechanical ventilation and cannot tolerate cuff deflation. Which of the following is an appropriate option to provide phonation?
    a. Change to TTS tube and use speaking valve
    b. Change to Speak EZ tracheal cannula
    c. Change to talking tracheostomy tube
    d. Change to cuffless tracheostomy tube and cap

    ANSWER: C. Option C is correct because it is the only method that provides cuff inflation, which is required in this case because this mechanically ventilated patient cannot tolerate cuff deflation. All of the other choices are incorrect because they do not provide or tolerate an inflated cuff.

4. Precautions with a fenestrated tracheostomy tube include all of the following EXCEPT:
    a. Fitting the tube to ensure the fenestration lies centrally within the airway
    b. Using a non-fenestrated inner cannula when suctioning is performed
    c. Shining a light within the tube to observe whether granulation tissue is present
    d. Using the fenestration for phonation within two days of tracheostomy placement

    ANSWER: D. All of the choices are correct except Choice D. Using the fenestration mechanism in an immature stoma can result in subcutaneous emphysema and an airway emergency. Choice A is a precaution because a proper fit of the tube prevents granulation tissue from forming. Choice B is a precaution because a suction catheter can get stuck within the fenestrated inner cannula. Choice C is a precaution because shining a light can detect the presence of granulation tissue within the fenestration.

5. Which of the following is the most appropriate choice for providing leak speech to a patient on continuous mechanical ventilation?
   a. Deflate cuff, increase tidal volume, increase inspiratory time
   b. Keep cuff inflated, decrease tidal volume, add PEEP
   c. Change to Blom tracheostomy tube, use speaking valve
   d. Change to fenestrated tube, inflate cuff, use speaking valve

   ANSWER: A. Leak speech is provided by deflating the cuff and increasing the tidal volume to compensate for the leak, and increasing the inspiratory time provides more time for inspiratory speech. Choice B is incorrect because cuff deflation and increased tidal volume are required, although using PEEP is optional. Choice C is incorrect because the Blom tube requires cuff inflation. Choice D is incorrect because a fenestrated tube is not needed to provide leak speech. In addition, the use of a speaking valve is not needed with a fenestrated tube.

Web Resources

The Airway Company, Shikani valve, Forest Hill, MD, www.thewairwaycompany.com.

Pulmodyne, Blom Tracheostomy Tube System, Indianapolis, IN, www.pulmodyne.com.

Passy-Muir, Passy-Muir valves, Irvine, CA, www.passymuir.com.

Technical Products, Inc. of Georgia, Speak EZ tracheal cannula, Lawrenceville, GA, www.tpi-ga.com.

TRACOE, Phon Assist, www.tracoe.com

Hood Labs, Eliachar valve, Pembroke, MA, www.hoodlabs.com

Boston Medical Products, Montgomery speaking valve, www.bosmed.com, www.trachs.com

Teleflex, Tucker tracheostomy tube, www.teleflex.com

References

1. Hoit JD, Banzett RB, Lohmeier HL, Hixon TJ, Brown R. Clinical ventilator adjustments that improve speech. *Chest*. 2003;124:1512-1521.
2. Leder SB. Importance of verbal communication for the ventilator-dependent patient. *Chest*. 1990;96(4):792-3.
3. Tolotti A, Bagnasco A, Catania G, Aleo G, Pagnucci N, Cadorin L, Zanini M, Rocco G, Stievano A, Carnevale FA, Sasso L. The communication experience of tracheostomy patients with nurses in the intensive care unit: A phenomenological study. *Intens & Crit Care Nurs*. 2018;46:24-31.
4. Pandian V, Bose S, Miller C, Schiavi A, Feller-Kopman D, Bhatti N, Mirski M. Exploring quality of life in critically ill tracheostomy patients: A pilot study. *ORL Head Neck Nurs*. 2014;32(1):6-13.
5. Freeman-Sanderson AL, Togher L, Elkins MR, Phipps PR. Quality of life improves with return of voice in tracheostomy patients in intensive care: An observational study. *J Crit Care*. 2016;33:186-191.
6. Kazandjian MS, Dikeman KJ. Communication options for tracheostomy and ventilator-dependent patients. In E. N. Myers & J. T. Johnson (Eds.), *Tracheostomy: Airway management, communication, and swallowing*. San Diego, CA: Plural Publishing, 2008.
7. Suiter DM, McCullough GH, Powell PW. Effects of cuff deflation and one-way tracheostomy speaking valve placement on swallow physiology. *Dysphagia*. 2003;18:284-292.
8. Leder SB, Ross DA. Investigation of the causal relationship between tracheostomy and aspiration in the acute care setting. *Laryngoscope*. 2000;110:641-644.
9. Bonnano PC. Swallowing dysfunction after tracheostomy. *Ann Surg*. 1971;174:129-133.
10. Logemann J. *Evaluation and Treatment of Swallowing Disorders*. San Diego, CA: College-Hill Press; 1983.
11. Nash M. Swallowing problems in the tracheostomized patient. *Otolaryngol Clin North Am*. 1988;21:701-709.
12. Ding R, Logemann JA. Swallow physiology in patients with trach cuff inflated or deflated: A retrospective study. *Head Neck*. 2005;27:809-813.

13. Amathieu R, Sauvat S, Reynaud P, Slavov V, Luis D, Dinca A, Tual L, Bloc S, Dhonneur G. Influence of the cuff pressure on the swallowing reflex in tracheostomized intensive care unit patients. *Brit J Anaesth.* 2012;109(4):578-583.
14. Holmberg EB, Hillman RE, Perkell JS. Glottal airflow and transglottal air pressure measurements for male and female speakers in soft, normal, and loud voice. *J Acoust Soc Amer.* 1988;84(2):511-529.
15. Bard MC, Slavit DH, McCaffrey TV, Lipton RJ. Noninvasive technique for estimating subglottic pressure and laryngeal efficiency. *Ann Otol Rhinol Laryngol.* 1992;101(7):578-582.
16. Hess DR. Facilitating speech in the patient with a tracheostomy. *Respir Care.* 2005;50(4):519-525.
17. Toremalm NG. A tracheotomy speech valve. *Laryngoscope.* 1968;78(12):2177-2182.
18. Saul A, Bergstrom B. A new permanent tracheostomy tube-speech valve system. *Laryngoscope.* 1979;89(6, Pt. 1):980-983.
19. Tippett DC, Vogelman L. Communication, tracheostomy and ventilator dependency. In Tippett DC, ed. *Tracheostomy and ventilator dependency.* New York: Thieme; 2000.
20. Fornataro-Clerici L, Zajac DJ. Aerodynamic characteristics of tracheostomy speaking valves. *J Speech Hear Res.* 1993;*36*:529-532.
21. Zajac DJ, Fornataro-Clerici L, Roop TA. Aerodynamic characteristics of speaking valves: An updated report. *J Speech Lang Hear Res.* 1999;42:92-100.
22. Shikani AH, French J, Sievens AA. New unidirectional airflow ball tracheostomy speaking valve. *Otolaryngol Head Neck Surg.* 2000;123(1):103-107.
23. Tippett DC, Siebens AA. Preserving oral communication in individuals with tracheostomy and ventilator dependency. *Amer J Speech Lang Pathol.* 1995;4(2):55-61.
24. Gross RD, Atwood CW, Grayhack JP, Shaiman S. Lung volume effects on pharyngeal swallow physiology. *J Applied Physiol.* 2003;95:2211-2217.
25. Barrazza GY, Fernandez C, Halaby C, Ambrosio S, SImpser EF, Pirzada MB. The safety of tracheostomy speaking valve use during sleep in children: A pilot study. *Am J Otolaryngol Head Neck Med Surg.* 2014;35:636-640.
26. Lichtman SW, Birnbaum IL, Sanfilippo MR, Pellicone JT, Damon WJ, King ML. Effect of a tracheostomy speaking valve on secretions, arterial oxygenation, and olfaction: A quantitative evaluation. *J Speech Hear Res.* 1995;38(3):549-555.
27. Dettelbach MA, Gross RD, Mahlmann J, Eibling DE. Effect of the Passy-Muir valve on aspiration in patients with tracheostomy. *Head Neck.* 1995;17(4):297-302.
28. Elpern EH, Okonek MB, Bacon M, Gerstung C, Skrzynski M. Effect of the Passy-Muir tracheostomy speaking valve on pulmonary aspiration in adults. *Heart Lung.* 2000;29(4):287-293.
29. Manzano JL, Lubillo S, Henriquez D, Martin JC, Perez MC, Wilson DJ. Verbal communication of ventilator-dependent patients. *Crit Care Med.* 1993;21(4):512-517.
30. Shikani AH, Dietrich-Burns K. Comparison of speech parameters and olfaction using different tracheotomy speaking valves. *Int Forum Allergy Rhinol.* 2012;2(4):348-353.
31. Prigent H, Lejaille M, Terzi N, Annane D, Figere M, Orlikowski D, Lofaso F. Effect of a tracheostomy speaking valve on breathing-swallowing interaction. *Intens Care Med.* 2012;38:85-90.
32. Morris LL, Bedon AM, McIntosh E, Whitmer A. Restoring speech to tracheostomy patients. *Crit Care Nurs.* 2015;35(6):13-28.

33. Shea SA, Hoit JD, Banzett RB. Competition between gas exchange and speech production in ventilated patients. *Biol Psychol.* 1998;49:9–27.
34. MacBean N, Ward E, Murdoch B, Cahill L, Solley M, Geraghty T, et al. Optimizing speech production in the ventilator-assisted individual following cervical spinal cord injury: A preliminary investigation. *Int J Lang Commun Dis.* 2009;44(3):382-393.
35. Hoit JD, Banzett RB. Simple adjustments can improve ventilator-supported speech. *Amer J Speech Lang Pathol.* 1997;6:87-96.
36. Hoit JD, Shea SA, Banzett RB. Speech production during mechanical ventilation in tracheostomized individuals. *J Speech Hear Res.* 1994;37:53-63.
37. Garguilo M, Leroux K, Lejaille M, Pascal S, Orlikowski D, Lofaso F, Prigent H. Patient-controlled positive end-expiratory pressure with neuromuscular disease: Effect on speech in patients with tracheostomy and mechanical ventilation support. *Chest.* 2013;143(5):1243-1251.
38. Passy V, Baydur A, Prentice W, Darnell-Neal R. Passy-Muir tracheostomy speaking valve on ventilator-dependent patients. *Laryngoscope.* 1993;102(6):653-658.
39. Mozart MJ, Stuart H. Subcutaneous emphysema caused by a fenestrated tracheostomy tube. *Anaesthesia.* 2001;56(2):191-192.
40. Orme RM, Welham KL. Subcutaneous emphysema after percutaneous tracheostomy—time to dispense with fenestrated tubes? *Anaesthesia.* 2006;61(9):911-912.
41. McGrath B, Lynch J, Wilson M, Nicholson L, Wallace, S. Above cuff vocalisation: A novel technique for communication in the ventilator-dependent tracheostomy patient. *J Intens Care Soc.* 2016;17(1):19-26.
42. McGrath B, Wallace S, Wilson M, Nicholson L, Felton T, Bowyer C, Bentley A. Effectiveness of above cuff vocalisation for ventilator-dependent patients with tracheostomies. *Brit J Anaesth.* 2018;120(5):e26.
43. Shahvari MBG, Kigin CM, Zimmerman JE. Speaking tracheostomy tube modified for swallowing dysfunction and chronic aspiration. *Anesthesiology.* 1977;46(4):290-291.
44. Leder SB, Traquina DN. Voice intensity of patients using a Communi-Trach I cuffed speaking tracheostomy tube. *Laryngoscope.* 1989;99:269-274.
45. Nomori H. Tracheostomy tube enabling speech during mechanical ventilation. *Chest.* 2004;125(3):1046-1051.
46. Adam SI, Srinet P, Aronberg RM, Rosenberg G, Leder SB. Verbal communication with the Blom low profile and Passy-Muir one-way tracheotomy tube speaking valves. *J Communic Dis.* 2015;56:40-46.

7

Care of the Patient with a Tracheostomy

by Linda L. Morris

Objectives

- Demonstrate proper procedure for cleaning the inner cannula and stoma
- Explain proper suction procedure to prevent complications
- Outline maintenance of cuff pressures within a safe range
- Prescribe a schedule of interval tracheostomy tube changes to prevent infection
- Differentiate tracheostomy care between hospital and home

Introduction

The tracheostomy patient requires vigilant care, especially in the first several postoperative days. Meticulous maintenance of the tracheostomy tube can prevent many complications. This chapter discusses the care required for the patient with a tracheostomy, including maintaining the tube, cleaning the inner cannula and stoma, stabilizing the cuff, mobilizing secretions, and caring for other tracheostomy devices such as the T-tube. In addition, considerations for patients at home will also be reviewed, including managing home emergencies.

MAINTENANCE OF THE TRACHEOSTOMY TUBE

The scope of maintenance of the tracheostomy tube can be divided into, first, securing the tracheostomy tube, and, equally important, routine cleaning of the apparatus. General care of the tracheostomy patient includes ensuring the presence of everyday as well as emergency supplies at all times. Inherently, there should be complete familiarity with the parts of the tube as well as the overall care of the tube and the patient. Bedside supplies (listed in **Table 7.1**) should include an extra tracheostomy tube of the same size and one size smaller, an obturator of appropriate size and type, a suction source with appropriately sized suction catheters, a manual resuscitation bag, and an oxygen source if needed.[1,2] Additional supplies include dressings, tracheostomy tube holders or cotton twill tape, and tracheostomy cleaning kits.

Table 7.1. Bedside Supply Kit
Extra tracheostomy tube of same size
Extra tracheostomy tube one size smaller
Obturator
Suction catheters
Manual resuscitation bag and face mask
Suction source, tubing
Oxygen source
Tracheostomy dressings (drain sponges)
Tracheostomy cleaning kits

SECURING THE TRACHEOSTOMY TUBE

The first step in proper tracheostomy care is to ensure the security of the tube. After initial placement, most surgeons prefer to suture the tracheostomy tube in place.[3] This is commonly done with a suture at each of the four corners of the neck flange in addition to snugly applied twill tape. This technique often makes taking care of the stoma challenging in the first postoperative week. However, the security of the tube during this time is a higher priority. Two groups have proposed more secure suturing techniques that differ from this conventional practice. Nouraie and others[4] described a four-point technique done closer to the pivot point on the neck flange, while Liew, Gibbins, and Oyarzabal[5] described securing the tracheostomy with two sutures through the central superior part of the neck flange. Both groups reported that their methods allow better care of the stoma, provide for easier replacement of stoma dressings, and function with different neck flange materials. Liew and coauthors reported that over the course of 10 years, their method has avoided tube dislodgement in the immediate postoperative period.[5] Rolls and Gardner[6] suggest an alternate securing method using shoulder epaulettes, created with Elastoplast and white tape, where there is concern for skin or blood flow of the neck vessels.

Most authors suggest that tracheostomy ties be secured snugly, allowing only one finger depth under the tracheostomy holder. Cotton twill tape is often used to secure the tracheostomy tube, especially in the early postoperative period. Twill tape does not slack when secured in place, but over a longer period of time, it may cut into the neck of the wearer or fray at the ends.[7] A study of tracheostomy securing devices by Dixon and Wasson[8] showed that Velcro holders were more comfortable, easier to use, and took significantly less time to apply. However, they may also degrade over time, especially when washed in hot water.[7] In fact, one manufacturer (Dale) specifically reported that their product should not be washed. While there is no consensus on the best device to use for anchoring the tracheostomy tube, tube security should be the priority in the early postoperative period. After the stoma and tract have matured, the clinician can then consider comfort as well as tube security.

When the tracheostomy tube can move within the airway, the tip intermittently comes in contact with the trachea. Patient discomfort and coughing can result and are more pronounced with a rigid tube and a wider angle. The continued contact of the tube within the trachea may cause erosion of the trachea and the formation of granulation tissue within the airway. This granulation tissue can also occur in the suprastomal area, where the connection of the neck flange repeatedly comes into contact with the stoma. The resultant granulation tissue can fall back into the airway and create a partial obstruction.[9] One way to assist in decreasing movement of the tube within the airway is to ensure the snugness of the tracheotomy ties.

Most authors state that the first tracheostomy tube change should be done at the end of the first postoperative week, which marks the transition from an immature to a mature tracheostomy. It usually takes 5–7 days for the tract to heal and mature.[10] If inadvertent decannulation were to occur during this time, the tissue planes would collapse, thus making simple reinsertion essentially impossible. It is inadvisable to attempt the reinsertion of a tube through an immature stoma because of the high likelihood of creating a false passage and failing to adequately ventilate the patient.

Clinical Scenario

A 42-year old woman received a tracheostomy because of acute respiratory failure after a complicated abdominal surgery. She now has a dual-cannula cuffed tube and currently remains on mechanical ventilator support. The tube is secured in place with 4 sutures: one placed in each corner of the neck flange.

Over the next few days, a large amount of dried blood and secretions have accumulated around the neck flange, and the nurses have found it difficult to clean the stoma because the neck flange is snugly sutured to the skin.

By the seventh postoperative day, the patient is weaned from mechanical ventilation, and the surgeon changes the tracheostomy tube to another cuffed, dual-cannula tube. The nurses now clean the stoma and apply a drain sponge around the tube to collect secretions and cushion the flange against the skin.

Care of the Inner Cannula

There is wide variation on the recommended frequency for cleaning or changing the inner cannula, but most authors suggest two to three times per day. Though cleaning may be required as often as every two hours, this frequency was challenged in one study, which suggested inner cannulas do not need to be changed often, if at all.[11] Sixty patients were studied over three days to determine whether the interval of changing the inner cannula had an impact on tube obstruction or colonization. One group of patients had the inner cannula changed every 24 hours, while the other group did not have the inner cannula changed at all over a three-day period. Surprisingly, the researchers found no difference on both outcome measures. The study had some limitations, however. All patients were suctioned in the hour before the inner cannula was examined, thus limiting the accurate interpretation of obstruction versus patency. Another limitation was the lack of defining the postoperative period in which the study took place. Results may differ between postoperative days 1–3 compared to postoperative days 10–12. Finally, the results could not be universally applied to all patients since the investigation was a small pilot study of only 60 patients in one surgical ICU. Comorbid conditions with large amounts of secretions—for example, pneumonia—might produce different results.

Hettige and colleagues[12] recommended the use of a tracheostomy bundle of interventions that includes checking the inner cannula every 2-4 hours. Outcomes of the tracheostomy bundle demonstrated a significant decrease in critical incidents from 58 to seven over a two-year period.[13] Another group studied the outcomes of a tracheostomy bundle and found significantly improved rates of decannulation and tolerance of oral feeding.[14]

The inner cannula should be cleaned or changed when needed as long as it is inspected at least two to three times per day. Disposable inner cannulas are a convenience for the nursing staff; however, they can be a significant added expense for patients at home. Insurance coverage may be insufficient for home medical care and supplies such as disposable inner cannulas.[15] Currently, the Medicare allowance is 30 inner cannulas per month and should be considered before discharging patients with tracheostomies.

Procedure for Cleaning the Inner Cannula

The inner cannula must be regularly inspected and ideally cleaned using an aseptic technique. There are few studies that define the optimal frequency for cleaning or replacing the inner cannula. Cited frequency of cleaning has ranged from almost 16 times per day[16] to no cleaning at all.[11] Most hospital policies recommend cleaning inner cannulas about three times per day.

Before beginning the procedure, supplies should be gathered and prepared. Most tracheostomy cleaning kits (**Figure 7.1**) are sterile and contain all necessary supplies, including two small containers, stoma dressing (or drain sponge), cotton twill tape, a small bottle brush, cotton-tipped swabs, pipe cleaners, a drape, and gloves. Hydrogen peroxide (3%) and sterile water or saline are used for cleaning plastic tracheostomy tubes but should not be used for metal, silicone, or nylon tubes. Cleaning instructions for tubes of the latter materials are discussed in the following instructions for standard plastic tubes.

Figure 7.1 TRACOE Tracheostomy cleaning kit

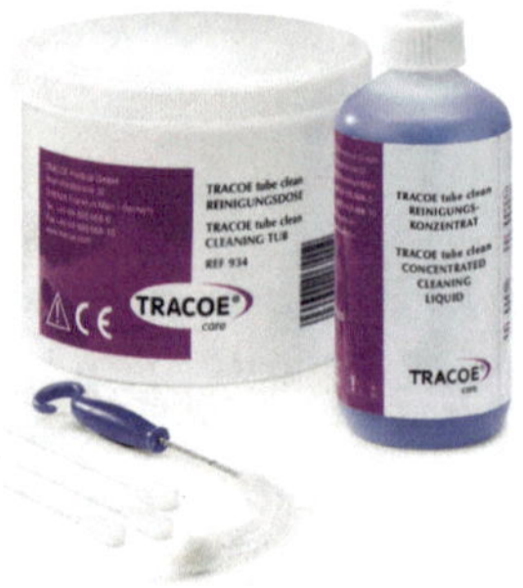

TRACOE tracheostomy tube cleaning kit

To clean plastic tubes, first fill one container with enough sterile water or saline to completely immerse the inner cannula. Fill the second container with the same amount of 3% hydrogen peroxide. Some practitioners prefer to use hydrogen peroxide diluted to a 1:1 solution with sterile water or saline.[17] The solution will be used to soak the inner cannula, and the diluted hydrogen peroxide solution will take a longer time. Other practitioners prefer to use saline alone.

It is important to minimize the movement of the tracheostomy tube during manipulation in order to prevent discomfort and coughing. The tube should be steadied using the thumb and forefinger of one hand to stabilize the neck flange while the other hand removes the inner cannula. Small movements of the tube from the outside create large movements within the trachea, especially if the tube is rigid and has a wide angle. The inner cannula should be placed in a container of either hydrogen peroxide, a hydrogen peroxide/saline solution, or simply a saline solution and allowed to soak for 3–5 minutes in order to soften and dissolve the accumulated secretions. During this interval, the stoma can be cleaned with cotton swabs dipped in saline.

After the inner cannula has soaked in the peroxide bath, the secretions should be sufficiently loosened for cleaning. The small bottle brush can then be used to scrub the inside as well as the outside of the cannula. The point of contact of the 15-mm connector with the shaft of the cannula generally harbors secretions and should be scrubbed carefully. After all debris is removed, the inner cannula should be rinsed in sterile water and shaken free of water droplets. Alternatively, pipe cleaners can be used to dry the inside of the inner cannula. The inner cannula is then locked in place within the outer cannula while once again stabilizing the neck flange.

One Swedish study[18] demonstrated the superior efficacy of a cleaning method utilizing decontamination with chlorhexidine-alcohol followed by rinsing with sterile saline. The study was intended to create clinical evidence in support of a new national guideline compared to standard practice. In Sweden, common practice for cleaning the inner cannula utilized warm water with mild detergent. However, a national guideline recommended decontamination via an additional step of rinsing the inner cannula with chlorhexidine-alcohol followed by sterile saline. A study was undertaken to examine the difference in bacterial counts between the two methods. The authors studied 47 patients using a crossover design and cultured the inner cannulas before and after each cleaning procedure. Before the decontamination step, all but three samples had bacterial colonization. Median counts were 10,000 cfu/ml (colony-forming units per milliliter) for silver cannulas, 52,500 cfu/ml for Portex cannulas, 17,000 cfu/ml for Shiley cannulas, and 100,000 cfu/ml for TRACOE cannulas. Following decontamination using detergent and chlorhexidine-alcohol, five of 48 inner cannulas grew up to 160 cfu/ml; after using detergent alone, only one of 49 inner cannulas grew up to 10 cfu/ml. Furthermore, cleaning with both methods resulted in a near total elimination of all organisms. The same group[19] performed a six-month study of material wear of polymeric tubes and found that all tubes exposed in the trachea for 3-6 months showed signs of material wear. They recommended that these tubes be changed before three months of wear.

Another study[20] compared different methods of cleaning tubes. They studied PVC tubes and silicone tubes from three different manufacturers to determine the effectiveness of the cleaning process. They used five different cleaning solutions: 3% bleach, chlorhexidine, peroxide, Polident, and saline (control). They found that all methods were effective in decreasing the counts of staph aureus, with bleach and chlorhexidine being more effective. All methods except Polident were effective in decreasing counts of pseudomonas. Surface integrity was intact with all treatments.

The same group studied repeated reprocessing of tracheostomy tubes. They cleaned the tracheostomy tubes with household detergent, then soaked the tubes in bleach. The tubes were then reprocessed 0, 10, or 20 times and exposed to either *Pseudomonas aerogenosa* or *Staphylococcus aureus*. They found that tubes that were reprocessed 20 times had significantly higher levels of *S. aureus* biofilm development. They concluded that higher levels of growth were due to degradation of the tube that facilitated bacterial growth.[21]

Leonhard and colleagues[22] studied the reprocessing of tubes using one of four methods: manual brushing and rinsing with tap water, manual brushing followed by disinfection with a glutaraldehyde solution, manual brushing followed by machine-based cleaning in a dishwasher, and manual brushing followed by ultrasound cleaning. They found that manual brushing with tap water reduced colonization by 102 cfu/ml, but complete microbial reduction was achieved only with chemical or machine-based disinfection, and an ultrasound yielded no further reduction after manual brushing.

Tracheostomy tubes with disposable inner cannulas were developed in the late 1980s with the intent of saving significant nursing time. Johnson, Wagner, and Sigler[16] compared the time to clean the inner cannula versus simply replacing it with a new one. They found that standard care of the inner cannula required over five minutes, while changing a disposable inner cannula took less than one minute. Even though disposable inner cannulas are popular in hospitals, the cost of supplies and insurance coverage may prohibit their use at home.

One of the primary benefits of plastic dual cannula tracheostomy tubes is that the inner cannula can be removed and cleaned while leaving the outer cannula in place within the airway. This may not be the case for tubes made of other materials.

Cleaning Metal Tracheostomy Tubes

Peroxide and enzyme cleaners should be avoided with sterling silver and stainless-steel tubes. These solutions cause silver tubes to discolor, stain, and tarnish; in stainless steel, they cause the solder connection joints to weaken and the surface to pit and stain. Rather, the manufacturers recommend that metal tracheostomy tubes be removed and cleaned daily by soaking in mild dishwashing liquid for one hour to soften and loosen mucus. A flexible tracheal brush should be used to clean the inside of the tube; a soft toothbrush can be used to clean the outside of the tube and the neck flange. Dry heat sterilization is not recommended, and the tubes should not be exposed to temperatures above 204°C (400°F). The recommended use for patients at home is to place the tube in a pan of tap water and boil for 30 minutes, followed by wiping dry the cooled tube.

Cleaning Silicone Tracheostomy Tubes

The manufacturers' recommendations state that the Bivona tracheostomy tubes and Provox LaryTubes (made of silicone) should be cleaned with a mild detergent. Because of its porous nature, silicone tends to absorb cleaning products, so those cleaning products should not be used.

Cleaning Nylon Tracheostomy Tubes

Nylon tracheostomy tubes such as the Air-Lon™ should be soaked in warm soapy water for a few minutes to loosen any dried mucus. A flexible tracheal brush can be used to clean the inside of the tube, and a soft toothbrush can be used to clean the outside of the tube and the neck flange. The

Air-Lon™ tube can be autoclaved, boiled, gas sterilized, or soaked in a cold germicidal solution that does not contain phenol or formic acid as a base.

Care of the Tracheostomy Tube Cuff

It is important to minimize pressure against the trachea from the air-inflated cuff for several reasons. Proper inflation of the cuff can ensure an adequate delivery of tidal volume and prevent loss of air around the cuff, thus preventing hypoxemia. Inadequate cuff inflation has also been implicated in the development of ventilator-associated pneumonia. Alternatively, hyperinflation of the cuff can result in ischemia of the trachea, which can lead to tracheomalacia, tracheal stenosis, and tracheal necrosis. Cuff pressures above capillary perfusion pressure (25 cm H_2O or 20–30 mm Hg) for a prolonged time have been associated with ischemia and necrosis of the trachea.[17,23] By contrast, cuff pressures below 20 cm H_2O have been associated with the leakage of oropharyngeal secretions around the cuff and are thought to contribute to ventilator-associated pneumonia (VAP).[24,25]

There are three primary acceptable methods to ensure adequate cuff pressure: direct measurement of cuff pressure through manometry, minimal occlusive volume, and the minimal leak technique. Direct measurement of cuff pressure can be done intermittently with a manual pump manometer, or continuously with an electronic manometer. The advantage of the electronic version is that it monitors cuff pressure as well as automatically regulates the pressure within the cuff and provides alarms to warn of leaks or overpressure.

Several studies have considered palpation of the cuff as a technique to estimate pressure; however, its accuracy has been disappointing. Faris and colleagues[26] asked experienced physicians and respiratory therapists to estimate cuff pressure by palpation and compared this value to a manometer measurement. Even the most experienced clinicians were accurate only 61% of the time. Guisti and colleagues[27] conducted a similar study with nurses in a simulation lab. They found that nurses incorrectly estimated cuff pressure 68% of the time. Stewart, Secrest, Norwood, and Zachary[28] asked nurse anesthetists to use their usual cuff estimation techniques and compared these values with direct cuff manometry. They found that less than 31% of the nurse anesthetists inflated the cuff within the ideal range. Fernandez, Blanch, Mancebo, Bonsoms, and Artigas[29] demonstrated that experienced physicians and nurses accurately estimated high cuff pressures only 69% of the time, normal cuff pressures 58% of the time, and low cuff pressures 73% of the time. Hoffman, Parwani, and Hahn[30] showed that experienced faculty in emergency medicine were only 22% sensitive for detecting overinflation of the cuff. In that study, the average cuff pressure measured more than 93 cm H_2O (9.3 kPa), and 90% of the participants inflated the cuff to more than 120 cm H_2O (12 kPa). The investigators concluded that the inability to detect overinflated cuffs is not related to years of experience.

Morris, Zoumalan, Roccaforte, and Amin[31] compared two hospitals using two different techniques for cuff inflation. One hospital used balloon palpation while the other used manometry. The study followed a total of 115 patients and found an overall overinflation rate of 38%, which, incidentally, was equal at both hospitals. They suggested the use of manometry alone did not prevent overinflation of the cuff and that more vigilant cuff monitoring practices were indicated.

Historically, high-pressure cuffs were exclusively found on tracheostomy tubes; routine cuff deflation was common practice to relieve pressure against the trachea. Intermittent cuff deflation provided an opportunity for reperfusion of the tracheal mucosa, but there was no evidence that capillary blood flow was restored. In addition, routine cuff deflation was not well tolerated in hemodynamically unstable patients. Therefore, deep oropharyngeal suctioning should be done prior to cuff deflation to remove accumulated secretions above the cuff. Cuff deflation should also be timed with exhalation to prevent the aspiration of secretions above the cuff. A positive-pressure breath can also be used to blow secretions upward into the pharynx so they can be suctioned.[17,32]

Alcan and others[33] demonstrated that cuff pressure varies with patient positioning. They measured 25 patients on mechanical ventilation who were first placed in a baseline position with the head of the bed elevated 30 degrees, with a neutral head position. Cuff pressure was then adjusted to 25cm H_2O. The patients were then moved into 16 different positions and the cuff pressure was measured after each position change. Of the total 400 measurements, 2.5% were below 20 cm H_2O; 50.3% were between 20-30 cm H_2O; and 47.3% were above 30 cm H_2O. The investigators recommended that cuff pressure should be measured after changing a patient's position and adjusted to be within the recommended range.

Duguet and colleagues[34] studied nine mechanically ventilated patients to evaluate a prototype device that maintained constant pressure within endotracheal tube cuffs. Continuous measurements of cuff pressures were taken when the cuffs were maintained by the device and when they were not. The investigators randomly ordered the sequence of measurements, varying days when the prototype device maintained constant pressure with days when constant cuff pressure was not maintained, yet was continuously monitored. The target cuff pressure was set at 22–28 cm H_2O. On control days, cuff pressure ranged from 30–50 cm H_2O for 29% of the time and from 15–30 cm H_2O for 56% of the time. On prototype days, cuff pressure was maintained at 15–30 cm H_2O for 95% of the time. The study showed that cuff pressure was successfully controlled with minimal human intervention. Another single-institution study showed reduced rates of microaspiration of gastric contents, tracheobronchial bacterial concentration, and VAP with the use of a continuous cuff management device.[35]

Accumulated secretions above the cuff have been implicated in the development of VAP and, therefore, should be suctioned regularly in order to prevent seepage around the cuff. Some tracheostomy and endotracheal tubes have a separate suction channel for this purpose.

Using intermittent and continuous suctioning schedules, one study[36] compared the quantity of secretions removed from conventional tracheostomy tubes to those with a suction channel. The purpose of their benchtop study was to determine if an above-the-cuff suction channel could decrease tracheal aspiration. They compared standard Shiley tubes to Portex Blue Line Ultra Suctionaid tubes, which include a suction channel. Tubes of similar outer diameter were placed in a simulated tracheal model, and donor human saliva was used because of its unique rheology and viscoelastic properties. Each cuff was inflated to 30 cm H_2O, and 10 ml of human saliva was placed above the cuff. The amount of saliva that migrated past the Shiley tubes with no suction was approximately 8.5 ml. A similar amount of saliva migrated past the cuff of the Portex tubes when no suction was applied.

Changing the Tracheostomy Tube

Most papers report the first tracheostomy tube change should take place on the seventh postoperative day. At this time, the tissue tract is considered mature. The first tube change is usually done by the surgeon who placed the tube, who typically signs off on the case afterward. Ideally, care should then be transferred to another practitioner who will provide follow-up for the tracheostomy.

There is anecdotal evidence that tracheostomy tube changes with the open surgical technique can be safely performed earlier than the fifth day. However, there are no randomized, controlled studies to identify the minimum safe interval following tracheostomy placement.

One of the biggest risks during the early postoperative period is inadvertent decannulation—an emergency requiring orotracheal intubation with an endotracheal tube. The rationale for orotracheal intubation is the lack of a mature tract and the collapse of tissue planes, which form an impediment to the emergency replacement of the tracheostomy tube. Refer to chapter 10 for a detailed discussion of inadvertent decannulation.

After the early postoperative period, the entire tracheostomy tube should be changed on a regular basis in order to prevent infection, obstruction of the tube, and other complications associated with an indwelling airway device. An additional goal for this procedure in children is to keep up with their physical growth. Manufacturers' recommendations suggest entire tube changes every one to two months. However, one study[9] suggested that routine tracheostomy tube changes should take place more often. The author found that implementing a new policy of tracheostomy tube changes every two weeks decreased the number of surgical interventions required for the removal of granulation tissue. He further suggested that tracheostomy tubes should be changed as potential sources of infection when sepsis is present. Some patients have reported success with daily tracheostomy tube changes and cleaning while rotating the use of two primary tubes.

In January 2016, the Centers for Medicare and Medicaid Services (CMS) introduced a radical change. Previously in the US, CMS covered replacement tracheostomy tubes every month, but changed their policy to replace tubes every three months. While not all insurance companies have yet followed suit, it is essential to teach patients and caregivers how to clean not only the inner cannulas, but also clean and reuse the tubes themselves. Discharge and home care for the tracheostomy patient should include clear awareness of their insurance provider's coverage of specific items. Further details about discharge and home care is discussed in chapter 12.

CARE OF THE STOMA

A healthy stoma should be clean and dry, with pink edges, though in the early postoperative period it is normal to see dried blood around the stoma. Any redness, swelling, or pus is abnormal. A small amount of blood should be expected with each tracheostomy tube change, especially when a cuffed tube is inserted or removed. However, if frank blood continues to be evident, the clinician may need to explore the wound to ligate or cauterize a leaking blood vessel or possibly apply packing.

The constant exposure of the stoma to secretions can be irritating to the skin, much like diaper rash. Secretions left in place around the stoma become dried and encrusted quickly. In addition, moist secretions can act as irritants to the skin, so the stoma must be cleansed regularly and kept dry. If continued redness occurs, a thin layer of zinc oxide can be used as a moisture barrier to protect the skin and allow healing. A precut drain sponge should be applied around the stoma until secretions have significantly decreased. This dressing should be changed at least twice per day,[37,38] or whenever secretions begin to collect. This can be challenging in the early postoperative period, as the priority during that time is the security of the tube.

In the hospital, 3% hydrogen peroxide is often used to clean around the stoma and soften encrustations. It can be applied full or half strength to a cotton swab to cleanse the skin around the tracheostomy tube, underneath the neck flange along the entire circumference of the stoma, and particularly along the point of connection with the neck flange. For long-term use, however, saline-dipped cotton swabs are recommended. Patients at home are taught to use saline or tap water to gently cleanse the stoma. All excess moisture should be removed with another cotton-tipped applicator or gauze pad, followed by a tracheostomy dressing.

The stomal dressing has a dual purpose: to collect secretions and to cushion the neck flange from direct contact with the skin. There is no evidence of the optimal material for the stomal dressing, but the primary goal should be to keep the neck dry and free of secretions. Hydrophilic absorbent dressings can be used in patients with large amounts of secretions, but their effectiveness over gauze dressings has not been demonstrated in tracheostomy patients. One Japanese group used an absorbent dressing (Aquacel) on five patients and reported favorable results,[39] but there is a need for randomized studies comparing various methods of dressing the stoma. The major goal is timely replacement of the dressing when it becomes soiled or moist with secretions, which occasionally may necessitate several dressing changes per day.

Nurses and respiratory therapists may sometimes find it difficult to change the dressing, especially in patients with cervical collars or large, thick necks. Regular dressing changes promote skin integrity and help to prevent infection.[40] Failure to cleanse the stoma could result in inflammation or infection. Two critical care nurses invented a new device called the Tracheostomy Dressing Applicator (TDA). Use of the TDA is shown in **Figure 7.2**. The TDA was designed to assist caregivers in applying tracheostomy dressings more quickly and efficiently while minimizing discomfort and potential injury to the patient. Initial pilot testing reported easier and quicker dressing changes by nurses and respiratory therapists. Morris and colleagues[41] validated those results by conducting a randomized trial comparing the effectiveness of the TDA compared to the standard method of dressing change. Follow-up questionnaires completed by nurses and patients revealed that the TDA made dressing changes easier than the standard method, and lessened perceived discomfort. The dressing change was also easier than the standard method in patients with thick, short, or obese necks.[41] Intuitively, the recommended frequency for dressing changes should depend on the volume of stomal secretions.

Figure 7.2 Proper use of the Tracheostomy Dressing Applicator (TDA)

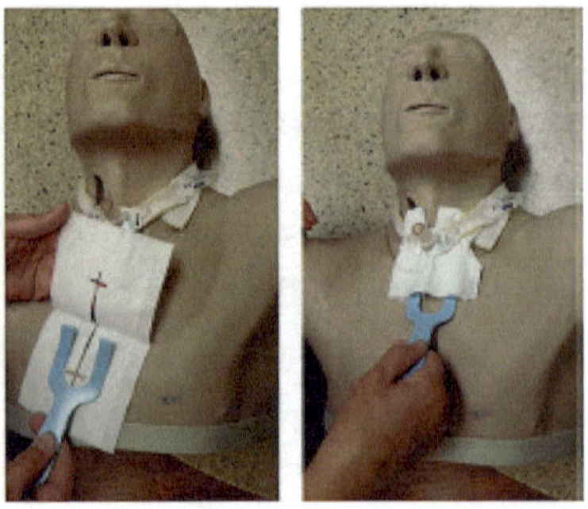

On the left, a drain sponge (pre-split gauze) is opened, and the TDA is inserted between the two layers. On the right, the dressing is pulled snugly around the TDA and then slides under the neck flange.

Photo courtesy of Marie Spitzer and Jeanne Hanneman, www.trachcare.net

Internal and external traction forces can create stomal erosion. The inward pressure of the neck flange against the skin can create erosion of the stoma from the outside. This is most often seen in tracheostomies with a rigid neck flange, as they tilt along one plane. This erosion can be exacerbated in patients with severe neck flexion, as in kyphosis. Excessive outward traction from the ventilator circuit is also a significant problem because it can erode the stoma from the inside. Any additional rotational force, or torque, can also exacerbate this problem. Care must be taken to support the ventilator circuit to prevent this outward traction and torque. There are also devices on the market, like the Shiley Stronghold, that support the connection of the ventilator circuit with the tracheostomy tube.

Occasionally, a large surgical incision is necessary, which can result in stomal discomfort and excessive drainage. One common option is to pack the wound with iodoform gauze. Hotter and Warfield[3] recommended frequent wound packing with cloth ribbon impregnated with 15% sodium chloride (Mesalt). Surgicel can also be used to pack the wound. These approaches offer the advantages of absorbing secretions, keeping the wound dry, and providing a bacteriostatic/bacteriocidal medium.

Mobilization of Secretions

Airway mucus is a viscoelastic gel composed of water, carbohydrates, proteins, and lipids. It is a product of the goblet cells of the airway epithelium and submucosal glands.[42] The volume of mucus secretion is between 10–100 ml per day in a healthy person. In instances of mucus hypersecretion or damage to the epithelial ciliary mechanism, cough is critical for effective bronchial hygiene.[43] Patients unable to cough effectively should be suctioned to prevent obstruction, decrease work of breathing, improve oxygenation and ventilation, and remove bacteria.[44,45] Blackwood appropriately described the goal of suctioning as maximizing the removal of secretions and minimizing hazards.[46] Two papers reviewed the impact of secretion management for patients on mechanical ventilation, albeit the studies involved patients intubated with endotracheal tubes.[47,48] One study examined the suctioning of secretions in pediatric tracheostomy patients.[44] Conclusions are likely applicable to any type of artificial airway, as the principles of secretion management apply to all airway devices.

Suctioning

The problem of secretion retention often begins in the ICU due to a confluence of additive factors. The patient is confined to bed and is relatively immobile. Atelectasis develops, and the coughing reflex is impaired and impeded by endotracheal or tracheostomy tubes. Fluid restriction and diuresis lead to thickened secretions. Finally, comorbid conditions compound the presence of secretions.

Suctioning is not without risk. Numerous complications may result from the suctioning procedure, including cardiac arrhythmias, hypoxemia, atelectasis, bleeding, and infection. Most of these complications can be prevented by meticulous attention to detail and technique.

There are no studies that identify whether the suctioning experience is different in tracheostomies versus endotracheal tubes, but numerous studies have discussed suctioning in general. An adequate explanation of the procedure is essential prior to suctioning. Patients report that suctioning is a painful procedure,[48-50] but it is essential to prevent the accumulation of secretions and promote adequate ventilation. Patients have described the suctioning procedure as "hell on earth,"[51] a feeling of choking or breathlessness,[52] a "frightening and unpleasant experience,"[53] and "horrific" and "terrifying."[51] Peruzzi and Smith[54] recommended that sedation and pain relief could lead to a reduction in stress, anxiety, and pain as well as increased effectiveness of the procedure itself.

Clinical Scenario Cont'd

The patient has remained ventilator-dependent, and she requires frequent suctioning.

Frequency of Suctioning

It is commonly held that suctioning should be done only as needed, rather than on a routine schedule. However, one small study of 14 patients showed no significant variation in complications between patients suctioned routinely and those suctioned as needed.[55] Pedersen and colleagues[48] reported that a number of studies have shown a decreased internal diameter of the airway because of the formation of a biofilm and the accumulation of secretions.[56-58] One group[48] further defined a suctioning frequency of every eight hours in order to reduce the accumulation of secretions and airway occlusion. The American Association of Respiratory Care (AARC) initially recommended that patients may require suctioning at a minimum frequency,[59] but their 2010 guidelines recommended suctioning only when secretions are present.[60]

Kost[10] described the clinical signs that require suctioning, which included visible secretions, audible gurgling, coarse or diminished breath sounds, dyspnea, increased airway pressures, and unexplained desaturation. Though the aforementioned list is intuitive, one must not overlook the importance of suctioning in order to check the patency of the tracheostomy tube, particularly in patients who do not produce secretions on their own due to inadequate physical strength or a neurological impairment of the normal cough reflex. These patients do not produce the usual cues of gurgling or visible secretions within the tube. Frequently, however, secretions are present deep within the airway of these patients, and they must be externally stimulated in order to produce secretions. External stimulation includes suctioning, turning, and regular physical mobility such as range-of-motion exercises. When used in combination on a regular basis, these maneuvers can effectively prevent inspissation of secretions and tube obstruction.

Size of Suction Catheter

The size of the suction catheter should be large enough to effectively remove secretions but small enough to prevent unnecessary obstruction. The effectiveness of the catheter is directly related to its size, with larger catheters being more effective. It is recommended that the catheter be no more than half the internal diameter of the tube. This allows space around the outside of the suction catheter for air to pass to the lungs during suctioning.[48] Odell and others[61] introduced a formula for determining the appropriate size of a suction catheter:

(Endotracheal or tracheostomy tube size in mm – 2) × 2 = size of French catheter in mm.

However, Singh and others[62] suggested using a catheter that is less than ½ the internal lumen, rather than the internal diameter.

Size of suction catheter [Fr] = (tube size in mm – 1) x 2

According to the latter formula, a patient with a size 8 tracheostomy tube should be suctioned with no greater than a 14 French suction catheter.

Application of Suction

It must be remembered that when suction is applied, secretions as well as oxygen are removed from the tracheobronchial tree. The application of suction using high negative pressure for a prolonged period of time could result in trauma to the trachea in addition to hypoxemia and cardiac arrhythmias. These effects can be lessened by hyperoxygenation prior to or during suctioning. It is recommended that suction be applied for less than 12 seconds, only upon withdrawal of the catheter, and with a suction pressure of less than -80 to -120 mm Hg.[10,63] Studies of suctioning focus on defining the optimal pressure to remove secretions while reducing the risks of hypoxia, atelectasis, and tracheal damage.[48,55] Most studies used a suction pressure of -80 to -120 mm Hg,[63] and, in general, higher negative pressure removed secretions more effectively. The safety of higher suction pressures depends on appropriately sized suction catheters to avoid the aforementioned risks. Tenaillon[58] recommended that a pressure of -200 to -300 mm Hg could be used safely with optimal-sized suction catheters. However, Pedersen and colleagues[48] conducted a systematic review of 77 studies and recommended a more cautious approach. They advised -200 mm Hg as the acceptable upper limit. While higher suction pressures are tolerated in patients who have adequate oxygen reserves and hemodynamic profiles, a more cautious approach is advisable for those who do not.

The mobilization of secretions is not limited to suctioning alone, but extends to methods for loosening, thinning, and facilitating the removal of secretions. The basis of mobilization begins with keeping the secretions thin, which is accomplished best with adequate fluid intake. Although a high-humidity tracheostomy collar is effective in providing humidity for comfort, it is not a substitute for adequate hydration. Strategies for the humidification of airways will be discussed elsewhere in this chapter. Patients should be encouraged to drink plenty of fluids. If they are not able to take fluids orally, then additional fluids should be given enterally or parenterally unless otherwise contraindicated.

Oxygenation

Oxygenation is part of the suctioning procedure and is used to avoid hypoxia and its sequelae. Oxygenation can be accomplished prior to, during, and after the procedure. Preoxygenation is frequently used in the immediate postoperative period, but its use tends to diminish over time. Most studies on preoxygenation were done on patients with endotracheal tubes, though it is not known whether a tracheostomy tube would decrease preoxygenation requirements.[64]

One source advises against using preoxygenation with manual resuscitation bags in patients with tracheostomies for head and neck cancer.[18] The authors reported that although preoxygenation with the manual resuscitation bag helped increase inspiratory volume and mobilize secretions, it also placed stress on the anastomosis of the surgical wound. When patients were able to take deep breaths on their own through a tracheal mask, hyperoxygenation with a manual resuscitation bag was not necessary.

Hyperoxygenation is the delivery of oxygen at a greater concentration than the patient is already receiving, up to 100% concentration.[55,56,65,66] Hyperoxygenation is advisable when the patient is critically ill and requires full ventilator support. The benefit from hyperoxygenation is not clear in patients who do not require ventilator support; therefore, its use is directed by clinical need.

Hyperinflation

Hyperinflation is the delivery of a tidal volume greater than that generated mechanically or spontaneously.[55,65] Hyperinflation can be accomplished by adjusting ventilator settings or with a manual resuscitation bag. A common method is the use of 150% of the preset tidal volume for at least three breaths.[63,66] Hyperinflation has been shown to decrease atelectasis and increase functional residual capacity, but the degree of hyperinflation necessary to prevent complications is not well defined.[65]

Some studies separate hyperinflation from oxygenation, although, in practice, hyperinflation is usually used with hyperoxygenation. Stone and colleagues[67] studied the effects of hyperinflation delivered by a ventilator on oxygenation and hemodynamic values. The investigators delivered three consecutive hyperoxygenation/hyperinflation breaths with randomly selected tidal volumes (12, 14, 16, and 18 ml/kg of body weight). Significant increases in mean arterial pressure, pulmonary artery pressure, and cardiac output were recorded during all hyperinflation/suctioning sequences and for all tidal volumes. No incidents of hypoxia were noted with any of the hyperinflation/suctioning sequences.

Depth of Suctioning

Depth of suctioning has also been studied, primarily in neonates and children, but there are a few adult studies. Shallow suctioning is placing the tip of the suction catheter no further than the depth of the airway, and deep suctioning is anything beyond that point. Numerous studies have recommended introducing the suction catheter to the level of the carina, and then withdrawing 1–2 cm before applying suction.[48] In a national sample of pediatric centers, 71.2% of nurses reported inserting the catheter until it met resistance.[66] A Cochrane meta-analysis of deep versus shallow suctioning in infants and children examined the evidence but did not offer an evidence-based preference for one method over the other.[68] However, in patients with large amounts of secretions, deep suctioning may be necessary. One Iranian study in 74 patients[70] examined the effect of deep versus shallow suctioning on heart rate and blood pressure in adults. While they found no significant difference in these two variables, they did find that shallow suctioning required more passes of the suction catheter in order to clear the airway. Thus, they recommended deep suctioning in order to prevent further complications.

Bleeding

Occasionally, mild bleeding occurs as a result of tracheal irritation and erosion during suctioning. This mild bleeding should not prevent suctioning but, rather, should be a cue to switch from standard suction catheters to soft rubber catheters to prevent continued irritation. Complete healing of tracheal lesions has been reported in as little as 24 hours when using softer suction catheters. However, one should be aware that these red rubber suction catheters cannot be used in a patient with a latex allergy, as latex is a product of rubber.

Open Versus Closed Suction Systems

There has been some debate about the use of open versus closed suction systems. Closed suction systems have gained popularity and are used frequently in the ICU while patients are on mechanical ventilation. Their widespread use has gained favor because of their convenience and containment of secretions. There is less concern for hypoxemia and desaturation because the ventilator circuit is not disconnected while suctioning takes place. One cautionary meta-analysis[63] showed that simultaneous insufflation of oxygen with suctioning in closed systems increased hypoxemia.

Most studies comparing open and closed suction systems show no difference in rates of VAP.[71-73] One Turkish study[74] found that closed suction systems resulted in a greater degree of colonization but did not have an effect on the development of VAP.

One animal study compared the effectiveness of secretion removal between the two methods.[75] They found that open suction systems were more effective in removing thick as well as thin secretions no matter what type of ventilator mode was used. Combes, Fauvage, and Oleyer[76] also investigated both infection and effectiveness and found that closed suction systems decreased the rate of VAP but had a volume of tracheal aspirate similar to open systems. Another animal study concluded that desaturation is greater in open suction systems, though this did not exacerbate lung injury over time.[77]

In a review conducted by Maggiore and colleagues,[78] the most frequent complications with open and closed suctioning were related to desaturation and hemorrhagic secretions, and PEEP was the only variable related to desaturation. They suggested that closed suction systems should not be considered routine but should only be used in those patients with higher oxygen requirements and levels of PEEP. Pedersen and others[48] reviewed the evidence and did not find one method superior to the other. The National Health Service systematic review[79] found that there were no significant differences between open and closed suction systems.

Seymour and colleagues[80] studied the recovery times of vital signs and hemodynamic parameters using the closed suction system on mechanically ventilated patients. Spontaneously breathing patients on pressure support mode were compared to those who were heavily sedated or paralyzed on volume-controlled continuous or intermittent mandatory ventilation. The median post-suctioning recovery time was greater than five minutes for minute volume, tidal volume, and respiratory rate. Heart rate, mean arterial pressure, and oxygen saturation increased after suctioning but were not clinically important. Furthermore, post-suctioning changes persisted longer in those breathing spontaneously on pressure support ventilation. The overall conclusion was that the timing of suctioning should be considered when assessing readiness to wean or extubate.

Although convenient, closed suction systems add a great deal of bulk, weight, and traction to the ventilator circuit.[63] Traction or torque on the tracheostomy tube and stoma can have numerous deleterious effects. First, it can shift the position of the tracheostomy tube within the airway and create a leak of air around the cuff. This shifting in position can also move the tip of the tube in contact with the posterior wall of the trachea, resulting in erosion and stenosis. Second, the torque can twist the tube itself inside the trachea and create friction against the endotracheal wall. If these problems are not corrected early, they can create erosion and enlargement of the stoma from the inside. The entire tracheostomy tube, including the cuff, may be visible. It is advisable to eliminate the added traction, whenever possible, and reserve the use of closed suction systems to patients whose hemodynamic status cannot tolerate an open suction system.

Saline Instillation, or Lavage

The use of saline lavage with suctioning has been a topic of great debate for many years. The instillation of 2–10 ml of normal saline, followed by manual ventilation with a resuscitation bag, has been used for loosening and thinning secretions just prior to aggressive suctioning. It was also thought that saline lavage helped lubricate the suction catheter and dislodge bacteria from the biofilm inside the endotracheal tube.[46,48,81,82] Numerous studies have been conducted over the years to evaluate the benefits of saline lavage and its effect on vital signs, oxygenation, airway pressures, infection, and amount of secretions.

Most studies do not favor the use of saline instillation; in fact, most have found detrimental effects.[83-85] Ackerman and Gugerty[86] studied the effect of saline lavage on oxygen saturation and reported significant decreases after suctioning. Patients who received a prior bolus of saline had a much greater fall in saturation compared to those who did not receive a bolus. O'Neal and others[82] used a crossover study design to quantify patients' perceptions of dyspnea with suctioning. Patients self-rated their level of dyspnea using a visual analog scale. They were randomized to two groups involving suctioning with or without saline. There was no difference in the level of dyspnea between the groups. However, the investigators found a significant correlation between age and level of dyspnea, with older patients experiencing higher levels of dyspnea with the use of saline.

No studies have demonstrated that saline instillation actually loosens or thins secretions. Nevertheless, it has been shown to promote vigorous coughing.[48,87] One study showed that less than 19% of the volume of saline was returned with suctioning.[88] Perhaps the unfavorable effects of saline can be attributed to its characteristics. Blackwood[46] reported that the earliest mention of the instillation of saline was questioned by Demers and Saklad[89] "because mucus and water do not mix, even after vigorous shaking."

Gray, MacIntyre, and Kronenberger[90] published one of the few studies to conclude that no apparent detrimental effects resulted from saline instillation. The investigators found that suctioning with and without instillation resulted in no differences in heart rate, respiratory rate, blood pressure, PaO_2, $PaCO_2$, or pH. In addition, there was no difference in peak airway pressure, minute ventilation, saturation, or forced vital capacity. Interestingly, the investigators noted that material suctioned after saline lavage weighed more than that suctioned without saline, and they concluded that the major effect of saline instillation was to stimulate a forceful cough.

Despite the lack of evidence showing its benefit, saline lavage is still widely practiced on a routine basis and is even advocated by some authors.[18,91,92] A national survey of pediatric centers in 1996 showed that 96.2% of nurses reported the use of an irrigant for suctioning, primarily normal saline.[66] Schwenker, Ferrin, and Gift[93] reported the differences between nurses and respiratory therapists regarding the use of saline lavage: 64% of nurses rarely used saline, while 71% of respiratory therapists commonly used it. A later study surveying 27 centers across the United States reported that saline lavage was commonly practiced by 26% of nurses and 51% of respiratory therapists. One reason saline lavage is used frequently is because the technique is still taught in schools.[94] Another study showed that 67% of respiratory therapists in a large acute-care hospital used saline lavage occasionally, and 24% used it routinely. There was no correlation between its use and the level of education or experience of the therapist. Sixty percent of therapists reported learning about the practice in school.[95]

A more recent study surveyed 180 ICU nurses and respiratory therapists regarding suctioning practices.[96] Both groups reported high use of saline lavage as well as decreased oxygen saturation, patient agitation, and increased volume of secretions. They found that 11.5% of respiratory therapists indicated they never used saline lavage, 49.4% used it rarely, 38.8% frequently, and 2.3% always. By contrast, nurses indicated that they used saline lavage in all patients at least some of the time, with 57.8% using it rarely, 41.0% using it frequently, and 1.2% always. The National Health Service[79] provided a systematic review of 95 studies of suctioning and found that there was contradictory evidence regarding benefits of saline lavage.

Paratz and Stockton[76] did a systematic review of 17 papers on saline lavage and found little evidence of benefit, but also minimal evidence of safety risk. Wang and colleagues[83] conducted a meta-analysis, including five randomized controlled studies including 337 patients. They concluded that saline instillation before suctioning does not benefit patients and reduces oxygen saturation for up to five minutes after suctioning. They admitted that the studies they reviewed had low quality and recommended additional studies of large-scale randomized controlled trials.

Caruso and colleagues[98] advocated the use of saline instillation as a means to decrease the incidence of VAP. This was a blinded, controlled study where 262 patients were divided into two groups: a saline group that received 8 ml of saline before tracheal suctioning and a control group that did not. The authors found that the incidence of confirmed VAP was significantly lower in the saline group, although clinical suspicion was the same in both groups. There was no difference between the groups in tube obstruction or atelectasis. The authors concluded that the decrease in VAP could be a result of the improvement in secretion removal, which is primarily due to cough stimulation. They also suggested that frequently rinsing the tube with saline could have reduced biofilm. No apparent effect was noted on mortality, mechanical ventilation, or length of stay. The authors acknowledged the study's limitations, including single-center design and not blinding the respiratory therapists, who performed all of the suctioning.

The AARC guidelines[60] recommended against routine use of saline lavage but acknowledged that its benefits may be in enhanced secretion clearance through cough stimulation[90] as well as decreased VAP.[98] Saline lavage has limited effectiveness in mobilizing, but not thinning, mucous plugs, especially when used in combination with hyperoxygenation, vigorous hyperinflation, and deep suctioning. Its use should be limited to cases in which standard methods have proven ineffective. Preventive measures such as hydration, humidification, and physical mobility should be provided to prevent mucous plugs from obstructing the airway.

Airway Humidification and Secretions

Mucous membranes often require added moisture because the tracheostomy tube bypasses the upper airway. Humidification can be provided by a tracheostomy collar, an HME, or atomized saline. Lack of adequate humidification can cause the trachea to develop squamous metaplasia, desiccation of the tracheal mucosa, and impaired ciliary function.[99] HMEs capture moisture in exhaled air to humidify inspired air. There are models that connect within the ventilator circuit and those that attach directly to the tracheostomy tube.

Humidity prevents the drying of secretions, but a standard measure of optimal humidity is lacking. Proposed measures of optimal humidity include secretion volume and consistency, frequency of suctioning, changes in airway resistance, incidence of airway occlusion, and the need for lavage. Humidity is provided differently for patients on mechanical ventilation from those who are not. Patients on mechanical ventilation require either an in-line HME or heated humidifier. A meta-analysis comparing these two methods of providing humidity in over 1,000 mechanically ventilated patients demonstrated a fourfold increase in the risk of occlusion with an in-line HME.[100] Branson[87] suggested HMEs should not be used in patients with retained secretions and their use should be limited to less than five days. There is no evidence to differentiate the effectiveness of humidification between heated and non-heated humidified tracheostomy collars.

In summary, the mainstay of secretion management rests on three primary interventions: suctioning, humidification, and physical mobility.

MOBILITY

Physical mobility is the third, but equally important, component of secretion mobilization. Physical movement of any kind helps mobilize secretions. Active or passive range-of-motion exercises for bedridden patients can be effective in mobilizing secretions, strengthening respiratory muscles, and improving cough ability. Although there have been no definitive studies to identify the optimal type or frequency of exercise, clinical experience has demonstrated that any type of movement is beneficial for the mobilization of secretions. Active or passive range of motion, frequent turning, and progressive ambulation are all recommended as early as possible. Clinicians may be reluctant to provide mobility to their patients for a variety of reasons, including time constraints or fear of dislodging tracheostomy tubes or other medical devices.

One study published by Morris and others[101] demonstrated benefit from initiating an early mobility program for patients with acute respiratory failure in the ICU. Their mobility therapy program was run by a dedicated team comprised of a critical care nurse, a nursing assistant, and a physical therapist. The protocol included four levels of activity. Level I consisted of passive range of motion administered three times per day to all joints except shoulder extension and hip flexion, which were limited by the patient's position in bed. In Level II, patients were sufficiently alert to participate in therapy and progressed to active range of motion with assistance. In addition to passive range of motion, patients were placed in a sitting position for at least 20 minutes three times a day. In Level III, sitting at the edge of the bed was added to the previous regimen. In Level IV, patients also got out of bed and transferred to a chair for a minimum of 20 minutes per day.

The early mobility therapy program showed a significant decrease in the number of days patients were confined to bed rest, as well as length of stay in the ICU and the hospital. The number of bedrest days was significantly shorter in the therapy group compared to the control (5 versus 11 days) group. Additionally, the length of stay in the ICU was significantly shorter (5.5 in the therapy group compared to 6.9 days in the control group), whereas the overall hospital length of stay was 11.2 days versus 14.5 days, respectively. Finally, there was a near-significant decrease in the incidence of VAP in the therapy group (3%) compared to the control group (7.9%). Paradoxically, the rate of deep vein thrombosis was higher in the therapy group at 5.4%, compared to 1.8% in the control group, although the difference was not significant. There were no incidents of cardiopulmonary compromise or inadvertent removal of any invasive device. This study did not report if this protocol made a difference in the numbers of tracheostomies performed or the time to tracheostomy.

The results of this study demonstrated that the benefits of early mobility outweigh the risks and can make a dramatic difference in length of stay. However, further research is needed to determine the optimal type of therapy, the frequency of therapy, and other outcomes that can be influenced by early mobility.

CLINICAL SCENARIO CONT'D.

The patient continues to be ventilator-dependent and has begun a program of physical therapy, as well as deep breathing and arm exercises. This has resulted in improved cough strength, enabling her to mobilize more secretions on her own and require less suctioning.

ORAL CARE

Poor oral hygiene has been implicated in the development of VAP. Several factors are related to the development of VAP, and they include the colonization of dental plaque, bacterial colonization of the oropharynx, the development of biofilm around the walls of the tube, and accumulation of subglottic secretions around the inflated cuff.

Treatment for VAP is targeted antibiotic therapy in addition to bundled preventative steps as recommended by the Institute for Healthcare Improvement (IHI). Bundled care for mechanically ventilated patients includes elevating the head of the bed, daily sedation vacations, and prophylaxis for peptic ulcer disease and deep venous thrombosis. The elevation of the head of the bed to 30–45 degrees can prevent aspiration of gastrointestinal contents and/or oropharyngeal secretions. Daily ventilator weaning trials coupled with decreased sedation have been shown to lessen time on mechanical ventilation.

Currently, oral care is not included in the ventilator bundle, but it has been adopted in nursing practice as an effective quality measure for the prevention of VAP. Recommended oral care includes toothbrushing, chlorhexidine oral swabbing, and deep subglottic suctioning above the cuff. Several studies have shown that oral decontamination with chlorhexidine decreased rates of VAP with no effect on mortality or length of stay.[102-105] Sona and investigators[106] demonstrated that toothbrushing every 12 hours decreased VAP rates by 46%. Fields[107] demonstrated that toothbrushing every eight hours eradicated VAP for the duration of the study. Bouza and colleagues[108] showed that continuous aspiration of subglottic secretions decreased VAP in patients undergoing major heart surgery. Tsai, Chang, and Lin[109] found that intermittent suctioning of oral secretions prior to each position change decreased rates of VAP from 11% to 2.6% and decreased ICU length of stay from 27.6 to 20.3 days. Interestingly, there is no evidence to show an advantage of continuous over intermittent aspiration of secretions on the development of VAP. Thus, regular oral care and suctioning of subglottic secretions are recommended for patients with tracheostomies.

It is important to distinguish between infection and colonization. Brook[110] reported that 100% of his pediatric patients with long-term tracheostomies were colonized with bacteria within the upper airway. Because most patients with chronic tracheostomies become colonized, it is usually not necessary to treat a positive culture unless there are other signs of active infection, such as leukocytosis, fever, or infiltrates on a chest x-ray.

OTHER TRACHEAL APPLIANCES

Care of the T-Tube

T-tubes are placed to support a weak or damaged trachea (**Figure 7.3**) caused by conditions such as tracheal stenosis, laryngotracheal injuries, tracheal reconstruction, or segmental resection. The T-tube consists of three lumens: the upper intraluminal limb, the lower intraluminal limb, and the external limb. In some cases, it may be necessary to shorten one or both of the intraluminal limbs in order to ensure a proper fit. If the required lengths are known prior to surgery, the manufacturer should be approached to customize the length. Customized kits are also available to cut, taper, and smooth the internal limbs.

Figure 7.3 T-tubes (Hood labs)

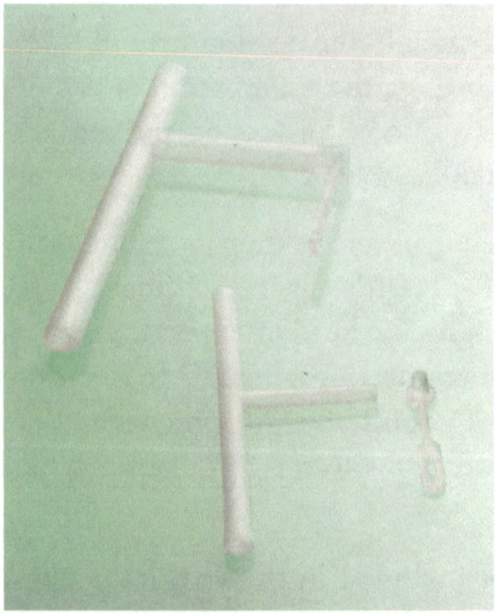

Hood Labs, (Pembroke, Massachusetts)

Generally, the T-tube should be plugged at all times to allow the natural humidification of the upper airway as well as normal phonation. Open T-tubes can promote dry secretions, which have a greater potential for tube obstruction. During the first few postoperative weeks, manufacturers recommend that 1 to 2 ml of saline be instilled into the lumen up to three times daily. The extraluminal limb should be cleaned with a hydrogen peroxide-soaked cotton-tipped swab.

Frequent suctioning several times a day is recommended during the early postoperative period after placement of a T-tube. One source stated that suctioning is not necessary after the initial postoperative period.[111] However, manufacturers recommend suctioning twice daily. The suction catheter should be small enough that it is easily inserted into the T-tube to traverse both the upper and lower limbs. To suction the lower limb, the extraluminal limb should be bent gently upward and the catheter should be directed caudad (**Figure 7.4**). To suction the upper limb, the extraluminal limb should be bent downward and the catheter should be directed cephalad. To avoid mucosal irritation, the suction catheter should not be advanced beyond the level of the intraluminal limbs.

Figure 7.4 Lifting limb of T-tube for suctioning

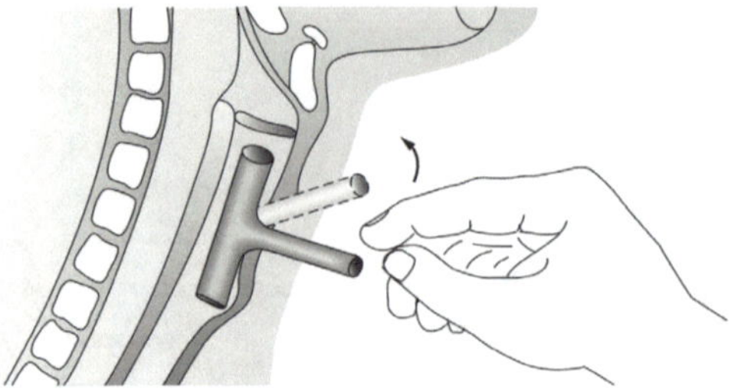

Suctioning the T-tube. Note that the external limb is lifted up to straighten the tube and allow suctioning of the lower intraluminal limb. Alternatively, the external limb is pulled downward to suction the upper intraluminal limb.

A separate 15-mm adapter can be ordered for use when positive-pressure ventilation is needed with a T-tube.[112] An alternative option is to replace the narrow lumen stent with a standard tracheostomy tube, but this approach should be considered carefully in terms of the patency of the airway. Wouters, Byreddy, Gleeson, and Morley[113] presented a stimulating case discussion of the challenges presented by the T-tube when planning anesthetic management for a surgical procedure. Early removal of the T-tube may leave the tracheal graft unsupported. If positive-pressure ventilation is required, a simple solution recommended by the manufacturer is to occlude the upper limb of the T-tube with a small balloon catheter. It is necessary to first tilt the external limb downward and then insert the catheter cephalad and ensure the balloon remains within the T-tube. When the balloon is inflated, a closed system is achieved. Another option is to use a T-tube device called the Hebeler tube, which has a built-in balloon around the upper intraluminal limb.

When a patient has a T-tube in place, emergency equipment, including a smaller cuffed tracheostomy tube and obturator, should be readily available. A curved hemostat should also be available to retrieve any pieces of the tube in case emergency removal is required. As the patient recovers from anesthesia, it is recommended to keep the external lumen plugged if possible. If plugging is not possible, then humidified air or oxygen should be administered through the external lumen.

Postoperative care includes lavaging the tube and cleansing the stoma three times daily with a 1:1 solution of peroxide and saline. The stoma should also be inspected for redness or edema. The ring washer on the external limb should also be monitored for inward or outward movement. Any movement of this washer can indicate edema or posterior displacement.

Care of the Tracheal Cannula

A tracheal cannula is designed to provide a secondary airway instead of a standard tracheostomy tube. It fits within the stoma and abuts the anterior tracheal wall. It is effective for long-term use for up to six months, and then it should be replaced. However, the tracheal cannula cannot be used for positive-pressure ventilation or for patients at risk of aspiration.

After the surgical procedure to insert the cannula, it is recommended that the faceplate be left in place for up to 10 days or until the incision is healed. The skin under the faceplate or ring washer should be cleaned twice per day with cotton-tipped applicators soaked in a 1:1 solution of hydrogen peroxide and saline. When the cannula is not needed for access, it can be plugged.

NUTRITION

Adequate nutrition is important to support wound healing and the strength required to do the work of breathing. It is commonly held that "whenever the gut works, use it." Enteral feeding eliminates the problems associated with parenteral nutrition, especially infection. However, enteral feeding should be administered with caution in the patient with a tracheostomy.

The effectiveness of the swallowing reflex must be determined prior to beginning oral feeding. The prolonged presence of an artificial airway can interfere with glottic function by applying mechanical pressure against the vocal cords. Vocal cord edema, or temporary paresis, can result. Most often these issues resolve over time, but in a few cases, full function of the glottis does not return.

All patients should initially be considered at risk for aspiration when given enteral feedings. Patients should be placed with the head of their bed elevated at least 30 degrees or higher. The cuff of the tracheostomy tube should be inflated if there is a question of airway protection. A common practice had been to add blue food dye to enteral feedings to detect aspiration through the tube. However, several studies described severe consequences of prolonged use of blue dye, including enteral bacterial infections, diarrhea, systemic dye absorption, and death. The incidence of toxicity was higher in septic patients.[114-116] Consequently, the American Association of Critical Care Nurses (AACN) banned the use of blue dye mixed with enteral feedings,[117] although blue dye may still be used as part of a test of swallowing function.[118]

Continuous Versus Intermittent Feedings

Small-bore enteral feeding tubes are preferred over larger-bore nasogastric tubes. The smaller diameter reaches farther into the alimentary tract, making aspiration less risky, which is supported by guidelines.[119] An important consideration with enteral feedings should be the regular assessment of residual volumes. Guidelines suggest that, in the absence of other signs of intolerance, one should provide enteral feeding unless the gastric residual volume is greater than 500 mls.[119] Enteral feedings should never be initiated until proper placement of the feeding tube has been confirmed. Local policies should govern the optimal method of assessing their proper placement.

CARE PATHWAYS

The National Confidential Enquiry into Patient Outcome and Death (NCEPOD)[120] published their findings through a national quality improvement effort in the UK. Their primary aim was to explore factors surrounding insertion and subsequent management of tracheostomies. During the 11-week study period, 2,546 tracheostomies were placed. They found that 85.4% of hospitals delivered training programs in accordance with clinical consensus guidelines. Nearly 64% of hospitals had a protocol in place to help patients communicate. Fifty-four percent of hospitals had a resuscitation policy in place for tracheostomy patients. Less than half of the hospitals had a resuscitation policy for neck breathers. Only 21.2% of hospitals provided regular audits of tracheostomy care, and nearly 64% reported an expected level of competency of staff caring for the tracheostomy. Recommendations included capnography and a difficult airway cart in the critical care unit, training programs for staff in blocked and displaced tubes as well as difficult tube changes, and staff competencies for care and resuscitation.

One group[121] tested a care pathway and nursing education program to improve tracheostomy outcomes. They found that standardizing tracheostomy care resulted in increased patient readiness for hospital discharge and decreased their readmission rates for issues related to the tracheostomy.

CARE OF THE PATIENT AT HOME

Patients going home with a tracheostomy require much pre-planning and at-home care. Family members must be taught the steps of care and strategies to prevent complications. Capable patients should learn how to care for themselves. The goal of this teaching is for the patients and caregivers to feel safe at home and in the community.

In response to a high readmission rate, one group[122] developed a tracheostomy training program for caregivers of patients with tracheostomies, which was developed in response to a high readmission rate with head and neck cancer patients discharged with a tracheostomy. The T-CARES program (Tracheostomy Care Anxiety Relief through Education and Support), consisted of an 18-minute video demonstration, return demonstration, and skills assessment. Results showed a significant decrease in anxiety and increased competency in tracheostomy care.

CLINICAL SCENARIO CONT'D.

> The patient has made a great deal of progress, and now has a cuffless tracheostomy tube. Because of a major upcoming surgical procedure, the current plan is to discharge the patient home with the tracheostomy, with future decannulation planned after the procedure.
>
> The patient and family meet with the tracheostomy specialist to review care of the tracheostomy. The specialist uses a tracheostomy model to provide a demonstration of all procedures (suctioning, stoma cleaning, inner cannula cleaning, tube cleaning, changing dressing, etc.) Each family member and the patient are asked to do a return demonstration of each procedure. They are encouraged to assume all care of the tracheostomy tube with nursing supervision so they have the opportunity to feel comfortable with the care prior to discharge.
>
> The case manager reviews the list of required supplies and coordinates with the patient's insurance company and the home care supply company to ensure the supplies are delivered to the home prior to the patient's arrival.

Patient and family teaching should begin with a review of the normal anatomy and physiology of the airway. Reviewing the location of the esophagus related to the trachea can sometimes help patients and family members understand the need for a cuff on the tracheostomy tube when the patient's swallowing mechanism is not optimal.

Patients and family members need to have a list of supplies so they can plan timely replenishment of inventory. All home caregivers need to know the location of emergency supplies so they can be reached immediately. They need to know what type of tracheostomy tube patients have in place and what size suction catheters to use. They should also have an extra tracheostomy tube of the same size and one size smaller to manage inadvertent decannulation if it occurs.

Patients need to know that tracheostomy care at home can be done as a clean procedure, rather than the sterile technique they saw in the hospital. All care of the tracheostomy begins with thorough hand washing. Patients and family members should be taught to wash their hands before touching the tracheostomy and again after care is complete. Gloves can and should also be used, but not as a substitute for handwashing.

In addition to a review of anatomy and physiology, discharge teaching should also include care of the stoma, care of the inner cannula, suctioning, care of the cuff, and managing emergencies. Caregivers and patients should have a list of phone numbers to contact for support as well as general questions. These emergency phone numbers should include the primary care practitioner, the tracheostomy specialist, the home care company, and the number to summon emergency personnel (e.g., 911). Upon discharge, a phone call should be placed to alert the local fire department that the patient has a tracheostomy. This advance notification could facilitate the timely arrival of the paramedics in the event of an emergency when a tracheostomy patient in distress may not be able to speak.

It is best to conduct teaching sessions with the patient and all family members together, so they can all hear the same information at the same time and discuss it among themselves and with the health professional. Supplemental written information should also accompany a demonstration of the techniques because patients and family members are usually overwhelmed with the amount of information provided. They will need reinforcement and repetition in order to feel competent.

Patients and family members should also be taught how to use the manual resuscitation bag. It can be used to give extra breaths with suctioning when needed, but it can also be used in an emergency to deliver air and facilitate a cough.

One of the most difficult procedures for family members to master is suctioning. The procedure itself is overtly unpleasant, and they do not want to harm their loved one and are usually reluctant to cause any discomfort. It is advisable to inform family members that inefficient suctioning is a disservice to their loved one. Each suctioning attempt should be with the goal of mobilizing as great a volume of secretions as possible, thereby minimizing multiple passes of the suction catheter. Useful advice to family members is to provide deep suctioning on the first attempt at minimum. Deep suctioning retrieves a large amount of secretions and also facilitates a deep cough, which, in turn, mobilizes more secretions. Subsequent passes of the suction catheter can be determined based on the yield of the previous pass. The usual maximum for each episode is three passes, but this depends on the results. The patient is usually aware of the need for suctioning by the time of hospital discharge. From the patient's perspective, optimal breathing is the anticipated result of suctioning.

In the home setting, Medicare and most insurance companies provide for 90 suction catheters per month, averaging three per day. This may not be enough to manage large volumes of secretions. In contrast to the hospital setting, suction catheters can be reused all day in the home. The catheter should be rinsed thoroughly to remove obvious secretions from the inside by filling a small disposable paper cup with tap water and flushing the catheter. In addition, the outside of the catheter should be wiped clean to remove secretions. Then the catheter can be laid on a paper towel and allowed to air dry in between uses. At the end of the day, the catheter and the paper cup can be discarded.

Patients need to be taught to observe the quality of their secretions. Changes in color, quantity, odor, or thickness should be watched closely and reported promptly to their health care professional.

Patients also need to cleanse the stoma to keep it dry and free of secretions. In the hospital, they may have seen the nurse use hydrogen peroxide. However, long-term use of peroxide on the skin can produce irritation. For this reason, the stoma should be cleansed with cotton-tipped swabs dipped in tap water or saline. Patients and family members should be told to examine the stoma area for redness, swelling, bleeding, or pus. Any of these signs should be reported to their health care provider.

In the early postoperative period, patients are encouraged to keep a drain sponge around the stoma site to protect the skin from constant exposure to secretions. Also, a drain sponge helps cushion the neck flange against the skin of the neck. Only pre-split sponges should be used at the stoma site. Gauze dressings should not be cut because shreds may become embedded in the tissue and create inflammation.

Patients and family members should also be taught to clean the stoma and inner cannula on a regular basis. Depending on the patient's condition, a larger volume of secretions is often produced in the early postoperative period and tends to lessen over time. For this reason, care of the stoma and inner cannula is often done routinely up to three times per day in the hospital and can be decreased to twice per day when at home and secretions have diminished.

MANAGING HOME EMERGENCIES

Before emergency personnel are mobilized, patients and family members must begin efforts to manage an emergency (see **Table 7.2**). By far, most tracheostomy emergencies are the result of mucous plugs. Patients and family members should be aware that the best way to manage mucous plugs is to prevent them with adequate hydration to thin secretions and vigorous physical mobility to loosen secretions, strengthen respiratory muscles, and facilitate an effective cough to expel secretions.

Table 7.2. Managing Respiratory Emergency at Home
1. Remove inner cannula (clean if obstructed).
2. Suction deeply.
3. If no relief, contact emergency services.
4. Use manual resuscitation bag to provide rescue breaths.
5. Change entire tracheostomy tube (if tube is still obstructed and stoma is mature, remove tube and suction directly in the stoma).
6. Provide Heimlich maneuver.

The initial presenting symptom of a mucous plug is usually dyspnea or shortness of breath. The patient should first be taught to check his or her inner cannula, if present. After it is removed, it will be obvious if it is clogged with secretions; if it is, it should be cleaned or replaced. If removal of the inner cannula is not successful in resolving the dyspnea, the problem is still likely to be a mucous plug farther down in the tracheobronchial tree. If removal of the inner cannula does not relieve the shortness of breath, the patient should suction himself. If the patient is still short of breath after these two maneuvers, emergency help should be summoned. Meanwhile, there are other steps the patient can take. The manual resuscitation bag can be used to provide rescue breaths. Several small breaths can be delivered, followed by one or two large and forceful breaths. The purpose of the larger breaths is to promote a strong cough.

Patients and family members should be taught the Heimlich maneuver in order to help dislodge a mucous plug. If all of the aforementioned steps have not been successful, the entire tracheostomy tube should be changed. Often, a mucous plug is pulled out when the entire tracheostomy tube is changed.

ACTIVITIES OF DAILY LIVING

At home, patients should be able to assimilate well into usual family life. Outside of the care required for the tracheostomy, there are few restrictions. A tracheostomy need not restrict activities, but a few simple precautions are necessary. Patients can shower and bathe normally as long as care is taken to avoid splashing or spraying water into the tracheostomy. Several devices such as shower collars can be used if there is concern about splashed water. Of course, swimming and water sports are contraindicated.

Tracheostomy patients may be more sensitive to odors and inhalants. Perfume and cologne use may need to be restricted, and smoking should not be allowed in the home.

Patients with tracheostomies need to minimize their exposure to dust, other allergens, and pet hair. A stoma grid or filter can be used if there are concerns about inhaled particulate matter. Pets that sleep next to, or in close proximity to, patients may need to be relocated to minimize the inhalation of pet hair or dander. If patients will be exposed to environmental hazards, a filter or mask can be used to cover the tracheostomy.

Patients with tracheostomies who experience some discomfort with lack of humidity can use an HME. Misted saline (such as Ocean nasal spray) can be instilled into the tracheostomy and mucous membranes. Alternatively, patients can become comfortable simply by using a room humidifier..

SUMMARY

Patients with tracheostomies require vigilant care in order to prevent complications. The most common complication is the development of mucous plugs resulting from thickened secretions. Routine care includes cleaning the stoma and inner cannula as well as regular tube changes to prevent infection. Colonization is common but does not require treatment unless there are outward signs of infection.

When discharged home, patients and their family members require extensive teaching in order to become comfortable with daily care and emergency procedures. It is essential for all caregivers to ensure supplies and emergency equipment are always available and functional. With attention to proper care, patients with tracheostomies can live long and productive lives.

KEY POINTS

- During the first postoperative week, the security of the tracheostomy tube is a priority.
- The inner cannula, when present, should be cleaned regularly to prevent tube obstruction.
- Suctioning is a key intervention to remove secretions, stimulate a cough, and assess patency of the tracheostomy tube.
- Cuff pressures should be maintained at 20–25 cm H_2O to prevent overinflation or underinflation of the cuff.
- Routine tube changes should take place every 1–2 months.
- The mainstay of secretion management includes adequate hydration and humidity, suctioning, and physical mobility.
- Care of the tracheostomy patient at home starts with education, can be adequately achieved by clean technique (rather than sterile), and should be integrated into the daily routine.

Available Resources for the Tracheostomy Patient

There are many resources available for patients with tracheostomies and many more for the health care professional.

Patient Resources

Devices for laryngectomy patients, including HMEs, shower collars, phonating devices such as electrolarynx, and reference books. Luminaud, Inc. Retrieved 7/5/18, from http://www.luminaud.com.

Discussion forums for tracheostomy patients and caregivers. Tracheotomy.info: A community for tracheotomy wearers and the people who love them. Accessed July 26, 2020, from http://www.tracheotomy.info/index.php.

Information about oral cancer, American Head and Neck Society. Accessed July 26, 2020, from https://www.ahns.info/patient-information/

Pediatric tracheostomy information, advice for parents, and listserv. Aaron's Tracheostomy Page, Accessed July 26, 2020 from www.tracheostomy.com.

Tracheostomy products, featuring Moore tracheostomy tubes, Montgomery cannulas. Also features protective neckwear, shower protection, cleaning supplies, and accessories. Boston Medical Products, Inc. Accessed July 26, 2020 from http://www.trachs.com.

Professional Resources

Agency for Clinical Innovation (2013). Care of adult patients in acute care facilities with a tracheostomy: Clinical practice guideline. www.aci.health.nsw.gov.au. Accessed July 26, 2020.

Devices for laryngectomy patients. Atos Medical. Accessed July 26, 2020 from http://www.atosmedical.com.

Education and research forum for healthcare professionals regarding care of the tracheostomy patient, Accessed July 26, 2020, www.TrachResource.com.

Global Tracheostomy Collaborative, International organization dedicated to tracheostomy patient safety and quality outcomes. Accessed July 26, 2020, www.globaltrach.org.

Intensive Care Society, 2014, Standards for the care of adult patients with a temporary tracheostomy: Standards and Guidelines. Accessed July 26, 2020, https://www.ics.ac.uk/ICS/ICS/GuidelinesAndStandards/ICSGuidelines.aspx,

National Tracheostomy Safety Program, National Health Service (UK) effort to improve tracheostomy patient safety. Accessed July 26, 2020, www.tracheostomy.org.uk.

Passy-Muir speaking valves and educational materials. Passy-Muir, Inc. Accessed July 26, 2020, from http://www.passy-muir.com.

Pilling products catalog. Teleflex Medical. 2917 Weck Drive, Research Triangle Park, NC 27709.

Portex and Bivona tracheostomy products. Smiths Medical. Accessed July 26, 2020 from http://www.smiths-medical.com/products/tracheostomy.

Shiley tracheostomy products. Medtronic. Accessed July 26, 2020, from http://www.medtronic.com/covidien/en-us/products/tracheostomy.html

Tracheostomy and airway products, featuring Moore tracheostomy tubes, Montgomery cannulas. Boston Medical Products. Accessed July 26, 2020, from http://www.bosmed.com.

Tracheostomy Dressing Applicator (TDA), Accessed July 26, 2020, www.trachcare.net, info@trachcare.net.

Tracheostomy Review and Management Service (TRAMS). Multidisciplinary tracheostomy management program across three campuses and the communities surrounding Melbourne, Australia. Accessed July 26, 2020, from www.tracheostomyteam.org.

Review Questions

1. Tracheostomy cuff pressure above 26 cm H_2O can create significant complications, including:
   a. Ventilator-associated pneumonia, tracheal stenosis
   b. Tracheomalacia, tracheal stenosis, tracheal ischemia
   c. Leakage of oropharyngeal secretions around the cuff
   d. Sepsis, hypovolemic shock, tracheal stenosis

   ANSWER: B is correct because all these conditions are related to excessively high cuff pressures. Choices A and C are incorrect because VAP and leakage of secretions can result from excessively low cuff pressure. Choice D is not correct because sepsis and hypovolemic shock are not related to cuff pressure.

2. Continued exposure of the stoma to secretions can lead to which of the following?
   a. Ventilator-associated pneumonia, tracheal stenosis, stomal cellulitis
   b. Inflammation, loose tracheostomy ties
   c. Inflammation, stomal infection, cellulitis
   d. Mucous plugs, ventilator-associated pneumonia, rash

   ANSWER: C. All of the other choices can be complications of a tracheostomy, but not directly related to stomal secretions.

3. A 76-year-old man received a tracheostomy three weeks ago, and he has a dual cannula cuffed tracheostomy tube, size 8. The nurse reports that his secretions are thick and copious, and he requires frequent suctioning, but vital signs and oxygen saturation are stable with suctioning. What is the best way to suction this patient?
   a. Preoxygenate, saline lavage, insert suction catheter 4 cm, then apply suction as it is withdrawn
   b. Saline lavage with closed suction system, insert suction catheter until gentle resistance is felt, then apply suction as it is withdrawn
   c. Insert suction catheter until gentle resistance is felt, apply suction as catheter is withdrawn, oxygenate if needed
   d. Suction patient on a routine schedule using deep suctioning technique

   ANSWER: C. Preoxygenation and closed suction systems are not required for all patients. Saline lavage is not recommended for routine use. Deep suctioning is preferable to mobilize secretions and decrease the number of passes required. Suctioning cannot be scheduled and is provided as needed.

4. A patient received a tracheostomy three days ago, and the tube is sutured in place. A large amount of dried blood and secretions have collected around the stoma and under the neck flange. Which of the following is the appropriate action regarding cleansing of the stoma?
   a. Remove and replace the tracheostomy ties so the stoma can be adequately cleansed
   b. Change the tracheostomy ties to prevent possible infection
   c. Remove sutures to allow adequate visualization and cleansing of the stoma
   d. Delay thorough cleansing of the stoma until the first tracheostomy tube change

ANSWER: D. The priority during the early postoperative period is tube security. Any attempt to manipulate the tracheostomy tube during the early postoperative period presents a risk of tube decannulation/dislodgement and loss of the airway.

5. Patient and caregiver education should include which of the following?
   a. Sterile technique with suctioning, change tube daily
   b. Use of gloves can replace handwashing, keep tracheostomy ties snug
   c. Shallow suctioning using sterile technique, re-use suction catheters if needed
   d. Clean technique with suctioning, Heimlich maneuver, and keep stoma clean and dry

ANSWER: D. Choice A is not correct because sterile technique is required in the hospital, but not at home, and the tube should be changed at least monthly. Choice B is incorrect because handwashing is always required. Choice C is incorrect because shallow suctioning is less effective than deep suctioning.

REFERENCES

1. Seay SJ, Gay SL. Tracheostomy emergencies: Correcting accidental decannulation or displaced tracheostomy tube. *Amer J Nurs.* 2002;102(3):59-63.
2. Mitchell RB, Hussey HM, Setzen G, Jacobs IN, Nussenbaum B, Dawson C, Brown CA, et al. Clinical consensus statement: Tracheostomy care. *Otolaryngol Head Neck Surg.* 2013;148(1):6-20.
3. Hotte AN, Warfield K. Technique for promoting healing of complex tracheostomy wounds. *Otolaryngol Head Neck Surg.* 1997;11(6):693-695.
4. Nouraei SA, Nouraei SM, Upile T, Taylor M, Patel A, Sandhu GS. A four-point suture fixation technique for securing surgical tracheostomies. *Clin Otolaryngol.* 2008;33:196-199.
5. Liew L, Gibbins N, Oyarzabal M. How I do it: Securing tracheostomy tubes. *Eur Arch Otorhinolaryngol.* 2008;265(5):607, 608.
6. Agency for Clinical Innovation (ACI, 2013). Care of adult patients in acute care facilities with a tracheostomy: Clinical practice guideline. Retrieved from www.aci.health.nsw.gov.au/resources/clinical-guidelines. Accessed July 25, 2020.
7. American Thoracic Society. Care of the child with a chronic tracheostomy. *Amer J Respir Crit Care Med.* 2000;161:297-308.
8. Dixon L, Wasson D. Comparing use and cost effectiveness of tracheostomy tube securing devices. *Medsurg Nurs.* 1998;7(5):270-274.
9. Yaremchuk, K. Regular tracheostomy tube changes to prevent formation of granulation tissue. *Laryngoscope.* 2003;113:1-10.
10. Kost, KM. Tracheostomy in the intensive care unit setting. In Myers EN, Johnson JT eds. *Tracheotomy: Airway management, communication, and swallowing.* San Diego, CA: Plural Publishing; 2008:83-116.
11. Burns SM, Spilman M, Wilmoth D, Carpenter R, Turrentine B, Wiley B, Marshall M, Martens S, Burns JE, Truwit JD. Are frequent inner cannula changes necessary? A pilot study. *Heart Lung.* 1998;27(1):58-62.
12. Hettige R, Arora A, Ifeacho S, Narula A. Improving tracheostomy management through design, implementation and prospective audit of a care bundle: how we do it. *Clin Otolaryngol.* 2008;33:472-494.
13. Cetto R, Arora A, Hettige R, Nel M, Benjain L, Gomez CMH, Oldfield WLG, Narula AA. Improving tracheostomy care: A prospective study of the multidisciplinary approach. Clin Otolaryngol. 2011;36:482-488.
14. Mah JW, Staff II, Fisher SR, Butler KL. Improving decannulation and swallowing function: A comprehensive multidisciplinary approach to post-tracheostomy care. *Respir Care.* 2017;62(2):137-143.
15. Crimlisk JT, O'Donnell C, Grillone GA. Standardizing adult tracheostomy tube styles: What is the clinical and cost-effective impact? *Dimens Crit Care Nurs.* 2006;25(1):35-43.
16. Johnson JT, Wagner RL, Sigler BA. Disposable inner cannula tracheostomy tube: A prospective clinical trial. *Otolaryngol Head Neck Surg. 1988;*99(1):83-84.
17. Hudak M, Hickey MM. Nursing management of the patient with a tracheostomy. In Myers EM, Johnson JT eds. *Tracheotomy: Airway management, communication, and swallowing.* San Diego, CA: Plural Publishing, 2008.
18. Bjorling G, Belin A, Hellstrom C, Schedin U, Ransjo U, Alenius M, Johansson UB. Tracheostomy inner cannula care: A randomized crossover study of two decannulation procedures. *Amer J Infec Contr.* 2007;35:600-605.

19. Backman S, Bjorling G, Johansson UB, Lysdahl M, Markstrom A, Schedin U, Aune RE, Frostell C, Karlsson S. Material wear of polymeric tracheostomy tubes: A six-month study. *Laryngoscope*. 2009;119:657-664.
20. Silva RA, Carver RA, Ojano-Dirain CP, Antonelli PJ. Efficacy of disinfecting solutions in removing biofilms from polyvinyl chloride tracheostomy tubes. *Laryngoscope*. 2013;123:259-263.
21. Rodney J, Ojano-Dirain CP, Antonelli PJ, Silva RC. Effect of repeated tracheostomy tube reprocessing on biofilm formation. *Laryngoscope*. 2016;126:996-999.
22. Leonhard M, Assadian O, Zumtobel M, Schneider-Stickler B. Microbiological evaluation of different reprocessing methods for cuffed and un-cuffed tracheostomy tubes in homecare and hospital setting. *GMS Hygiene Infec Contr*. 2016;11:1-7.
23. Bernhard WN, Yost L, Joynes D, Cothalis S, Turndorf H. Cuff pressures in endotracheal and tracheostomy tubes. Related cuff physical characteristics. *Chest*. 1985;87:720-725.
24. Rello J, Sonora R, Jubert P, Artigas A, Rue M, Valles J. Pneumonia in intubated patients: Role of respiratory airway care. *Amer J Respir Crit Care Med*. 1996;154(1):111-115.
25. Sole ML, Penoyer DA, Su X, Jimenez E, Kalita SJ, Poallilo E, et al. Assessment of endotracheal cuff pressure by continuous monitoring: A pilot study. *Amer J Crit Care*. 2009;18(2):133-143.
26. Faris C, Koury E, Philpott J, Sharma S, Tolley N, Narula A. Estimation of tracheostomy tube cuff pressure by pilot balloon palpation. *J Laryngol Otol*. 2007;121(9):869-871.
27. Guisti GD, Rogari C, Gili A, Nisi F. Cuff pressure monitoring by manual palpation in intubated patients: How accurate is it? A manikin simulation study. *Austral Crit Care*. 2017;30:234-238.
28. Stewart SL, Secrest JA, Norwood BR, Zachary R. A comparison of endotracheal tube cuff pressures using estimation techniques and direct intracuff measurement. *AANA J*. 2003;71(6):443-7.
29. Fernandez R, Blanch L, Mancebo J, Bonsoms N, Artigas A. Endotracheal tube cuff pressure assessment: Pitfalls of finger estimation and need for objective measurement. *Crit Care Med*. 1990;18(12):1423-1426.
30. Hoffman RJ, Parwani V, Hahn I. Experienced emergency medicine physicians cannot safely inflate or estimate endotracheal tube cuff pressure using standard techniques. *Amer J Emerg Med*. 2006;24:139-143.
31. Morris LG, Zoumalan RA, Roccaforte JD, Amin MR. Monitoring tracheal tube cuff pressures in the intensive care unit: A comparison of digital palpation and manometry. *Ann Otol Rhinol,Laryngol*. 2007;116(9):639-642.
32. Shapiro BA, Harrison RA, Kacmarek RM, Cane RD. *Clinical Application of Respiratory Care* (3rd ed.). Chicago: Yearbook Medical Publishers, 1985.
33. Alcan AO, van Giersbergen MY, Dincarslan G, Hepcivici Z, Kaya E, Uyar M. Effect of patient position on endotracheal cuff pressure in mechanically ventilated critically ill patients. *Austral Crit Care*. 2017:30(5):267-272.
34. Duguet A, D'Amico L, Biondi G, Prodanovic H, Gonzalez-Bermejo J, Similowski T. Control of tracheal cuff pressure: A pilot study using a pneumatic device. *Intens Care Med*. 2007;33:128-132.
35. Nseir S, Zerimech F, Fournier C, Lubret R, Ramon P, Durocher A, Balduyck M. Continuous control of tracheal cuff pressure and microaspiration of gastric contents in critically ill patients. *Amer J Respir Crit Care Med*. 2011;184(9):1041-1047.

36. Coffman HMS, Rees CJ, Sievers AEF, Belafsky PC. Proximal suction tracheotomy tube reduces aspiration volume. *Otolaryngol Head Neck Surg.* 2008;138(4):441-445.
37. Dennis-Rouse MD, Davidson JE. An evidence-based evaluation of tracheostomy care practices. *Crit Care Nurs Q.* 2008;31(2):150-160.
38. Wright SE, Van Dahm K. Long term care of the tracheostomy patient. *Clin Chest Med.* 2003;24:473-487.
39. Tsunezuka Y, Suzuki M, Nitta K, Oda M. The use of fibrous wound dressing sheets made of carboxymethylcellulose natrium in the postoperative management of tracheostomy. *Kyobu Geka.* 2005;58(12):1063-1067.
40. Nance-Floyd B. Tracheostomy care: An evidence-based guide to suctioning and dressing changes. *Amer Nurs Today.* 2011;6(7):14-17.
41. Morris LL, Kuncis M, Perleberg D, Kuczek, A, Kashul K, Zabel D, Heinemann A, Semik P. New device makes tracheostomy dressing changes easier and more comfortable. *Rehabil Nurs* 2020;00(0), 00–00. doi: 10.1097/rnj.0000000000000302.
42. Rogers DF. Physiology of airway mucus secretion and pathophysiology of hypersecretion. *Respir Care.* 2007;52(9):1134-1146.
43. Rubin BK. Physiology of airway mucus clearance. *Respir Care.* 2002;47(7):761.
44. Ireton J. Tracheostomy suction: A protocol for practice. *Paediatr Nurs.* 2007;19(10):14–18.
45. Lewis RM. Airway clearance techniques for the patient with an artificial airway. *Respir Care.* 2002;47(7):808-817.
46. Blackwood B. Normal saline instillation with endotracheal suctioning: Primum non nocere (first do no harm). *J Adv Nurs.* 1999;29(4):928-934.
47. Branson RD, Campbell RS, Chatburn RL, Covington J. Endotracheal suctioning of mechanically ventilated adults and children with artificial airways. *Respir Care.* 1993;38(5):500-504.
48. Pedersen CM, Rosendahl-Nielsen M, Hjermind J, Egerod I. Endotracheal suctioning of the adult intubated patient: What is the evidence? *Intens Crit Care Nurs.* 2009;25(1):21-30.
49. Arroyo-Novoa CM, Figueroa-Ramos MI, Puntillo KA, Stanik-Hutt J, Thompson CL, White C, Wild LR. Pain related to tracheal suctioning in awake acutely and critically ill adults: A descriptive study. *Intens Crit Care Nurs.* 2008;24:20-27.
50. Puntillo KA, White C, Morris AB, Perdue ST, Stanik-Hutt J, Thompson CL, Wild LR. Patients' perceptions and responses to procedural pain: Results from Thunder Project II. *Amer J Crit Care.* 2001;10:238-251.
51. Sawyer N. Back from the twilight zone. *Nurs Times.* 1997;93(7):28–29.
52. Bergbom-Engberg I, Halijamae H. A retrospective study of patients' recall of respiratory treatment: Nursing care factors and feelings of security/insecurity. *Intens Care Nurs.* 1989;4(3):95-101.
53. Griggs A. Tracheostomy: Suctioning and humidification. *Nurs Stand.* 1998;13(2):49-53.
54. Peruzzi WT, Smith B. Bronchial hygiene therapy. *Crit Care Clin*; 1995;11(1):716-720.
55. Wood CJ. Can nurses safely assess the need for endotracheal suction in short-term ventilated patients, instead of using routine techniques? *Intens Crit Care Nurs.* 1998;14(4):170-178.
56. Glass CA, Grap MJ. Ten tips for safer suctioning. *Amer J of Nurs.* 1995;95(5):51-53.
57. Shah C, Kollef MH. Endotracheal tube intraluminal volume loss among mechanically ventilated patients. *Crit Care Med.* 2004;32(1):120-125.
58. Tenaillon A. Tracheobronchial suctions during mechanical ventilation. *Update Intens Care Emerg Med.* 1990;10:196-200.

59. Branson RD. Secretion management in the mechanically ventilated patient. *Respir Care.* 2007;52(10):1328-1347.
60. American Association of Respiratory Care Clinical Practice Guidelines. Endotracheal suctioning of mechanically ventilated patients with artificial airways. *Resp Care.* 2010;55(6):758-764.
61. Odell A, Allder A, Bayne R, Everett C, Scott S, Still B, West S. Endotracheal suction for adult non-head injured patients. A review of the literature. *Intens Crit Care Nurs.* 1993;9(4):274-278.
62. Singh NC, Kissoon N, Frewen T, Tiffin N. Physiological responses to endotracheal and oral suctioning in paediatric patients: The influence of endotracheal tube sizes and suction pressures. *Int J Crit Cor Care Med.* 1991;2(6):345-50.
63. Oh H, Seo W. A meta-analysis of the effects of various interventions in preventing endotracheal suction-induced hypoxemia. *J Clin Nurs.* 2003;12:912-924.
64. St. John RE, Malen JF. Contemporary issues in adult tracheostomy management. *Crit Care Nurs Clin N Amer.* 2004;16(3):413-430.
65. Day T, Farnell S, Wilson-Barnett J. Suctioning: A review of current research recommendations. *Intens Crit Care Nurs.* 2002;18(2):79-89.
66. Swartz K, Noonan DM, Edwards-Beckett J. A national survey of endotracheal suctioning techniques in the pediatric population. *Heart Lung.* 1996;25(1):52-60.
67. Stone KS, Preusser BA, Groch KF, Karl JI, Gonyon DS. The effect of lung hyperinflation and endotracheal suctioning on cardiopulmonary hemodynamics. *Nurs Res.* 1991;40(2):76-80.
68. Spence K, Gillies D, Waterworth L. Deep versus shallow suction of endotracheal tubes in ventilated neonates and young infants. *Cochrane Database Syst Rev.* 2003;3:CD003309.
69. Van de Leur JP, Zwaveling JH, Loef BG, Van der Shans CP. Endotracheal suctioning versus minimally invasive airway suctioning in intubated patients: A prospective randomized controlled trial. *Intens Care Med.* 2003;29(3):426-432.
70. Irajpour A, Abbasinia M, Hoseini A, Kashefi P. Effects of shallow and deep endotracheal tube suctioning on cardiovascular indices in patients in intensive care units. *Ir J Nurs Midwif Res.* 2014;19(4):366-370.
71. Niel-Weise BS, Snoeren RL, van den Broek PJ. Policies for endotracheal suctioning of patients receiving mechanical ventilation: A systematic review of randomized controlled trials. *Infec Contr Hospl Epidem* 2007;28(5):531-536.
72. Siempos II, Vardakas KZ, Falagas ME. Closed tracheal suction systems for prevention of ventilator-associated pneumonia. *Brit J Anaesth.* 2008;100(3):299-306.
73. Vonberg RP, Eckmanns T, Welte T, Gastmeier P. Impact of the suctioning system (open vs. closed) on the incidence of ventilation-associated pneumonia: Meta-analysis of randomized controlled trials. *Intens Care Med.* 2006;32(9):1329-1335.
74. Topeli A, Harmanci A, Cetinkaya Y, Akdeniz S, Unal S. Comparison of the effect of closed versus open endotracheal suction systems on the development of ventilatorassociated pneumonia. *J Hosp Infec.* 2004;58(1):14-19.
75. Copnell B, Tingay DG, Kiraly NJ, Sourial M, Gordon MJ, Mills JF, Morley CJ, Dargaville PA (2007). A comparison of the effectiveness of open and closed endotracheal suction. *Intens Care Med.* 2007;33:1655-1662.
76. Combes P, Fauvage B, Oleyer C. Nosocomial pneumonia in mechanically ventilated patients, a prospective randomized evaluation of the Stericath closed suctioning system. *Intens Care Med.* 2000;26(7):878-882.

77. Sakuramoto H, Shimojo N, Jesmin S, Unoki T, Kamiyama J, Oki M, Miya K, Kawano S, Mizutani T. Repeated open endotracheal suctioning causes gradual desaturation but does not exacerbate lung injury compared to closed endotracheal suctioning in a rabbit model of ARDS. *BMC Anesthesiol.* 2013;13:47. http://www.biomedcentral.com/1471-2253/13/47. Accessed July 25, 2020.
78. Maggiore SM, Jacobone E, Zito G, Conti G, Antonelli M, Proietti R. Closed versus open suctioning techniques. *Minerva Anestesiol.* 2002;68:360-364.
79. NHS Centre for Reviews and Dissemination. Suctioning adults with an artificial airway: A systematic review. York: University of York, 2017.
80. Seymour CW, Cross BJ, Cooke CR, Gallop RL, Fuchs BD. Physiologic impact of closed-suction endotracheal suctioning in spontaneously breathing patients receiving mechanical ventilation. *Respir Care.* 2009;54(3):367-374.
81. Hagler DA, Traver GA. Endotracheal saline and suction catheters: Sources of lower airway contamination. *Amer J Crit Care.* 1994;3(6):444-447.
82. O'Neal PV, Grap MV, Thompson C, Dudley W. Level of dyspnoea experienced in mechanically ventilated adults with and without saline instillation prior to endotracheal suctioning. *Intens Crit Care Nurs.* 2001;17:356-363.
83. Wang CH, Tsai JC, Su CL, Chen L, Lin CC, Tam KW. Normal saline instillation before suctioning: A meta-analysis of randomized controlled trials. *Austral Crit Care Nurs.* 2017;30:260-265.
84. Caparros AC, Forbes A. Mechanical ventilation and the role of saline installation in suctioning adult intensive care unit patients: An evidence-based practice review, *Dimens Crit Care Nurs.* 2014;33(4):246-253.
85. Raymond SJ. Normal saline instillation before suctioning: Helpful or harmful? A review of the literature. *Amer J Crit Care.* 1995;4(4):267-271.
86. Ackerman M, Gugerty BP. The effect of normal saline bolus instillation in artificial airways. *J Soc Otorhinolaryngol Head Neck Nurs.* 1990;14-17.
87. Branson RD. Secretion management in the mechanically ventilated patient. *Respir Care.* 2007; 52(10): 1328-1347.
88. Hanley MV, Raud T, Butler J. What happens to endotracheal instillations? [Abstract]. *Amer Rev Respir Dis.* 1978; 117(4, Pt. 2): 124.
89. Demers RR, Saklad M. Minimizing the harmful effects of mechanical aspiration. *Heart Lung.* 1973; 2(4): 542-545.
90. Gray JE, MacIntyre NR, Kronenberger WG. The effects of bolus normal-saline instillation in conjunction with endotracheal suctioning. *Respir Care.* 1990; 35(8): 785-790.
91. Johnson JT. Tracheostomy in patients with the obstructive sleep apnea syndrome. In Myers EN, Johnson JT (eds.). *Tracheotomy: Airway Management, Communication, and Swallowing.* San Diego, CA: Plural Publishing, 2008; 141-146.
92. Walvekar RR, Myers EN. Technique and Complications of Tracheostomy in Adults. In Myers EN, Johnson JT (eds.). *Tracheotomy: Airway Management, Communication, and Swallowing.* San Diego, CA: Plural Publishing, 2008.
93. Schwenker D, Ferrin M, Gift AG. A survey of endotracheal suctioning with instillation of normal saline. *Amer J Crit Care.* 1998; 7(4): 255-260.
94. Celik SA, Kanan N. A current conflict: Use of isotonic sodium chloride solution on endotracheal suctioning in critically ill patients. *Dimens Crit Care Nurs.* 2006; 25(1): 11-14.
95. French BA, Bauer BS. Incidence of normal saline lavage by RTs in a large acute care hospital. *Respir Care.* 2002; Open Forum Abstracts.

96. Leddy R, Wilkinson JM. Endotracheal suctioning practices of nurses and respiratory therapists: How well do they align with clinical practice guidelines? *Can J Respir Ther.* 2015; 51(3): 60-64.
97. Paratz JD, Stockton KA. Efficacy and safety of normal saline instillation: A systematic review. *Physiother.* 2009; 95(4): 241-250.
98. Caruso P, Denari S, Ruiz SAL, Demarzo SE, Deheinzelin D. Saline instillation before tracheal suctioning decreases the incidence of ventilator-associated pneumonia. *Crit Care Med.* 2009; 37(1): 32-38.
99. Epstein SK. Late complications of tracheostomy. *Respir Care.* 2005; 50(4): 542-549.
100. Hess DR. And now for the rest of the story [Letter]. *Respir Care.* 2002; 47(6): 696-699.
101. Morris PE, Goad A, Thompson C, Taylor K, Harry B, Passmore L, et al. Early intensive care unit mobility therapy in the treatment of acute respiratory failure. *Crit Care Med.* 2008; 36(8): 2238-2243.
102. Chan EY, Ruest A, Meade MO, Cook DJ. Oral decontamination for prevention of pneumonia in mechanically ventilated adults: Systematic review and meta-analysis. *BMJ*, 334(7599): 1-11.
103. Chlebicki MP, Safdar N. Topical chlorhexidine for prevention of ventilator-associated pneumonia: A meta-analysis. *Crit Care Med.* 2007; 35(2): 595-602.
104. Tantipong H, Morkchareonpong C, Jaiyindee S, Thamlikitkul V. Randomized controlled trial and meta-analysis of oral decontamination with 2% chlorhexidine solution for the prevention of ventilator-associated pneumonia. *Infec Control Hosp Epidem.* 2009; 29(2): 131-136.
105. Wip C, Napolitano L. Bundles to prevent ventilator-associated pneumonia: How valuable are they? *Curr Op Infec Dis.* 2009; 22(2): 159-166.
106. Sona CS, Zack JE, Schallom ME, McSweeney M, McMullen K, Thomas, J, et al. The impact of a simple, low-cost oral care protocol on ventilator-associated pneumonia in a surgical intensive care unit. *J Intens Care Med.* 2009; 24(1): 54-62.
107. Fields LB. Oral care intervention to reduce incidence of ventilator-associated pneumonia in the neurologic intensive care unit. *J Neurosci Nurs.* 2008; 40(5): 291-298.
108. Bouza E, Perez MJ, Munoz P, Rincon C, Barrio JM, Hortal J. Continuous aspiration of subglottic secretions in the prevention of ventilator-associated pneumonia in the postoperative period of major heart surgery. *Chest.* 2008; 134(5): 938-946.
109. Tsai H, Chang S, Lin F. Intermittent suction of oral secretions before each position change may reduce ventilator-associated pneumonia: A pilot study. *Amer J Med Sci.* 2008; 336(5): 397-401.
110. Brook I. Bacterial colonization, tracheobronchitis, and pneumonia following tracheostomy and long-term intubation in pediatric patients. *Chest.* 1979; 76(4): 420-424.
111. Wahidi MM, Ernst A. The Montgomery T-tube tracheal stent. *Clin Chest Med.* 2003; 24: 437-443.
112. Jessup B, Stephan N. What nurses need to know and teach their patients about the care and maintenance of the Montgomery Safe-T-Tube. *ORL Head Neck Nurs.* 1993; 11(3): 23-27.
113. Wouters KMA, Byreddy R, Gleeson J, Morley AP. New approach to anaesthetizing a patient at risk of pulmonary aspiration with a Montgomery T-tube in situ. *Brit J Anaesth.* 2008; 101: 354-357.
114. Acheson D. FDA Public Health Advisory. *Reports of blue discoloration and death in patients receiving enteral feedings tinted with the dye, FD&C Blue No. 1.* Retrieved 7/5/18, https://www.fda.gov/forindustry/coloradditives/coloradditivesinspecificproducts/inmedicaldevices/ucm142395.htm. 2003.

115. Bell R, Fishman S. Eosinophilia from food dye added to enteral feedings [Letter]. *NEJM.* 1990; 322: 1822.
116. Maloney J, Metheny N. Controversy in using blue dye in enteral feedings as a method for detecting pulmonary aspiration. *Crit Care Nurs.* 2002; 22: 84-86.
117. American Association of Critical Care Nurses. AACN Practice Alert: Dye in enteral feeding. Retrieved from http://www.aacn.org/WD/Practice/Docs/Dye_in_Enteral_Feeding_4-2005.pdf. 2005.
118. Fiorelli A, Ferraro F, Nagar F, Fusco P, Mazzone S, Costa G, DiNatale D, Serra N, Santini M. A new modified Evans blue dye test as screening test for aspiration in tracheostomized patients. *J Cardiothor Vasc Anesth.* 2017; 31: 441-445.
119. Martindale RG, McClave SA, Vanek VW, McCarthy M, Roberts P, Taylor B, et al. American College of Critical Care Medicine, ASPEN Board of Directors. Guidelines for the provision and assessment of nutrition support therapy in the adult critically ill patient: Society of Critical Care Medicine and American Society for Parenteral and Enteral Nutrition: Executive summary. *Crit Care Med.* 2009; 37(5): 1757-1761.
120. National Confidential Enquiry into Patient Outcome and Death (NCEPOD). A review of the care received by patients who underwent a tracheostomy, 2014. http://www.ncepod.org.uk/2014tc.html. Retrieved 7/18/18.
121. Colandrea M, Eckardt P. Improving tracheostomy care deliver: Instituting clinical care pathways and nursing education to improve patient outcomes. *ORL Head Neck Nurs.* 2016; 34(1): 7-16.
122. Loerzel VW, Crosby WW, Reising E, Sole ML. Developing the tracheostomy care anxiety relief through education and support (T-CARES) program. *Clin J Oncol Nurs.* 2014; 18(5): 522-527.

8

Tracheostomy in the Pediatric Patient

by Karen Watters

Objectives

- Explore differences in indications for tracheostomy in children versus adults
- Detail the perioperative management of the pediatric tracheotomy procedure, including technique and choice of tubes
- List common complications and their management
- Evaluate developmental considerations for pediatric tracheostomy
- Explain timing and technique of phonation in a child with a tracheostomy
- Differentiate the decannulation process in a child compared to an adult

Introduction

Clinical Scenario

DJ was born at 24 weeks gestation, weighing 580 grams, and was intubated at birth. At three months of age, he remained intubated with severe bronchopulmonary dysplasia and pulmonary hypertension. Extubation trials were unsuccessful despite maximal non-invasive ventilatory support. After a multidisciplinary meeting with his medical providers and caregivers, a tracheostomy was placed at four months of age. A 3.5 mm pediatric cuffed tracheostomy tube was placed. He returned to the ICU for post-operative tracheostomy care.

In this chapter, we will discuss the increased incidence of tracheostomy placement over the last decade in infants and children. The decision-making process in tracheostomy placement in children will be outlined. The indications and the surgical procedure for tracheostomy will be described, as well post-operative care and potential adverse events. Considerations specific to children with tracheostomy will be discussed, including the importance of multidisciplinary tracheostomy care and the transition to the home setting.

PEDIATRIC TRACHEOSTOMY EPIDEMIOLOGY

Tracheostomy placement after a period of prolonged ventilation in adult ICUs is a routine clinical intervention.[1] It is very different in the pediatric setting, where tracheostomy is much less commonly performed. Studies report an incidence of tracheostomy in 2% of pediatric ICU patients.[2] There is also no consensus regarding the timing of tracheostomy placement in a child. Premature infants are often intubated for up to three months or longer before the decision is made to proceed with tracheostomy.[3,4] Despite this, the incidence of pediatric tracheostomy has been steadily increasing over the last decade in tandem with the improved survival of premature infants and children with complex medical conditions. The majority of pediatric tracheostomies are placed in the first year of life, with approximately 50% of them placed in infants under six months of age.[5]

DECISION FOR TRACHEOSTOMY AND ITS CARE

The decision to place a tracheostomy in a child can be challenging. The medical complexity of the child, long-term care needs, future prognosis, and caregiver support are important factors to discuss in the decision-making process. A large number of children require a tracheostomy for years, and frequently a lifetime.[6, 7] Less than 50% of children who have a tracheostomy will ultimately be decannulated.[6-8] Nowadays, children who have a tracheostomy placed have chronic complex medical conditions and are frequently ventilator-dependent. Consequently, this requires complex long-term hospital care and/or labor-intensive homecare. Caregivers need to be fully informed of the demands of caring for a child with a tracheostomy.[9] In children with life-limiting medical conditions or profound neurological disabilities, the decision to place a tracheostomy can be both controversial and ethically challenging.

Communication with the caregivers and the patient, when appropriate, is important as early as possible in the decision-making process. The caregiver's ability to comprehend the implications of a tracheostomy in their child should be assessed. Intense support is required for caregivers who will need to be appropriately trained to care for their child with a tracheostomy. A family-centered approach is optimal. Caregivers and patients should be provided with information about tracheostomy tubes, the labor-intensive care required, and potential complications. Any alternatives that may exist for their child should also be discussed. Caregivers should meet with the tracheostomy education team at the hospital to gain a more comprehensive understanding of short-term and long-term needs and expectations, including eventual transition to home or long-term care. A meeting between the family contemplating a tracheostomy for their child and a family who already has a child with a long-term tracheostomy can provide valuable insight into the care required and the decision-making process.

INDICATIONS FOR PEDIATRIC TRACHEOSTOMY

The indications for tracheostomy in children are in parallel with the improved survival of premature infants and children with chromosomal abnormalities and neurological impairements.[8,10] An analysis of 917 children (0-18 years) who underwent tracheostomy from 36 children's hospitals between 2002-2007, demonstrated that chronic lung disease (56%), neurological impairment (48%), and upper airway anomaly (47%) were the most common comorbid conditions.[5] Table 8.1 summarizes the indications for tracheostomy in the pediatric population.

Table 8.1. Indications for Tracheostomy in the Pediatric Patient

1. Airway Obstruction	Congenital • Craniofacial Anomalies • Bilateral Vocal Cord Paralysis • Tracheomalacia • Laryngeal Anomaly • Neoplasm Acquired • Subglottic Stenosis • Trauma
2. Assisted Ventilation	Bronchopulmonary Dysplasia Chronic Lung Disease Neuromuscular Disease Congenital Central Hypoventilation
3. Pulmonary Hygiene	Chronic Lung Disease Neuromuscular Disease Recurrent Pneumonias

The three indications for tracheostomy are discussed below.

Upper Airway Obstruction

The introduction of vaccinations to Haemophilus Influenzae Type B and Diphtheria almost completely eliminated the need for tracheostomy secondary to infectious upper airway obstruction.[4,11] Nowadays, upper airway obstruction is usually secondary to acquired subglottic stenosis in premature infants who have prolonged endotracheal intubation and/or congenital upper airway abnormalities in premature infants with genetic diagnoses.[12,13]

Failure to Extubate/Ventilatory Dependence

The increased survival of premature infants has led to a cohort of infants requiring tracheostomy for long-term ventilator support for bronchopulmonary dysplasia and chronic respiratory failure. In 2016, 9.8% of 3,945,875 live births in the United States were preterm with 2.76% (N=108,906) being less than 34 weeks and 0.68% (N=26,832) less than 28 weeks gestational age.[14] Thirty-nine percent of pre-term infants less than 28 weeks develop some degree of bronchopulmonary dysplasia or chronic lung disease of prematurity.[15] Duration of endotracheal intubation prior to tracheostomy in infants is not clearly defined. Infants tolerate prolonged periods of intubation without the severity of sequelae experienced by adults. Often, preterm infants are intubated for up to three months before a tracheostomy is considered.[4]

Pulmonary Hygiene

Tracheostomy is frequently placed in children with chronic neurological impairment, congenital heart disorders and lung disease to facilitate airway clearance and pulmonary hygiene.[5]

Pre-Operative Considerations and Surgical Technique

Anatomy

Pediatric tracheostomy should only be performed by a surgeon with advanced training or experience in pediatric airway management, particularly in a small infant or child with atypical anatomy. It is important to be aware of the indication for tracheostomy, especially if an upper airway or tracheal anomaly is present.[16] This may make entry into the airway more difficult with subsequent posterior tracheal wall injury. The increasing incidence of comorbid conditions such as congenital heart disease, craniofacial syndromes, and congenital anomalies of the larynx, trachea, esophagus, or chest wall may significantly increase the complexity and risks of the surgical procedure.

There are a number of pertinent anatomical differences in the pediatric larynx that should be considered prior to placing a tracheostomy in a child.[17,18] The infant larynx is higher and more anterior in the neck, and its size is only one third of an adult larynx. The cartilages in the infant larynx and trachea are more pliable and softer. The neck can also be much shorter and fatter. The hyoid bone overlies the thyroid cartilage in infants, making landmarks considerably more difficult to palpate. The cricoid is the narrowest part of the airway in an infant, measuring only 4 mm in internal diameter compared to 14-16 mm in the adult. The cricothyroid membrane is very short. Emergency placement of an airway through the cricothyroid membrane in a small child may result in damage to the vocal cords. Differentiating the trachea from the great vessels may be challenging at times, and it is important that the surgeon stays midline. Cervical extension of the thymus gland may obstruct access to the trachea or may mask the presence of a high riding innominate artery. Pleural apices may extend into the cervical paratracheal space, increasing potential for pneumothorax or pneumomediastinum.

Surgical Technique

Pediatric tracheostomies are performed by open surgical technique. Percutaneous tracheostomy technique in children is not commonly performed and is reported infrequently, primarily only in older children/adolescents.[19, 20]

A horizontal midline skin incision is made midway between the sternal notch and cricoid cartilage. The subcutaneous fat plane is divided, and the strap muscles are retracted laterally. If the isthmus of the thyroid gland is across the upper tracheal rings, it must be divided or pushed superiorly to expose the upper tracheal rings. Lateral stay sutures are then placed vertically on either side of the tracheal incision; these are maintained until after the first tracheostomy tube change.[21] In small infants and children, a vertical incision is made in the trachea, typically between rings 2 through 4. The endotracheal tube is visualized by the surgeon and is slowly withdrawn by the anesthesiologist under direct vision to just below the vocal cords. The tracheostomy tube is inserted into the trachea, and its position is confirmed. When the patient is adequately ventilated through the tracheostomy tube, the endotracheal tube is removed.

The position of the tracheostomy tube above the carina is confirmed by flexible tracheoscopy. In some cases, the tracheostomy is "matured" by advancing cutaneous flaps to the pre-tracheal fascia along the inferior and/or lateral borders of the stoma.[22] The tube is typically secured with Velcro ties.

Tube Selection

Pediatric tracheostomy tubes come in a variety of sizes and materials. It is important to select an appropriately sized tube before placement. The age, weight, and medical condition of the child, as well as the indication for tracheostomy, help to select the appropriate tube. In contrast to adult tubes, pediatric tracheostomy tubes do not have inner cannulas (**Figure 8.1**). The connector on all pediatric tracheostomy tubes is the universal standard 15-mm outer diameter to connect to ventilation equipment.

Figure 8.1 Shiley tracheostomy tube

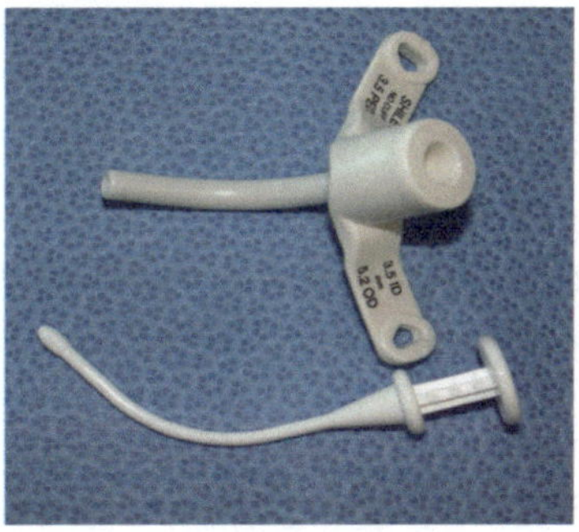

A Shiley pediatric tracheostomy tube with obturator. Note, there is no inner cannula.

Tube Size

Tracheostomy tubes come in a number of sizes, which are chosen on the basis of age of the child, and, if intubated, the size of the endotracheal tube used. Tracheostomy tubes have three dimensions: inner diameter, outer diameter, and length (**Figure 8.1**). Tube sizing is based on the ISO system, with the tube size denoting the internal diameter of the tracheostomy tube. Sizes range from 2.5 to 5.5. The length of the tube is measured from the flange to its tip. Pediatric tracheostomy tubes come in two size types based on different lengths, such as neonatal and pediatric. Neonatal tubes are shorter, ranging from 30 to 36 mm, and are typically used in small infants. Pediatric tubes are longer, starting at 38 mm in length, and are used in toddlers and older children. If a longer tracheostomy tube is needed, extended length tubes are available for pediatric sizes 4.0-5.5.

Custom-length tracheostomy tubes can also be ordered, and are more frequently used nowadays in infants with severe tracheomalacia. Adjustable-length pediatric tubes are available, but should be used with extreme caution and only in an ICU setting. Patient movement and other factors can affect tube depth relative to the flange, causing the tube to inadvertently become too long or too short. In general, an adjustable-length tube should only be used to determine the ideal cannula length needed to secure the airway while a custom-length tube is obtained. Other available custom modifications include flange angle and shape, angle of the shaft, and position of the cuff on the shaft. "Flex-tend" ™ tubes have a longer external connector to the flange and are useful in small infants with short necks (**Figure 8.2**). In a number of institutions, many tube types are no longer a custom order. When considering a specific custom tube type, consultation with a tracheostomy specialist or pediatric otolaryngologist is recommended prior to ordering.

Figure 8.2 Bivona Flextend

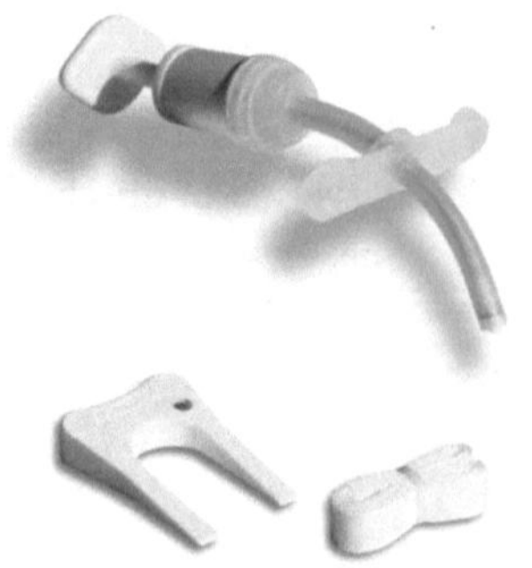

Flex-tend Bivona™ pediatric tracheostomy tube

Photo courtesy of Smiths Medical

Tube Material

An ideal tube should be flexible to prevent pressure on any portion of the neck or airway, have a thin wall thickness to maximize the internal diameter, and maintain structural integrity to prevent kinking or collapse. Pediatric tracheostomy tubes are usually plastic and made of polyvinylchloride, polyurethane, silicone, or metal reinforced silicone.[23] Polyvinyl chloride, which is rigid, is used in Shiley ™ tubes. Bivona ™ tubes, which are silicone, are softer and relatively inert. However, they may need to be reinforced with wire and may have restrictions on use in MRI equipment, although the majority of non-custom silicone tubes are now MRI compatible.

Cuffed Tubes

A cuffed tube is indicated in children requiring mechanical ventilation as well as select patients with chronic aspiration.[24] Cuff types include tight to shaft (TTS), high volume, low-pressure, and foam. TTS tubes are inflated with sterile water, whereas high-volume, low-pressure and foam cuffs are inflated with air.[23] The most commonly used cuffed type in children is the TTS cuff (Bivona ™), which remains flush with the outer diameter of the tube when deflated, thus preventing stoma trauma during insertion or removal. In children who do not require cuff inflation during the day, the TTS cuff can be deflated sufficiently to allow for speech. Foam cuffs are rarely required in children, but can be used in cases where minimal leak is optimal, such as oscillating ventilation or when extremely high-pressure ventilation is required.

Cuff pressures should be closely monitored to avoid overinflation. Overinflation may misalign the tube in the airway and cause the tube to become obstructed at the tip when angled against the tracheal wall. An overinflated cuff may create abnormal contact points in the airway, leading to the formation of granulation tissue, ulceration, and stenosis. Direct visualization of the tracheostomy tube in the airway via flexible tracheoscopy can greatly aid with its positioning on cuff inflation and ensure the tube is in a good position above the carina. Occasionally, a cuff does not inflate in a symmetric way, which may also cause it to be malpositioned in the airway. Prolonged overinflation of a cuff can lead to "tracheomegaly," or tracheal dilatation.[25] Use of minimal leak technique to minimize cuff pressures can determine adequate cuff inflation.

Tracheostomy Tube Ties

Available tracheostomy tube ties include synthetic fleece-like material with a Velcro fastener, cotton twill tape, and metal chain. The Velcro fastener types are most commonly used as they are disposable and facilitate easy removal in an emergency.

POST-OPERATIVE TRACHEOSTOMY CARE

A child with a new tracheostomy is managed post-operatively in the ICU. A chest radiograph is customarily performed, though may not be necessary in some patients.[26] If there is any concern for respiratory distress, a chest radiograph is mandatory to ensure there is no evidence of pneumothorax, pulmonary edema, or subcutaneous emphysema. Ventilator settings may also need to be changed after the tracheostomy.

A "fresh" tracheostomy is considered a "critical airway" until the stoma or fistula tract from the skin to the trachea is healed, even in a child with a structurally normal upper airway. If the tube becomes dislodged during the immediate post-operative period, there is a risk of development of a false passage when it is being replaced. This would result in loss of the airway with subsequent subcutaneous air, pneumothorax or pneumomediastinum, respiratory compromise, and an inability to ventilate. In infants and small children, sedation is typically administered to prevent them becoming agitated and pulling out the tube prior to the first tube change. A plan for managing the airway in the event of accidental decannulation should be reviewed with the ICU team on arrival with the child and documented at the bedside. Documentation of the airway management plan should include whether the child can be mask ventilated, intubated by standard methods, or requires the need for any special equipment, tubes, or techniques to establish ventilation.

Secretions from the tracheostomy are frequently increased and often bloody in the first few post-operative days. Regular suctioning should be performed as needed. Humidification is essential to prevent crusting and mucus plugging. Stoma care may include a thin dressing under the outer edges of the flange where ties are attached to prevent pressure sores or skin breakdown. The skin should be closely monitored under the flange and the ties for signs of skin breakdown or infection. The stoma site should be cleaned with normal saline. Stoma care varies between institutions, but it is essential for healing.

Tracheostomy ties should be tight enough to allow only one finger's width under the tie. If ties are too loose, there is a risk of improper positioning and accidental decannulation. Ties that are too tight cause skin breakdown and infection. Loose ties increase risk of improper positioning and accidental decannulation. Two people should be present when adjusting ties: one person to hold the tube securely in place, while the second person adjusts or changes the ties and examines the underlying skin. At the discretion of the surgeon who placed the tracheostomy, ties can be changed if they become excessively soiled in the early post-operative period.

The first tracheostomy change is typically performed five days post-operatively while the patient is still in the ICU, and it is usually performed by the surgical team who placed the tube.[23] It is important that necessary equipment be readily available at the bedside (**Table 8.2**).[27] This should include the obturator of the tracheostomy tube that is in place, spare tracheostomy tubes of the same size and smaller, appropriately sized suction catheters, saline, endotracheal tubes, scissors, and lubricant. Other items may be requested, including a complete operative tracheostomy tray at the discretion of the surgical team.

Table 8.2. Tracheostomy Tube Change Equipment
Tracheostomy tube with obturator
Half size smaller tracheostomy tube
Lubricant
Tracheostomy Ties
Gauze (wet and dry to clean stoma)
Syringe (to inflate cuff)
Ambu bag (with tracheostomy and face mask connector)
Oxygen
Blanket (rolled to extend neck in infants)

Once the first tube change has been successfully performed, routine tracheostomy care can now begin, and the family tracheostomy education can also start, with subsequent changes being performed by the family.

TRACHEOSTOMY RELATED COMPLICATIONS

Children who have tracheostomy are a medically complex population and likewise have a high risk of associated morbidity and mortality. It can be a challenge to address these risks with caregivers prior to tracheostomy placement. The mortality rate in children who have tracheostomy is high, especially in those under one year of age and those who require long-term ventilation, reportedly as high as 2.2-59%.[4,28] Almost 8% of children do not survive to discharge following tracheostomy placement, with the majority of these deaths being secondary to underlying medical conditions.[4,5] Up to 38% of children may experience a tracheostomy-related event in the first two years following tracheostomy.[9] These events may include tracheostomy tube obstruction, accidental decannulation, tracheostomy-related hemorrhage, stomal issues, tracheal stenosis, and tracheoesophageal fistula. Tracheostomy-related adverse events can be prevented by the institution of a comprehensive tracheostomy education program for all providers and caregivers caring for such children.

Tube Obstruction

Thick secretions in a small child can easily occlude the tracheostomy tube. This can be minimized through humidification, and regular suctioning when required. Secretions may increase significantly during acute respiratory illness, whether viral or bacterial in nature, and these should be aggressively managed with pulmonary hygiene, nebulized medications, and antibiotics, if necessary. Acute obstruction of a tracheostomy tube is an emergency. If a mucous plug is not removed with suctioning, the tracheostomy tube should be immediately changed. If changing the tracheostomy tube does not relieve the obstruction, bag ventilation through the tube should be performed. Additional supports should be immediately called for. If available, flexible tracheoscopy can be performed through the tube to assess its position in the airway and patency of the airway. If ventilation continues to be unsuccessful through the tracheostomy tube, a different tube (endotracheal tube) may be placed in the stoma. If the patient continues to deteriorate, oral mask ventilation or endotracheal intubation may be necessary. The stoma needs to be covered during attempts at oral mask ventilation to prevent leakage of air. It is thus highly important to be aware of the initial indication for tracheostomy, noting the patency of the airway above the tracheostomy. If intubation from above is not possible and the patient is deteriorating, rescue breaths may be delivered through the stoma.

Accidental Decannulation

Accidental decannulation is responsible for the majority of tracheostomy-related deaths in children.[2,29] Accidental decannulation may occur at any time, such as during routine tracheostomy care or when the child is sleeping or playing, in which case the tube should be immediately replaced. If the same size tracheostomy tube cannot be replaced, a tube one size smaller should be used. If the latter is not possible and the child is in distress, bag mask ventilation should be performed until additional help arrives. Steps similar to those described for tracheostomy tube obstruction should be performed, including orotracheal intubation if necessary.

Stomal Problems/Granulation Tissue

Moisture from oral or tracheal secretions may become trapped under the flange or within the neck creases. These trapped secretions increase the potential for skin breakdown and infection, including candida infections, as well as pressure-related skin and wound complications. This is particularly common in infants who have relatively shorter and more flexed necks when compared to older children. Stomal granulations can be managed conservatively with silver infused dressings (e.g., Mepilex AG ™) or topical steroid ointment (**Figure 8.3**). If granulation interferes with tracheostomy tube changes, they can be cauterized or surgically removed. Ensuring the optimal choice of tracheostomy tube size, flange type, and tube material may reduce risks of pressure-related injuries.

Figure 8.3 Stoma granulation

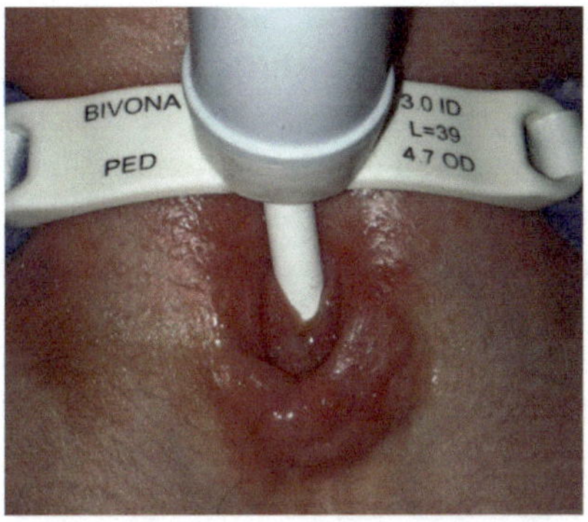

Stoma granulation and skin irritation

Suprastomal granulations may occur secondary to pressure from the tracheostomy tube on the superior border of the stoma on the tracheal side (**Figure 8.4**). Suprastomal granulations may need to be removed if they are occluding the airway or causing bleeding; otherwise, they are not routinely removed during endoscopy unless decannulation is planned in the near future.[30] Repeated excision of suprastomal granulation can weaken the suprastomal cartilage with subsequent suprastomal collapse, which may need to be surgically repaired. Granulation tissue may also form in the trachea at the site of the tip of the tracheostomy tube. Here, it can cause obstruction of the tube and bleeding with suctioning. If non-obstructive, it may be possible to apply topical steroid drops to the granulation tissue. If obstructive, surgical excision of the granulation is needed. A shorter or longer length tracheostomy tube may also help to minimize trauma at the level of the granulation tissue, and bypass it to prevent airway obstruction.

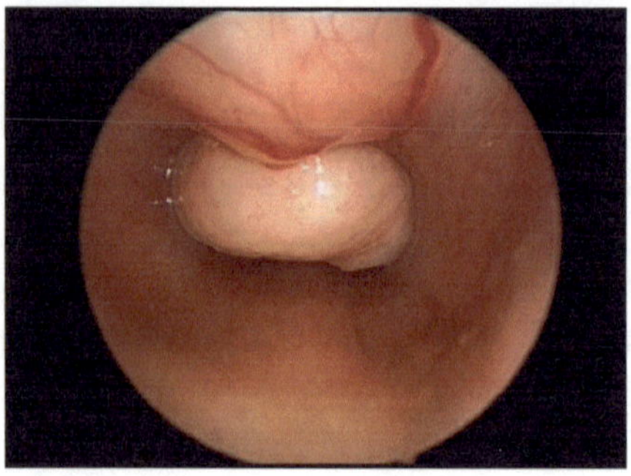

Figure 8.4 Suprastomal granuloma

Bleeding

Bleeding from the tracheostomy tube is most frequently secondary to suction trauma or inflammation of the trachea. This is managed with adequate humidification and avoiding the application of suction beyond the tip of the tracheostomy tube. Antibiotics may be needed if tracheitis is present. Recurrent bleeding may also be caused by the tube eroding the posterior wall of the trachea into the esophagus.

Excessive or brisk bleeding may be indicative of a tracheo-innominate fistula. Although rare, pediatric patients experience twice the number of tracheo-innominate hemorrhage events, in comparison to adults with tracheostomy.[31] This is presumably associated with closer proximity of the tracheostomy tube to the innominate artery. Risk of tracheo-innominate fistula and hemorrhage is also associated with a high-riding innominate artery course or inferior extension of the tracheostomy incision below the fifth tracheal ring. A tracheo-innominate fistula is life-threatening, and urgent intervention is required by a thoracic or general surgeon. The bleeding may be temporarily stopped with tamponade by placing a cuffed endotracheal tube in the stoma, inflating the cuff to maximal and retracting it back to the level of the stoma. Sentinel tracheo-innominate bleeds frequently occur in the preceding days prior to massive hemorrhage, where the latter is associated with a high mortality.

Subglottic/Tracheal Stenosis

Surgical technique is critical in reducing rates of subglottic and glottic stenosis.[32,33] Use of a vertical midline incision through 2-3 cartilage rings significantly reduces suprastomal tracheal collapse and subsequent airway stenosis cephalad to the stoma site. When a horizontal or tracheal window incision is used, the curve of the tracheostomy tube can exert pressure on the superior aspect of the tracheostomy incision, thus causing collapse of the anterior tracheal wall, known as suprastomal collapse. If this collapse is obstructive, it may need to be surgically corrected to allow for decannulation.

Distal tracheal stenosis can be caused by the tip of the tracheostomy tube against the trachea. Management of the granulation tissue and an appropriately sized tracheostomy tube, whether shorter or longer than the site of the stenosis, may be used to treat this.[34] If available, a pediatric otolaryngologist, pulmonologist, or tracheostomy specialist should be consulted to help determine the appropriate tube length. If the area of irritation is stenotic and not too mature, balloon dilatation with steroid injection can be used.

Developmental Considerations

Speech and Language Delay

Tracheostomy placement has been demonstrated to negatively impact phonation, vocal quality, and articulation skills in children. Infants and young children with tracheostomy are at increased risk for speech and language delay. Ideally, the child should be able to pass enough air up around the tracheostomy tube to allow for voice production; however, depending on the size of the tube and the size of the child's airway, there may not be significant space to allow for adequate airflow resulting in an inability to vocalize. Reduced clearance around the tracheostomy tube may also prevent airflow to the glottis. Speech and language evaluation, with initiation of speech, language, and communication therapy as indicated, is essential for all children with a tracheostomy.[35,36] Evaluation and initiation of therapy should start even before the child reaches the age of vocalization. The introduction and use of sign language may significantly improve communication and reduce frustration experienced by both the child and caregivers.

Speech delay may be more prominent in children who are ventilator-dependent and require a cuffed tracheostomy tube or in those children who do not have a patent airway above the tracheostomy tube. Evidence of suprastomal collapse or other upper airway anomalies, including subglottic stenosis and vocal cord paralysis, will also delay vocalization. For children who require ventilator support only at night, a Bivona™ TTS (Tight To Shaft) cuffed tube can be used with the cuff deflated when the child is awake to allow for voice.

Speaking valves, such as the Passy-Muir™ valve, can also be used in children (**Figure 8.5**).[35] Use of a speaking valve requires that the patient is medically stable, has suitable airway patency above the level of the tracheostomy, and sufficient clearance between the tracheostomy tube and the trachea. Some centers advocate early application of speaking valves, even in the NICU setting. The speaking valves are one-way valves designed such that air can enter the airway through the tracheostomy on inspiration, but on expiration, the air is expelled up around the tracheostomy tube and through the larynx and upper airway. Children who have increased tracheal secretions may not be suitable for use of these valves until secretion clearance improves through the upper airway.

Figure 8.5 Passy-Muir Speaking Valve

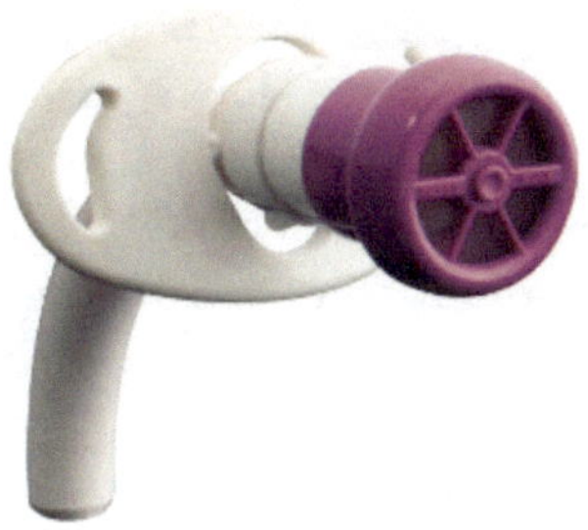

Pediatric tracheostomy tube with Passy Muir™ speaking valve

Prior to speaking valve use, the patient should be first evaluated by an otolaryngologist to assess airway patency and medical readiness, and then evaluated by a speech language pathologist to determine safety with speaking valve trials. Measuring trans-tracheal pressures can assess upper airway patency and suitability for valve use. The child must be able to tolerate tube occlusion and the passage of air around the tube. Should the child become distressed with a speaking valve in place, the valve should be immediately removed. When using speaking valves in children, it is important that caregivers are educated on how they function, as well as informed that they should never use them when the child is sleeping/napping or unsupervised.

Speaking valve use with a cuffed tube should be avoided. Applying a speaking valve to a patient with an inflated cuff will prevent the patient from exhaling, leading to a rapid onset of distress, possible pneumothorax, and, ultimately, death if the problem is not quickly identified and the valve immediately removed. In-line speaking valves are available for use in ventilator-dependent patients who do not require cuff inflation for adequate ventilation; however, they are much more commonly used in pediatric patients.

Speaking valves help to improve phonation, vocal intensity, pitch, and intonation, resulting in improved vocal quality and volume, allowing for increased communication with the child and a reduction in their frustration. Airflow around the tracheostomy tube also increases subglottic pressures, facilitating vocal fold closure with resultant improved cough response and airway clearance. With increased airflow through the mouth and nose, taste and smell are enhanced. The ability to close the vocal folds and increase subglottic pressures also helps to protect the airway against aspiration and may improve swallowing function..

Swallowing Impairment

The presence of a tracheostomy tube in a child may contribute to feeding difficulties. Due to its location, the tube may fix the larynx in a more stationary position, causing a reduction in laryngeal elevation during swallowing. The underlying medical comorbidities necessitating tracheostomy placement may also contribute to swallowing dysfunction. Neuromuscular problems cause motor weakness, reduced reflexes, and discoordination of the swallowing mechanism. Early involvement by a pediatric feeding therapist is essential for feeding and swallowing evaluation and intervention.

Prior to initiating oral feeding, the child's medical team should ensure there are no contraindications and the child is medically stable to begin oral feeding assessment. Children who have experienced prolonged periods of intubation frequently demonstrate oral aversion, swallowing discoordination with subsequent feeding difficulty, oropharyngeal dysphagia, and problems managing oral secretions. They may require intensive oromotor and feeding therapy. Many require enteral tube feeding by nasogastric tube or placement of a gastrostomy tube. A feeding and swallowing evaluation by a pediatric speech language pathologist is needed to assess readiness for oral feeding as well as develop a plan to safely introduce oral feeding.[36,37] If there is a concern regarding aspiration and pulmonary health of the child, the medical team may recommend deferring the initiation of oral feeding in order to optimize post-natal pulmonary development. Prior to initiating oral feeding, a fiberoptic endoscopic evaluation of swallowing (FEES) or modified barium swallow (MBS) may be indicated if there is a clinical concern for aspiration.

TRACHEOSTOMY CARE

Tracheostomy Tube Changes

The first tracheostomy tube change following surgical placement is traditionally done by the surgical team at approximately day five post-operatively.[23] At this time, they can assess for complications and confirm the stoma is healing. Once the first tracheostomy tube change has been safely performed and the stoma has healed adequately, caregivers can be taught how to change the tube. They must be comfortable with performing tube changes before their child can be discharged. Pediatric tracheostomy tube changes are usually more frequent than in adults because their tubes lack an inner cannula. Tubes are changed, at minimum, once a month. In some patients, tracheostomy tubes may be changed weekly or twice a month.

Safe tracheostomy tube changes are an important part of tracheostomy care. Tracheostomy tube changes should be approached in a calm, methodical manner and done when the child is awake and most cooperative. Routine tracheostomy tube changes should be performed during the day, in case there is difficulty, and also when another caregiver is available to assist, if possible. Supplies and emergency equipment should be prepared and checked prior to any change.[23] Supplies include the obturator of the tube in place, a spare tracheostomy tube, a smaller size tracheostomy tube, tracheostomy ties, dressing, suction catheters, suction machine, humidity devices, and monitors, if indicated. In the hospital setting, a "time-out" is frequently performed prior to a tracheostomy change to ensure the correct tube is being placed and no one has any concerns. A checklist is helpful. The new tracheostomy tube should have the obturator inserted. A second tube one half-size smaller should be immediately available. If a cuff is present on the tube, it should be checked to confirm its integrity. The suction machine should be turned on with an appropriately sized catheter attached, and tracheostomy ties and dressings should be prepared. Supplemental oxygen or bag ventilation should be available. It is important to be prepared for any emergency, such as a difficult insertion, inability to replace the tube, or respiratory distress.

Proper hand hygiene should be performed before any manipulation of the tracheostomy tube, unless it is an emergency. To minimize the risk of vomiting or aspiration during the tube change, at least two hours should have passed after the last feeding. The role of the partner should be determined. One must always communicate with the partner, be prepared for the worst, and remain calm, especially during an emergency. The infant and younger child should be in supine position with the neck extended in neutral position (chin pointing toward the ceiling) in a setting with good lighting. A small rolled towel or blanket can be placed behind the shoulder blades to allow adequate extension of the neck. The tracheostomy tube to be removed is suctioned, if necessary.

The primary caregiver then deflates the cuff, if present, and replaces the tube with a new one with the obturator in situ. The obturator is removed, and the child's breathing is assessed by watching for respiratory efforts and chest wall motion. The partner helps to maintain correct position of the child, while providing comfort and performing tracheostomy site care. This site care includes cleaning the peristomal area and neck skin, while the tube is held in place by the primary caregiver. The ties are then applied, secured, and checked for correct tension; they should be tight enough to ensure the tube does not become dislodged, typically allowing one finger breadth beneath them. If the ties are too tight, they will pinch the skin. If a problem occurs during the change, the partner is able to call for help, obtain emergency supplies, and provide assistance.

The skin around the stoma should be cleaned daily with sterile saline or water. Areas of the neck can be cleaned with mild soap and water. The skin on the back of neck should also be inspected daily to ensure the ties are not causing irritation or skin breakdown.

Suctioning

A clean technique should be used for suctioning in the home setting. Suctioning is usually performed on an "as needed" schedule. Infants and young children with small lumen tracheostomy tubes are at risk for mucous plugs within the tube and regular suctioning is required. For patients with chronic aspiration, poor pulmonary hygiene, or inability to cough, suctioning may be required more frequently. In the hospital setting, especially in the ICU, a sterile technique is typically used for suctioning. In the period following tracheostomy placement, tracheal mucus production is increased, and suctioning may be required every two hours to keep the tube clear of mucus and any residual post-surgical sero-sanguinous drainage.

Suction depth is determined by the length of the tracheostomy tube. The suction catheter is inserted to a prescribed depth, just slightly beyond the tube tip. Suction is applied, and the suction catheter may be rolled as it is slowly withdrawn. Excessive suctioning or suctioning too deeply can cause tracheal irritation with the development of ulceration, granulation tissue, and subsequent bleeding. Suctioning may also induce bronchospasm or hypoventilation. The quantity, color, and consistency of suctioned material should be observed. A change in quantity, odor, or color of mucus may suggest infection. Blood-stained secretions are not normal, and suggest tissue trauma or infection, which require further evaluation. In rare cases, minor bleeding is the sentinel-bleeding event prior to a major life-threatening hemorrhage. For this reason, all bleeding from the tracheostomy warrants further evaluation.[31]

Humidification

Air entering the tracheostomy tube is not humidified by the upper respiratory tract, and, thus, humidification is necessary to keep secretions thin and aid in muco-ciliary clearance. Thick secretions and mucous plugs can occur when humidification is not adequate and can cause obstruction of the tracheostomy tube or lower airway, resulting in respiratory distress.

Humidification is provided via in-line humidification, humidified tracheostomy collar, or a heat moisture exchanger (HME) , also referred to as an artificial nose. Humidification warmed to 37 degrees Celsius is used for in-line ventilator humidifiers. Nebulized saline can also be used to aid in thinning mucus when secretions are thick. Inhaled medications may be administered through the tracheostomy tube using an adapter or a spacer.

Water Precautions

Water or particulate matter should not be allowed to enter the tracheostomy tube. There is no natural mechanism to prevent this happening. When bathing, the child should be supported upright in shallow water and should never be unsupervised. Covering the tube with an HME or a cap, if tolerated, may significantly reduce the quantity of water that might enter the airway; however, water may still pass around the outside of the tube into the airway. Children with tracheostomy tubes in place should never be submerged in water, and extreme caution should be taken with any kind of water activities.

Tracheostomy Home Care

Caregivers must be satisfactorily trained in tracheostomy care prior to home discharge.[38] The majority of tracheostomy complications take place in the home environment. Caregiver education usually begins prior to the tracheostomy being placed. After the first tracheostomy tube change, bedside education can begin, as long as the stoma is healing and the child's medical condition allows. Caregivers can then start to do tube changes.

Caregivers need to demonstrate competent skills in tracheostomy tube care (suctioning, stoma cleaning, humidification) and be able to perform tube changes in both routine and emergency situations, such as accidental decannulation. It is important that caregivers are aware of the signs of respiratory distress that may indicate the tracheostomy tube needs to be changed urgently, and also be aware of conditions when they should return to the hospital urgently or contact emergency services. This is particularly important in children who are ventilator-dependent, because such children have a high incidence of readmission back to the hospital in the months following home discharge. Graf and colleagues reported a 63% 180-day readmission rate of children with tracheostomy following discharge from an acute hospital setting, and a 13% 180-day all-cause mortality rate.[39]

The majority of institutions have standardized protocols for tracheostomy education and designated specialist tracheostomy educators (nurses, respiratory therapists) to deliver and help simplify caregiver education. Caregivers are also encouraged to teach other adults in the home setting about tracheostomy care. In the majority of institutions, caregivers of children with tracheostomy are trained in cardiopulmonary resuscitation.[25] If a child requires home care nursing, this should be established prior to the child being discharged home. Local emergency services and the electric company in the child's neighborhood should also be contacted prior to discharge and made aware that a child with a tracheostomy is being discharged home. The individual needs of the child and caregivers must be determined prior to the child's discharge home.[40] Parents who care for tracheostomy-dependent children experience significant caregiver burden and increased associated caregiver costs.[41]

DECANNULATION

There are no standardized guidelines for pediatric tracheostomy management or decannulation. Recent studies have attempted to define clinical predictors of successful decannulation.[42,43] A child is considered suitable for a trial of decannulation if the original indication for the tracheostomy has resolved or has been corrected, or if the patient is tolerating a speaking valve or capping during waking hours. It is also important that the child is managing their secretions, has an effective cough to clear secretions, and does not need frequent suctioning. The tracheostomy is initially downsized to the smallest tube suitable for the child's age.[44]

A capped sleep study, if feasible, is recommended to help determine readiness for decannulation.[42,45,46] In a patient tolerating full-time capping while awake, the absence of significant obstructive sleep apnea or central apnea, with a capped tracheostomy tube within the airway, is felt to be a good predictor of successful decannulation. The child's airway should be formally evaluated in the operating room, via direct laryngo-bronchoscopy, to ensure the upper airway is patent and tracheo-bronchomalacia, if previously present, is no longer significant.[47] The child's tonsils and adenoids should be assessed to ensure they are not enlarged, as this may contribute to obstructive sleep apnea that would only manifest itself once the tracheostomy tube is capped, or at any point after its removal. Vocal cord motion should also be assessed in the awake child with flexible laryngoscopy. If the child has a difficult airway or is difficult to intubate, a plan for airway management for future surgeries should be made prior to tracheostomy removal.

The staged process of initially downsizing the tracheostomy tube, and the use of a speaking valve or cap, allows the child to adjust to breathing through the nose and oral cavity. The child may also have some degree of anxiety related to the fear of the tracheostomy removal, especially if it has been present for a number of years.[48] It is important to address this fear, otherwise it may result in decannulation failure. Decannulation in children is performed in a monitored setting, and the child is observed overnight to ensure there is no respiratory distress. When the tube is removed, an occlusive dressing is placed over the stoma. In the majority of children, the stoma closes spontaneously. However, in some children, the stoma may persist and require surgical closure. If so, this should be done no sooner than 6-12 months after decannulation to ensure the child is tolerating decannulation.

Multidisciplinary Team Approach

In the past decade, the number of children having tracheostomy has increased, as has their medical complexity.[49] Such children are usually cared for by multiple medical providers, resulting in fragmented care due to a lack of communication. This may result in suboptimal tracheostomy care. Studies have shown that care can be significantly improved through the establishment of multidisciplinary tracheostomy care.[50-52] Multidisciplinary teams help to establish standardized protocols of care, and ultimately reduce tracheostomy-related adverse events. Most of the reports in the literature are related to adult tracheostomy care. However, Adobe and colleagues reported that a multidisciplinary approach in children being cared for at an airway center can result in measurable improvements in outcomes.[53] After the institution of an enhanced tracheostomy education program, weekly clinical care conferences, and implementation of an institutional consensus for care, they demonstrated that the mean length of stay, in children under one year of age, was reduced from 36 to 27 days for those discharged to home. A standardized decannulation protocol resulted in successful decannulation in 71% of the first attempts.

Airway Surveillance

A child with a tracheostomy should be seen on a regular basis at a multidisciplinary tracheostomy clinic, if available. The age of the child, chronicity of the tracheostomy and associated medical issues will dictate the frequency with which they need to be seen. During office visits, an endoscopic evaluation of the airway can be performed via flexible tracheoscopy to ensure there is no irritation or granulation tissue in the distal airway, and the tracheostomy size is adequate. The caregiver's emergency supplies should also be checked during these visits. There is no consensus on the timing of formal airway evaluation under anesthesia with direct laryngo-bronchoscopy.[54] If a child is having tracheostomy-related issues or bleeding, endoscopy should be performed on an urgent basis.

SUMMARY

Children who require tracheostomy tubes are some of the most medically complex patients, and they are not just small adults. There are a number of factors that should be considered prior to placement of a tracheostomy in a child, such as indication, anatomy, comorbidities, suitable tracheostomy tube and size, developmental issues (feeding and speech), and caregivers' needs. Multidisciplinary tracheostomy care improves the quality of care for children and their caregivers, and ultimately reduces adverse events.

KEY POINTS

- Children tend to have a tracheostomy placed earlier in life (majority in <1 year of age) and remain for prolonged periods (often a lifetime), as compared to adults.
- Indications for tracheostomy in children differ from adults. There is no set criteria for prolonged length of intubation prior to tracheostomy, particularly in premature infants.
- Children with tracheostomy have a high incidence of adverse events, primarily due to their underlying chronic medical conditions.
- Pediatric tracheostomy tubes come in many different sizes as well as neonatal and pediatric lengths. They also do not have inner cannulas and are more prone to mucous plugging and occlusion.
- Tracheo-innominate fistula, although rare, is more common in the pediatric age group and can be associated with a high-riding innominate artery.
- It is essential to involve the speech language pathologist for early assessment and intervention related to speech, communication, feeding, and swallowing.
- Contraindications to speaking valve use include cuff inflation, upper airway stenosis, distal tracheomalacia, and inability to manage secretions.
- A multidisciplinary approach is important in the care of children with tracheostomy. It can help to standardize tracheostomy care protocols, provide education to both staff and caregivers, reduce tracheostomy-related adverse events, and ultimately improve the care that a child with tracheostomy and his caregivers receive.

REVIEW QUESTIONS

1. With respect to the laryngeal anatomy of an infant, which of the following statements is correct?
    a. The infant larynx is similar in size to an adult larynx.
    b. The infant larynx is more pliable than the adult larynx.
    c. The infant larynx is lower in the neck than the adult larynx.
    d. The vocal cords are the narrowest part of the airway in an infant.

    ANSWER: B. There are a number of anatomical differences between the pediatric and adult larynx that need to be considered when placing a tracheostomy in an infant.[17] The infant larynx is one third the size of the adult larynx and is higher in the neck than the adult larynx. The narrowest part of the infant larynx is the cricoid.

2. Which of the following statements is correct with respect to pediatric tracheostomy tubes?
    a. Pediatric tracheostomy tubes do not have an inner cannula.
    b. A pediatric-length tube is shorter than a neonatal-length tube.
    c. The external diameter of a size 3.5 mm pediatric tube is standard across different brands of tracheostomy tubes.
    d. Cuffed pediatric tubes are not available.

    ANSWER: A. In contrast to adult tracheostomy tubes, pediatric tubes do not have an inner cannula. It is therefore important to routinely change the tracheostomy tube in a child to prevent crusting and mucous plugging.

3. Contraindications to use of a speaking valve in a child include all of the following EXCEPT:
    a. Laryngeal atresia
    b. Ability to cap the tube
    c. High trans-tracheal pressures
    d. An inflated cuff

    ANSWER: B. If a child is tolerating capping of the tube, a speaking valve can be trialed. In fact, a speaking valve is usually trialed prior to capping trials. A speaking valve should never be trialed in a child with severe upper airway obstruction or if a cuffed tube is present with the cuff inflated.

4. Decannulation can be considered in all of the following EXCEPT:
    a. The indication for tracheostomy tube has resolved.
    b. The child is tolerating capping during waking hours.
    c. The child will not tolerate non-invasive ventilation for management of severe obstructive sleep apnea.
    d. The child successfully passed a capped sleep study.

    ANSWER: C. If the child does not tolerate non-invasive ventilation for management of severe obstructive sleep apnea and there are no other treatment options, decannulation cannot be considered.

5. Which of the following statements is INCORRECT?
    a. The majority of devastating tracheostomy complications occur in the home setting.
    b. If a child with a tracheostomy tube successfully passes a capping trial, there is no need for a formal swallow evaluation.
    c. Local emergency services should be contacted prior to a child with a tracheostomy being discharged to the home setting.
    d. A multi-disciplinary approach to tracheostomy care in children can help reduce adverse events.

ANSWER: B. The presence of a tracheostomy tube in a child may contribute to feeding difficulty. The location of the tube may tether it to the larynx, causing laryngeal elevation during swallowing. The underlying medical comorbidities may also contribute to swallowing dysfunction. Therefore, a feeding and swallowing evaluation by a pediatric speech language pathologist is needed to assess readiness for oral feeding as well as develop a plan to safely introduce oral feeding.[36,]

REFERENCES

1. Veenith T, Ganeshamoorthy S, Standley T, et al. Intensive care unit tracheostomy: a snapshot of UK practice. *Int Arch Med.* 2008;1:21.
2. Wood D, McShane P, Davis P. Tracheostomy in children admitted to paediatric intensive care. *Arch Dis Child.* 2012;97(10):866-869.
3. Principi T, Morrison GC, Matsui DM, Speechley KN, Seabrook JA, Singh RN, Kornecki A. Elective tracheostomy in mechanically ventilated children in Canada. *Intensive Care Med.* 2008;34:1498-1502.
4. Lewis CW, Carron JD, Perkins JA, Sie KC, Feudtner C. Tracheotomy in pediatric patients: a national perspective. *Arch Otolaryngol Head Neck Surg.* 2003;129(5):523-529.
5. Berry JG, Graham DA, Graham RJ, Zhou J, Putney HL, O'Brien JE, Roberson DW, Goldman DA. Predictors of clinical outcomes and hospital resource use of children after tracheotomy. *Pediatrics.* 2009;124:563-572.
6. Mahadevan M, Barber C, Salkeld L, Douglas G, Mills N. Pediatric tracheotomy: 17-year review. *Int J Pediatr Otorhinolaryngol.* 2007;71:1829-1835.
7. de Trey L, Niedermann E, Ghelfi D, Gerber A, Gysin C. Pediatric tracheotomy: a 30-year experience. *J Pediatr Surg.* 2013;48:1470-1475.
8. Carron JD, Derkay CS, Strope GL, Nosonchuk JE, Darrow DH. Pediatric tracheotomies: changing indications and outcomes. *Laryngoscope.* 2000;110:1099-1104.
9. Watters K, O'Neill M, Zhu H, Graham RJ, Hall M, Berry J. Two-year mortality, complications, and healthcare use in children with Medicaid following tracheostomy. *Laryngoscope.* 2016;126(11):2611-2617.
10. Hadfield PJ, Lloyd-Faulconbridge RV, Almeyda J, Albert DM, Bailey CM. The changing indications for paediatric tracheostomy. *Int J Pediatr Otorhinolaryngol.* 2003;67(1):7-10.
11. Dursun O, Ozel D. Early and long-term outcome after tracheostomy in children. *Pediatr Int.* 2011;53(2):202-206.
12. Berry JG, Graham RJ, Roberson DW, et al. Patient characteristics associated with in-hospital mortality in children following tracheotomy. *Arch Dis Child.* 2010;95:703-710.
13. Sidman JD, Jaguan A, Couser RJ. Tracheotomy and decannulation rates in a level 3 neonatal intensive care unit: A 12-year study. *Laryngoscope.* 2006;116(1):136-139.
14. Martin JA, Osterman MJK. Describing the Increase in Preterm Births in the United States, 2014-2016. *NCHS Data Brief.* 2018;(312):1-8.
15. Stoll BJ, et al. Neonatal outcomes of extremely preterm infants from the NICHD Neonatal Research Network. Eunice Kennedy Shriver National Institute of Child Health and Human Development Neonatal Research Network. *Pediatrics.* 2010;126(3):443-456.
16. Jackson, C. High tracheostomy and other errors: the chief causes of chronic laryngeal stenosis. *Surg Gynecol Obstet.* 1921;32:392-398.
17. Monnier P. Applied Surgical Anatomy of the Larynx and Trachea Springer. In: Monnier P. ed. *Pediatric Airway Surgery.* Management of Laryngtoracheal Stenosis in Infants and Children. Springer-Verlag Berlin Heidelberg, 2011:7-10.
18. Henick DH, Holinger LD. Laryngeal development. In: Holinger LD, Lusk RP, Green CG. (eds.) *Pediatric laryngology and bronchoesophagoscopy.* Lippincott- Raven, Philadelphia; New York, 1997:1-17.
19. Raju A, Joseph DK, Diarra C, Ross SE. Percutaneous versus open tracheostomy in the pediatric trauma population. *Am Surg.* 2010;76(3):276-278.

20. Gollu G, Ates U, Can OS, Kendirli T, Yagmurlu A, Cakmak M, Aktug T, Dindar H, Bingol-Kologlu M. Percutaneous tracheostomy by Griggs technique under rigid bronchoscopic guidance is safe and feasible in children. *J Pediatr Surg.* 2016;51(10):1635-1639.
21. Ruggiero FP, Carr MM. Infant tracheotomy: results of a survey regarding technique. *Arch Otolaryngol Head Neck Surg.* 2008;134(3):263-7.
22. Colman KL, Mandell DL, Simons JP. Impact of Stoma Maturation on Pediatric Tracheostomy-Related Complications. *Arch Otolaryngol Head Neck Surg.* 2010;136(5):471-474.
23. Mitchell RB, Hussey HM, Setzen G, et al. Clinical consensus statement: tracheostomy care. *Otolaryngol Head Neck Surg.* 2013;148(1):6-20.
24. Schroeder JW Jr, Schneider JS, Walner DL. The influence of peak airway pressure and oxygen requirement on infant tracheostomy. *Int J Pediatr Otorhinolaryngol.* 2012;76(6):869.
25. Keszler M, Nassabeh-Montazami S, Abubakar K. Evolution of tidal volume requirement during the first 3 weeks of life in infants <800 g ventilated with volume guarantee. *Arch Dis Child Fetal Neonatal Ed.* 2009;94(4):F279–82.
26. Genther DJ, Thorne MC: Utility of routine postoperative chest radiography in pediatric tracheostomy. *Int J Pediatr Otorhinolaryngol.* 2010;74(12):1397.
27. Gluth MB, Maska S, Nelson J, et al. Postoperative management of pediatric tracheostomy: Results of a nationwide survey. *Otolaryngol Head Neck Surg.* 1996;35:11-17.
28. Zhu H, Das P, Roberson DW, Jang J, Skinner ML, Paine M, Yuan J, Berry J. Hospitalizations in children with preexisting tracheostomy: A national perspective. *Laryngoscope.* 2015;125(2):462-468.
29. Tantinikorn W, Alper CM, Bluestone CD, Casselbrant ML. Outcome in pediatric tracheotomy. *Am J Otolaryngol.* 2003;24(3):131.
30. Chen C, Bent JP, Parikh SR. Powered debridement of suprastomal granulation tissue to facilitate pediatric tracheotomy decannulation. *Int J Pediatr Otorhinolaryngol.* 2011;75(12):1558.
31. Das P, Zhu H, Shah RK, Roberson DW, Berry J, Skinner ML: Tracheotomy-related catastrophic events: Results of a national survey. *Laryngoscope.* 2012;122:30-37.
32. Gallagher TQ, Hartnick CJ. Pediatric tracheotomy. *Adv Otorhinolaryngol.* 2012;73:26-30.
33. Song JJ, Choi IJ, Chang H, Kim DW, Chang HW, Park GH, et al. Pediatric tracheostomy revisited: a nine-year experience using horizontal intercartilaginous incision. *Laryngoscope.* 2015;125(2):485-492.
34. Arjmand, EM, Brenski AC. Advances in tracheostomy in the pediatric age group. *Adv Otolaryngol Head Neck Surg.* 2001;15:41-69.
35. Gereau SA, Navarro GC, Cluteria B, et al. Selection of pediatric patients for use of the Passy-Muir valve for speech production. *Int J Pediatric Otolaryngol.* 1996;35:11-17.
36. Baumgatener CA, Bewyer E, Bruner D. Management of communication and swallowing in intensive care: The role of the speech pathologist. *AACN Adv Crit Care.* 2008;19(4):433.
37. Gluth MB, Maska S, Nelson J, et al. Postoperative management of pediatric tracheostomy: Results of a nationwide survey. *Otolaryngol Head Neck Surg.* 1996;35:11-17.
38. Joseph RA. Tracheostomy in infants: Parent education for home care. *Neonatal Netw.* 2011;30(4):231.
39. Graf JM, Montagnino BA, Hueckel R, McPherson ML. Pediatric tracheostomies: A recent experience from one academic center. *Pediatr Crit Care Med.* 2008;9(1):96-100.

40. Graf JM, Montagnino BA, Hueckel R, McPherson ML. Children with new tracheostomies: Planning for family education and common impediments to discharge. *Pediatr Pulmonol.* 2008;43(8):788-94.
41. Hartnick CJ, Bissell C, Parsons SK. The impact of pediatric tracheotomy on parental caregiver burden and health status. *Arch Otolaryngol Head Neck Surg.* 2003;129(10):1065-9.
42. Robison JG, Thottam PJ, Greenberg LL, Maguire RC, Simons JP, Mehta DK. Role of polysomnography in the development of an algorithm for planning tracheostomy decannulation. *Otolaryngol Head Neck Surg.* 2015;152(1):180-4.
43. Prickett KK, Sobol SE. Inpatient observation for elective decannulation of pediatric patients with tracheostomy. *Otolaryngol Head Neck Surg.* 2015;141(2):120-125.
44. Kubba H, Cooke J, Hartley B. Can we develop a protocol for the safe decannulation of tracheostomies in children less than 18 months old? *Int J Pediatr Otorhinolaryngol.* 2004;68(7):935-937.
45. Cristea AI, Jalou HE, Givan DC, Davis SD, Slaven JE, Ackerman VL. Use of polysomnography to assess safe decannulation in children. *Pediatr Pulmonol.* 2016;51(8):796-802.
46. Gurbani N, Promyothin U, Rutter M, Fenchel MC, Szczesniak RD, Simakajornboon N. Using polysomnography and airway evaluation to predict successful decannulation in children. *Otolaryngology-Head and Neck Surgery.* 2015;153(4):649-655.
47. Wirtz N, Tibesar RJ, Lander T, Sidman J. A pediatric decannulation protocol: Outcomes of a 10-year experience. *Otolaryngol Head Neck Surg.* 2016;15:731-734.
48. Black RJ, Baldwin DL, Johns AN. Tracheostomy "decannulation panic" in children: Fact or fiction? *J Laryngol Otol.* 1984;98(3):297-304.
49. Funamura JL, Yuen S, Kosuke K, Gergin O, Adil E, Rahbar R, Watters K. Characterizing mortality in pediatric tracheostomy patients. *Laryngoscope.* 2016;127(7):1701-1706.
50. Garrubba M, Turner T, Grieveson C. Multidisciplinary care for tracheostomy patients: A systematic review. *Crit Care.* 2009;13:R177.
51. Cetto R, Arora A, Hettige R, Nel M, Benjamin L, Gomez CM, et al. Improving tracheostomy care: A prospective study of the multidisciplinary approach. *Clin Otolaryngol.* 2011;36(5):482-488.
52. Hettige R, Arora A, Ifeacho S, Narula A. Improving tracheostomy management through design, implementation and prospective audit of a care bundle: How we do it. *Clin Otolaryngol.* 2008;33:488-491.
53. Abode KA, Drake AF, Zdanski CJ, Retsch-Bogart GZ, Gee AB, Noah TL. A multidisciplinary children's airway center: Impact on the care of patients with tracheostomy. *Pediatrics.* 2016;137(2):e20150455.
54. Kharasch VS, Dumas HM, Haley SM, et al. Bronchoscopy findings in children and young adults with tracheostomy due to congenital anomalies and neurological impairment. *J Pediatr Rehabil Med.* 2008;1(2):137.

9

Care of the Patient with a Laryngectomy

by Heather Starmer, Itzhak Brook

Clinical Scenario

Mr. Jones is a 62-year-old fire fighter who has had extensive occupational exposure to smoke and other carcinogens. He noted changes in his voice and a chronic sore throat and cough that persisted for several months. As a result, he presented to an otolaryngologist who identified a large laryngeal mass. The patient completed diagnostic imaging and had a biopsy that revealed squamous cell carcinoma.

Objectives

- Elucidate the differences between tracheostomy and laryngectomy
- Describe the epidemiology of laryngeal cancer and outline common treatments
- Highlight the role of the speech-language pathologist in the care of patients with laryngeal cancer
- Illustrate methods of voice restoration following total laryngectomy
- Emphasize other changes following total laryngectomy relevant to patient rehabilitation

Introduction

It is not uncommon for tracheostomy and total laryngectomy to be confused with one another. While there are some similarities, marked differences must be acknowledged, particularly when considering rehabilitation. While both procedures result in surgical alteration of the airway, care providers must understand the primary difference between them; namely the presence or absence of the larynx. The patient who undergoes a total laryngectomy presents a clinical challenge because of the varied nature of the procedure related to the extent of disease. These patients are without a voice in the literal and figurative senses of the word.

The upper aerodigestive tract performs three critical and often interrelated functions: (a) respiration, (b) facilitation of safe swallowing, and (c) production of speech and voice. The most critical of these biologic functions is respiration. When any medical device or respiratory tube is introduced into the upper airway, all three functions must be considered; however, respiration is always primary, as it supports life.

Laryngeal cancer treatment may include surgical removal of the tumor with or without reconstruction, radiation therapy, and/or chemotherapy.[1] The clinician's first step is to define the nature of the tumor treatment and how it may affect the airway and its functions. In this chapter, we will review causes of laryngeal cancer, traditional treatments for laryngeal cancer, and rehabilitation of patients with laryngeal cancer. The role of the speech-language pathologist on the multi-disciplinary care team will be highlighted. Finally, other changes that may impact a patient's recovery and quality of life will be explored.

EPIDEMIOLOGY

Incidence of laryngeal cancer becomes more common with advanced age and is more common in men than in women. Smoking is a major risk factor, and reduction of smoking rates in recent years has led to a downturn in both incidence and mortality. The number of new cases of laryngeal cancer between 2013-2017 was 2.9 per 100,000 men and women annually.[2] In 2017, it was estimated that there will be 13,360 new cases of laryngeal cancer and an estimated 3,660 people will die of this disease.[2] The earlier cases are identified, the better the chance of surviving five years after diagnosis. Approximately half of patients are diagnosed at the local stage (i.e., the cancer is confined to the laryngeal region and has not spread to the lymphatic or circulatory system).[3] The five-year survival rate for localized laryngeal cancer is 76%.[3] With the decline in use of tobacco, a subsequent decline in incidence has been observed (2.4% reduction in incidence in the United States between 2005-2009).[4] Laryngeal cancer accounts for 1% of all cancers in men and 0.3% of all cancers in women.[3] Globally, the burden of laryngeal cancer is anticipated to increase by nearly 70% in developing countries between 2012-2030 and by ~20% in more developed countries.[5]

Squamous cell carcinoma is the most common form of laryngeal cancer, and the five-year survival rate, irrespective of disease stage, is 65%.[6] Laryngeal cancer is most frequently diagnosed in a 60- to 70-year-old with a long history of smoking and, frequently, alcohol abuse. However, it is manifesting in younger people without these risk factors.[7] Laryngeal cancer can metastasize to distant sites such as the lungs and liver. The risk of metastasis is higher in advanced stage tumors with nodal disease. The greatest risk of metastasis is in the first five years, and especially in the first two years after the cancer appears.[8]

SYMPTOMS OF LARYNGEAL CANCER

The presenting symptoms of laryngeal cancer are listed in **Table 9.1.**[9]

Table 9.1. Common Presenting Symptoms of Laryngeal Cancer
Sore throat and persistent cough
Change of voice or hoarseness that persists for greater than two weeks
Lump in the neck or a sore that does not heal
Difficulty swallowing
Pain when swallowing or ear pain
Difficulty breathing
Unintentional weight loss

TYPES OF LARYNGECTOMY

Although there are non-surgical ways to treat laryngeal cancer, this chapter will focus on surgical management. There are two categories of surgery for removal of laryngeal cancer: partial or total. Partial surgeries include removal of portions of the larynx, while total laryngectomy leads to removal of the entire larynx. While patients undergoing partial surgeries may require temporary tracheostomy, they typically do not require permanent alteration of the upper airway. In contrast, patients undergoing total laryngectomy will require a permanent stoma leading to perpetual neck breathing.

Partial Laryngectomy

The main goals of these procedures are to remove the cancer while avoiding a permanent breathing tube in the neck, preserving a suitable voice, and maintaining the ability to swallow.[10] Partial laryngectomy procedures are typically limited to early stage cancers in individuals with good baseline laryngeal function. The procedure can be performed through open surgical techniques or transoral approaches using lasers or robots.

There are several types of open partial laryngectomies:

- Laryngofissure with cordectomy: Following vertical splitting of the thyroid cartilage, the inside of the larynx is exposed, allowing the removal of vocal cord tumors. A temporary stent can be placed in the larynx for a few weeks to prevent scar band formation. A temporary tracheostomy tube may be required.
- Horizontal laryngectomy: The hemi-laryngectomy can be either supraglottic or supracricoid and can be performed with or without resection of the hyoid bone.[11] Following resection, the cricoid cartilage is sewn back up to the hyoid bone or to the hyoid bone and epiglottis, depending on what remains after resection of the tumor.
- Vertical hemi-laryngectomy, or fronto-lateral vertical partial laryngectomy: The thyroid cartilage is incised vertically following middle neck incision and the vocal cord and arytenoid on one side are removed. Up to 3/4 of the thyroid cartilage may be removed, and the resection can include a small part of the vocal cord on the opposite side as well. Reconstruction can be performed in various ways, including local flaps, staged procedures, and/or free flaps.

- Transoral laser microsurgery (TLM) with partial laryngectomy: This procedure is performed through the mouth using special laryngoscopes, instruments, and lasers. It is an option for small recurrent cancers after non-surgical therapy.[12] A laser is used to remove the tumor, attempting to achieve a margin of normal tissue around it. Associated procedures might include a tracheotomy, feeding tube placement or a neck dissection—sometimes performed a few weeks later as a staged neck dissection.
- Transoral robotic-assisted partial laryngectomy: As with transoral laser microsurgery, this procedure uses a robot to expose and remove a laryngeal tumor through the mouth. The purpose is to limit incisions and dissection of the neck.[13] The development of this procedure is ongoing.

Total Laryngectomy

While partial laryngectomy may avoid a permanent need for neck breathing, many patients with more advanced tumors may not have this option. Total laryngectomy is generally performed for the following reasons:[14]

- A large laryngeal cancer that has eroded through cartilage and other structures.
- Laryngeal cancer that recurs after previous treatment (i.e., radiation with/without chemotherapy)
- For prevention of aspiration (pneumonia) resulting from prior head and neck cancer surgery at sites other the larynx (i.e., hypopharynx, tongue base).
- Nonfunctional larynx, or inability to eat or drink because of pharyngeal or esophageal strictures.

During total laryngectomy, an incision is made in the central neck, typically extending to both sides to perform bilateral neck dissections. The larynx, lymph nodes (if needed), and one or both lobes of the thyroid gland are removed. Frozen sections of the edges/margins of the resected tissue are studied by the surgical pathologist before the surgery is complete to determine if cancer cells are left behind. A stoma is created by sewing the top part of the trachea directly to the skin. After a total laryngectomy, the patient breathes through the stoma. There is no longer a connection between the trachea and the mouth and nose.

Reconstruction procedures might include repair of the pharynx with primary closure or a flap if there is inadequate local tissue to close the pharynx. The flap is obtained from other parts of the body, including a pectoralis major flap, or free flap harvested from the radial forearm, lateral thigh, abdominal or scapula area.[15] Total laryngopharyngectomy includes removal of the entire larynx along with the entire pharynx. Reconstruction is always required following total laryngopharyngectomy due to the extent of resection.

Clinical Scenario Cont'd.

Mr. Jones is diagnosed with a T4N1 squamous cell cancer of the larynx. Because his tumor has spread to include the thyroid cartilage, a total laryngectomy is his best opportunity for a cure. He meets with the multidisciplinary team consisting of the surgical oncologist, medical oncologist, radiation oncologist, speech-language pathologist, and social worker in preparation for his upcoming surgery.

LARYNGECTOMY CARE TEAM

Following total laryngectomy, patients have a variety of needs and challenges that require the assistance of a multidisciplinary team. This team may include the surgeon, nursing staff, speech-language pathologist (SLP), dieticians, respiratory therapists, and many others. While the surgeon will take the lead in medical decision-making, the speech-language pathologist plays an important role on the team both prior to and following surgery. In the following section, we will discuss the role of the SLP in the care of the patient following laryngectomy.

PREOPERATIVE EDUCATION AND COUNSELING BY THE SLP

It is critical that patients undergoing total laryngectomy to receive thorough education and preparation prior to surgery. Patient uncertainty and anxiety is quite common prior to any surgery,[16] but perhaps more so in patients requiring total laryngectomy due to the profound impact on communication and appearance.[17,18] In many cases, the shock regarding the diagnosis and the need for the removal of the voice box may negatively impact the patient's ability to comprehend and recall information provided by the treatment team. Zeine & Larson[19] surveyed patients following laryngectomy regarding their preoperative education experiences. Results of the study revealed that 21% of patients did not realize their surgery would lead to loss of voice. Such outcomes stress the importance of the SLP, ensuring patient comprehension of the key information provided prior to surgery.

While much of the pre-operative information is reviewed by the surgical team, review of functional expectations after surgery is typically completed by the SLP. Consensus regarding what should be included in a pre-operative education session does not exist;[20] therefore, the clinician needs to evaluate the patient's current level of understanding, readiness for information, and ability to comprehend the information. A number of factors should be addressed whenever possible prior to surgery. One of the most important subjects to review is the anatomic and physiologic change following surgery, particularly in regard to communication, swallowing, and respiration. Additionally, the SLP should provide information about different communication options and the advantages and disadvantages of each. The SLP should educate the patient regarding the SLP's role on the team and the anticipated timeline for recovery and rehabilitation. Finally, the SLP should ensure that the patient and their family are aware of safety concerns following surgery. For patients who need higher levels of information, the SLP can also discuss pulmonary rehabilitation, olfactory rehabilitation, and different products that may be of benefit after surgery, such as hands-free speech valves. Data suggests that, in addition to the benefits in regards to patient anxiety, SLP consultation prior to laryngectomy may also positively impact length of hospital stay and reduce the need for unplanned readmissions.[21]

Multi-modal education should include visual information to highlight the structures that will be surgically removed while also discussing the physiology of breathing, communication, and swallowing prior to and following surgery. There are a number of high value resources the SLP can utilize for patient education, including anatomic diagrams made available by In Health Technologies (**Figures 9.1-9.5**) and Atos Medical. Additionally, a number of books such as *Self-Help for the Laryngectomee*[22] and *The Laryngectomy Guide*[23] may be available to both patients and clinicians at little to no charge. In addition, many patients find it beneficial to hear what the different communication options sound like. Use of audio and video demonstrations and/or patient visits can be extremely valuable for patients and their families.

Figure 9.1
Normal
Pre-laryngeal
Speech

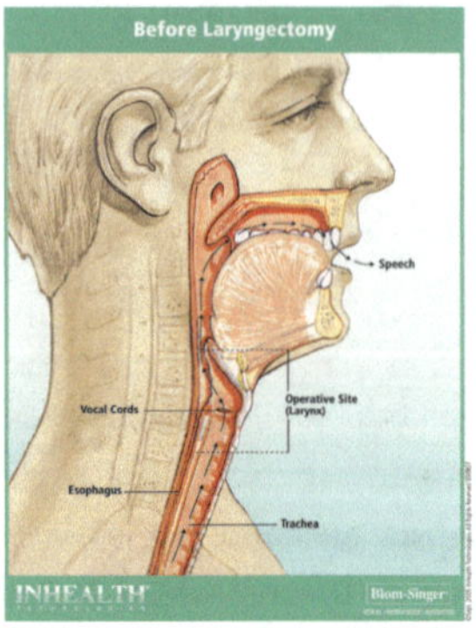

Figure 9.2
Post
Laryngectomy
Anatomy

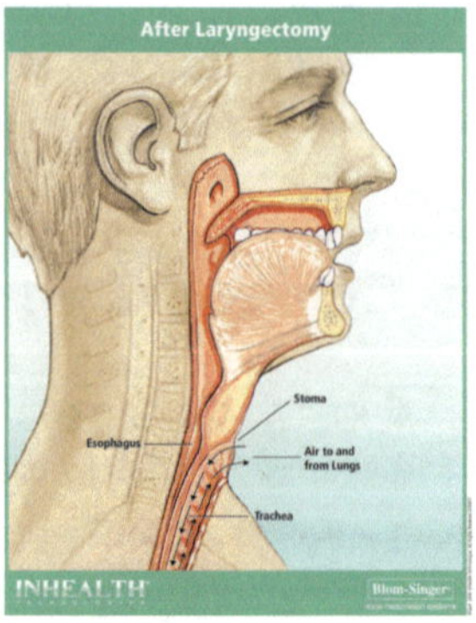

Figure 9.3

Electrolaryngeal
Speech

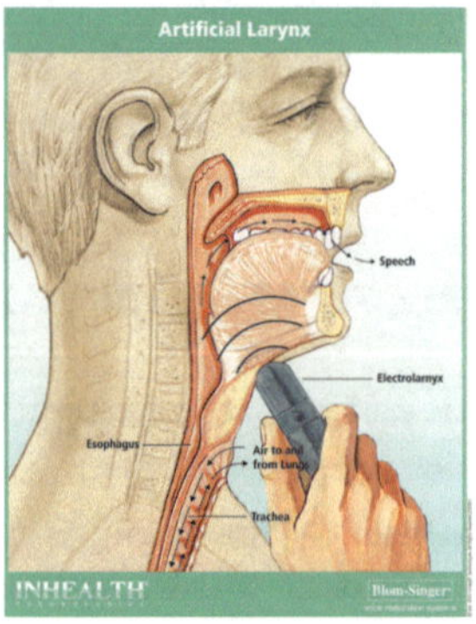

Figure 9.4
Esophageal
Speech

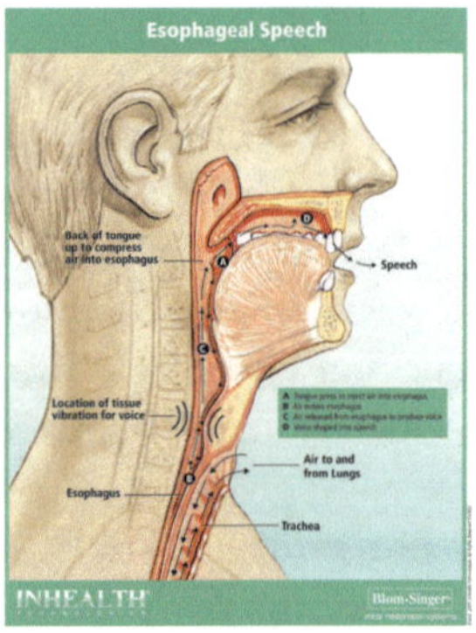

Figure 9.5
Tracheoesophageal
Speech

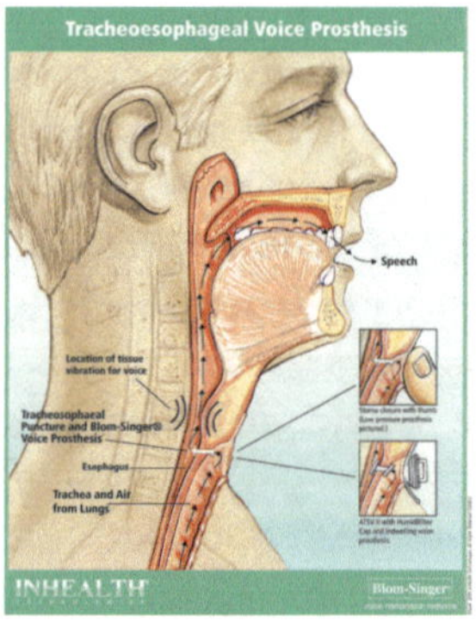

Images courtesy of
InHealth Technologies®
www.inhealth.com

In addition to providing the patient with education prior to surgery, the pre-operative consultation is an opportunity for the SLP to get to know the patient and their support team. Understanding a patient's baseline function and post-operative goals will help the SLP to target intervention appropriately. The SLP should assess articulation, voice and resonance, conversational intelligibility, and any unique factors such as dialect.[24] Additionally, the SLP may screen or assess cognitive communication function, which may also impact rehabilitation. Other factors that are important to note include social support, dynamics between the patient and their caregivers, patient engagement, and relative level of medical literacy, all of which may impact post-treatment rehabilitation. Finally, it is critical to ascertain the patient's personal functional goals following surgery. It is important to understand the unique communication needs of each patient so that treatment can be tailored toward those outcomes. In some cases, patients may indicate a preference for a communication option for which they are not well suited. In those instances, it is important for the SLP to discuss realistic expectations with the patient. Additionally, identification of preferred alternative means of communication prior to establishing alaryngeal speech should occur before surgery and may include use of written communication, pictorial communication boards, and text to speech applications. It is important to estimate the literacy level of the patient and the primary caregiver prior to surgery in order to select the most appropriate non-verbal options for early post-operative recovery.

In addition to education regarding communication following laryngectomy, it is critical that the patient understand the elementary changes in the respiratory system. Permanent stomal/neck breathing should be emphasized. The SLP should discuss typical functions of the upper airway, such as filtration, warming, and humidifying the air prior to reaching the lungs as well as how these functions are disrupted following laryngectomy. The SLP should discuss how use of heat and moisture exchange filters (HMEs) could help to restore a more normal respiratory climate.[25] The SLP should also discuss the need to keep the stoma moist and clean, and the patient should be referred to nursing or respiratory therapy for in-depth training on stoma care.

Finally, safety concerns after laryngectomy should be discussed during the preoperative education session. The stoma provides direct access to the trachea and lungs and provides a portal for entrance of environmental items such as particulates in the air, and more importantly, water. It is critical that patients understand that if the stoma is submerged in water, it can lead to drowning. Protection and covering of the stoma should be reviewed and options should be provided for activities like showering. Though slightly less critical, loss of smell may impact the patient's ability to detect warning smells such as smoke or natural gas. Patients should be encouraged to regularly change the batteries in these detection devices. Finally, the patient and their caregivers should be aware that rescue breathing must occur at the level of the stoma rather than the nose/mouth.[26] Patients should notify their local firehouse that there is a neck breather in their home. A medic alert bracelet is another effective way to communicate neck breather status to first responders. As previously mentioned, supplementary information can be provided by the care team prior to surgery as appropriate. Continued education will be integrated into post-operative rehabilitation therapies.

Clinical Scenario Cont'd.

Mr. Jones meets with the speech pathologist to discuss his upcoming surgery. He was previously under the impression that he would not be able to return to work after his surgery. His SLP discussed with him his communication needs at work, which typically included leading meetings and one on one communications. As he no longer is involved in active firefighting, but rather administrative management of his firehouse, he is relieved to know he will be able to return to work. He is reassured after seeing videos and speaking with another patient who has had a laryngectomy that he will be able to communicate well in the future.

Postoperative Rehabilitation

While pre-operative education is a critical aspect of patient preparation for surgery, early rehabilitation is equally vital to recovery.[27] Patients and their caregivers will likely have many questions about expectations and recovery. In addition to providing education, the SLP should ensure the patient is able to communicate basic wants and needs. While early communication may predominantly be non-verbal, early electrolaryngeal speech training should be offered within the first 1-2 days after surgery. The hospital stay is an opportune time for the SLP to initiate rehabilitation. Early electrolaryngeal training will focus on patient use as well as caregiver engagement to optimize comprehension. The intraoral adaptor will be used in the early stages of rehabilitation due to neck edema and healing.

During the hospital stay, the patient will begin to adapt to and manage post-operative changes. Adjusting to the changes in the respiratory system is often slow and frustrating for the patient. In order to prevent the stoma from closing, a soft silicone laryngectomy tube may be placed in the stoma following surgery. In most cases, this tube is temporary, although some patients will require its permanent use to maintain a patent stoma. Immediately after surgery, the patient will have an increase in tracheal mucus production that they may have difficulty clearing.[25] Tracheal suctioning will be provided by hospital staff, and the patient and caregivers should learn how to perform suctioning prior to hospital discharge. In many hospitals, nursing staff will take the primary role in training the patient to care for their stoma; however, in hospitals where nursing staff is less familiar and comfortable with this information, the SLP may need to assist with this training. It is critical that the patient and their caregivers demonstrate competency in airway management prior to discharge home, or they may require home health or temporary placement at a nursing facility. The patient must understand that keeping the stoma clean and clear is critical to breathing.

The SLP should consult with the surgeon to determine the appropriate timing of tracheoesophageal/esophageal voice restoration. Healing is typically more challenging after salvage laryngectomy (laryngectomy performed after prior radiation therapy) and may delay initiation of swallowing and esophageal/tracheoesophageal speech.[28,29] On average, patients are typically able to initiate tracheoesophageal or esophageal speech 1-2 weeks following surgery. In the following section, we will provide additional information regarding alaryngeal speech options.

Clinical Scenario Cont'd.

During his hospitalization, Mr. Jones and his wife are trained in how to care for his stoma and to provide suctioning. The SLP works with him daily to facilitate communication using the electrolarynx. With diligent practice, he is able to communicate well with family and staff. Because of his proactive rehabilitation, he is discharged home seven days after surgery, communicating and caring for his airway independently.

Methods of Speaking After Laryngectomy

Surgical removal of the larynx/vocal folds leads to absence of a sound source for production of speech. The primary goal of speech rehabilitation following laryngectomy is to establish an alternative sound source. This sound source may either be mechanical (electrolarynx) or physiologic (esophageal or tracheoesophageal speech).[30] Optimally, patients will become fluent in the use of electrolaryngeal and either esophageal or tracheoesophageal speech so that a back-up modality is available. The following section will expand on alaryngeal speech options, the pros and cons of each (**Table 9.2**), and rehabilitation with each modality.

Table 9.2. Pros and cons of alaryngeal communication options

	Pros	Cons
Electrolaryngeal speech	1. Can be initiated one day after surgery. 2. Best option if issues with upper esophageal sphincter (vibrating segment for other options). 3. Once acquired, does not require follow-up care from SLP.	1. Reduced speech intelligibility. 2. Reduced speech naturalness. 3. May not be readily accepted by communication partners. 4. Relies on an expensive device.
Tracheoesophageal speech	1. Provides the most natural, understandable communication. 2. Judged by most patients as most acceptable option.	1. Requires maintenance and upkeep. 2. Costs for devices can be a burden for patients with limited income. 3. May not be effective if issues with upper esophageal sphincter.
Esophageal speech	1. Does not rely on any device. 2. Once acquired, does not require follow-up care from SLP. 3. Lowest cost option.	1. Difficult to acquire even with extensive speech therapy. 2. Judged as unnatural appearing, due in part to behaviors for air insufflation. 3. May not be effective if issues with upper esophageal sphincter.

Electrolarynx

The electrolarynx (artificial larynx) is one alaryngeal speech option that may be offered to patients (**Figure 9.6**). While other options rely upon the upper esophageal sphincter (UES) as the source of sound, the electrolarynx (EL) uses an external, mechanized source of vibration. As such, the EL may be the only method of alaryngeal speech available to patients unable to achieve vibration of the UES. In addition, the EL serves as an immediate communication option for patients after surgery. Some patients may prefer the electrolarynx to tracheoesophageal (TE) speech due to the care, maintenance, and long-term dependence on the SLP associated with TE speech. Disadvantages to EL speech include the mechanical sound quality, reduced intelligibility with some listeners, and less natural speech.

Figure 9.6 Electrolarynx

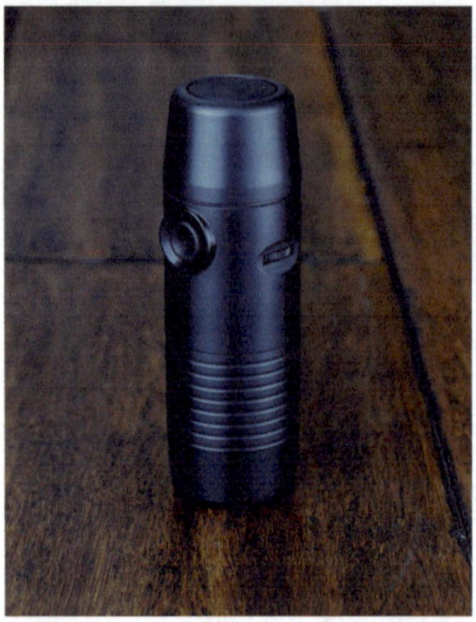

True Tone™ Electrolarynx

Used with permission from Griffin Laboratories, Inc.

Training with the electrolarynx includes three primary aims: device placement, timing, and over-articulation.[31] When the intraoral adaptor is used in the early post-operative period, it is important that the patient place the adaptor in an optimal position to achieve the most intelligible speech. If the adaptor is too anterior, the sound will spill forward without proper articulation/shaping of sounds. If the adaptor is too lateral, the buccal walls may dampen sound, thus impacting intelligibility. If the adaptor is too central, it may interfere with tongue movement for articulation. Thus, the optimal position for the adaptor in most patients will be approximately halfway back in the mouth, midway between the cheek and the center of the mouth. For neck placement, finding the "sweet spot" for vibration may take some effort, particularly if the patient has had radiation therapy. The goal is to find the placement that facilitates best resonance/amplification in the articulatory tract.

In addition to device placement, the patient will need to understand the importance of timing of turning the sound on and off and over-articulation. If the device is turned on prematurely, there will be non-meaningful sound that may negatively impact intelligibility. Alternatively, if the device is turned off too quickly, it may cut off final sounds critical to intelligibility. Over-articulation is similarly important to optimize intelligibility. Additional factors that may require SLP assistance include basic communication skills such as the listener looking at the EL speaker, use of context to facilitate understanding, and slowed speaking rate. Finally, some patients will continue typical respiratory patterns of exhaling when speaking. This may lead to audible rushes of air from the stoma, sometimes known as "stoma blast." Patients with noted stoma blast will need to be instructed to reduce expiratory forces when speaking. While the electrolarynx is an excellent option for some patients, the mechanical quality leads many patients to pursue more physiologic voice options such as tracheoesophageal voice.

Tracheoesophageal Speech

Tracheoesophageal (TE) speech is one alaryngeal voice option that uses the upper esophageal sphincter as the sound source for voice. A tracheoesophageal puncture is performed by the surgeon by placing a small opening in the wall between the trachea and the esophagus.[32] A one-way valve (TE prosthesis) is then placed in the puncture tract (**Figures 9.7, 9.8**). When the patient occludes the stoma, pulmonary air is shunted through the tracheoesophageal prosthesis (TEP) into the esophagus where it induces vibration of the upper esophageal sphincter. The major advantage of TEP is that it yields the most intelligible, fluent, natural sounding voice in contrast to other alaryngeal speech options.[33] While esophageal speech also uses the upper esophageal sphincter (UES) as the sound source, patients using a TEP rely on pulmonary air as their power source for speech production, rather than the limited air supply available in esophageal speech. This leads to greater fluency and longer utterance lengths.[34] A disadvantage of TE speech is the amount of care and maintenance required. The patient will need to clean and care for the prosthesis daily, which will need to be replaced at regular intervals.[35] For patients relying on the SLP for prosthesis changes, this may require clinic visits as frequently as once per month and on average every two to three months.[36] In addition, because this option relies on the upper esophageal sphincter as the sound source, patients with issues like stricture or narrowing of this region may not be able to achieve good voice.[37]

Figure 9.7 Blom Singer Voice Prosthesis

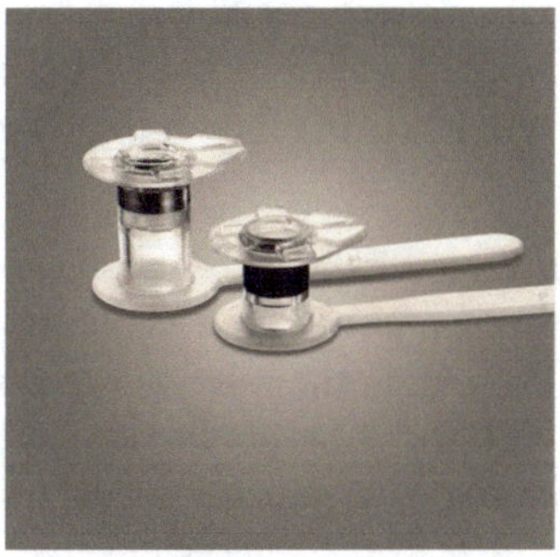

Image courtesy of InHealth Technologies® www.inhealth.com

Figure 9.8 Provox Voice Prosthesis

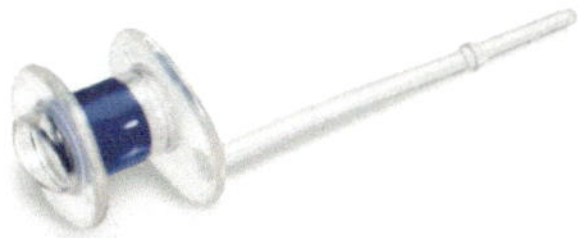

Image © Atos Medical AB and Chris Edghill

TE puncture may be performed at the time of the laryngectomy or at a later date. When performed at the time of laryngectomy, this is referred to as primary puncture. If the puncture is done at a later date, it is known as secondary puncture. Many surgeons will have preferences toward one or the other. In patients who will undergo secondary puncture, the SLP has the advantage of determining TE voice quality prior to the procedure.[38,39] This allows the patient and the clinicians to determine whether TE voice will be acceptable/functional. The technique used to ascertain voice prior to TE puncture is known as insufflation testing.[40] To perform the air insufflation test, a catheter is passed through the patient's nose into the esophagus just below the upper esophageal sphincter. The other end of the catheter attaches to a housing placed over the stoma. When the patient occludes this housing, pulmonary air is directed through the catheter to the UES. The patient is asked to phonate on a vowel and then to count. Fluent speech is defined as the ability to sustain phonation for 8-10 seconds on a single breath and produce 10-15 syllables on a single breath.[41] If the patient is not fluent or the voice quality is poor, the clinician can work with the surgeon to determine appropriate interventions prior to puncture to optimize outcomes.

Training with the TEP is multifaceted. First, the patient must learn to care for the device and monitor for any signs of problems with the prosthesis. We will discuss the details of prosthesis care and maintenance later in this chapter. In addition to caring for the device, the SLP will provide training to ensure the patient is able to communicate effectively.[42] This includes work on coordination of respiration, stomal occlusion, and phonation. Some patients will require more practice than others in the sequence of breathing in, covering the stoma, speaking, and uncovering the stoma. Some patients will also require SLP assistance in achieving good stomal occlusion. Use of mirrors and hand-over-hand guidance can be helpful. In patients presenting with a strained voice, the SLP should use strategies to facilitate more relaxed phonation. Finally, in patients who are struggling to produce functional TE voice, the SLP may need to evaluate the underlying cause of the problem. This often involves video-fluoroscopic imaging of the UES during phonation attempts to determine if there is restriction in vibration/airflow due to stricture or spasm of the muscles of the UES.[43]

Patients who establish fluent TE speech may be candidates for hands-free speech.[44] This is accomplished by placing a second valve at the level of the stoma. The valve remains open for respiration, but upon exhalation for speech, the valve is forced closed, thus occluding the stoma. The air then passes through the TEP for voice production. While the goal for many patients is hands-free speech, it can be challenging to acquire for several reasons. First, the patient must have an airtight seal with the interface used to hold the hands-free device.[45] If a seal is not possible, adequate pressure to close the valve will not be present. Because of the high pressures generated to close the valve, many patients cannot sustain hands-free speech for extended durations. Thus, many patients who use hands-free valves only do so in particular situations or for short durations.[46] The SLP will work with the patient to identify the most appropriate interface to allow for an airtight seal and the best duration of seal possible.

Clinical Scenario Cont'd.

Mr. Jones needs to perform public speaking on a regular basis. His therapist fits him with an adhesive baseplate and hands-free valve. Using this hands-free valve, he is able to speak more normally and reports feeling "more like a full person again."

There are many prosthesis options available to address different challenges that patients may encounter. It is important that the SLP providing care for patients with TEPs have knowledge of the different devices available and the indications for use so that thoughtful problem solving may be applied. The most common problem patients may experience with a TEP is leakage of esophageal contents through the center of the TEP.[47,48,49] This typically occurs when biological agents like bacteria and yeast build up on the valve of the prosthesis.[50]

The build-up of biofilm prevents the valve from closing, thus allowing esophageal contents (particularly thin liquids) to leak into the trachea. Options to address leakage through the prosthesis may use biofilm resistant materials, designs that inset the flap into the shaft of the prosthesis to minimize contact with esophageal contents, double valves, and/or magnets.[51] Prosthetic options are summarized in **Table 9.3**. While biofilm is the most common cause of leakage through the prosthesis, other issues within the esophagus can also lead to this untoward outcome. **Figure 9.9** provides a framework for troubleshooting leakage through the prosthesis.

Table 9.3. Prosthetic Options for Leakage Through the Prosthesis
Blom Singer Advantage
Blom Singer Dual Valve
Provox Vega
Provox Activalve

Figure 9.9 Algorithm-Options for Leakage Through Prosthesis

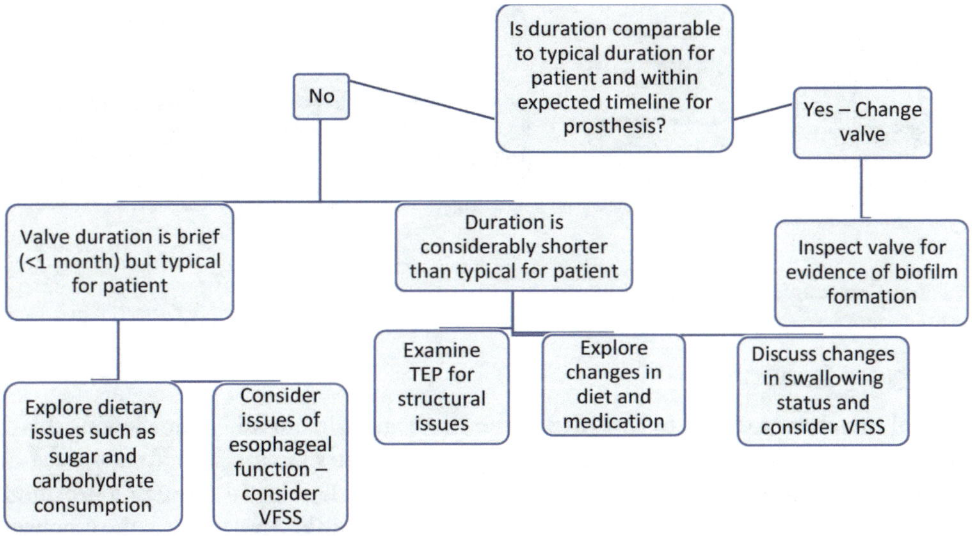

(VFSS-videofluoroscopic swallow study)

Another common problem encountered with TEP use is leakage around the prosthesis.[47,48,49] Leakage occurs when there is excessive space between the prosthesis and the surrounding tissue. Most commonly, this is the result of a prosthesis of excessive length pistoning in the tract leading to dilation of the tissue.[52] In most cases, downsizing to a smaller length prosthesis will solve this issue, but in some cases, additional interventions may be required.[53,54,55] **Figure 9.10** provides a framework for troubleshooting leakage around the prosthesis, and **Table 9.4** provides prosthetic solutions to leakage.

Table 9.4. Prosthetic Options for Leakage Around the Prosthesis
Blom Singer large esophageal flange
Blom Singer large tracheal flange
Provox XtraSeal
Provox XtraFlange

Figure 9.10 Algorithm-Options for Leakage around Prosthesis

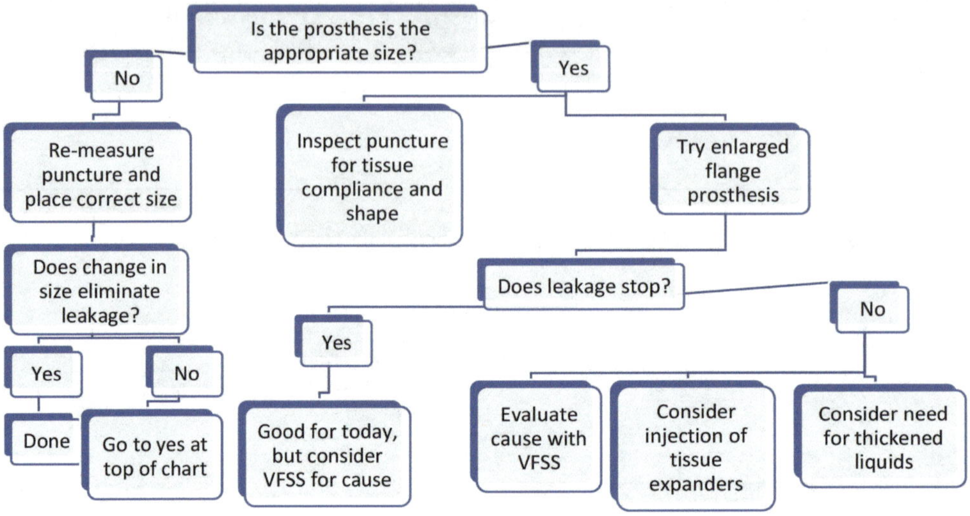

(VFSS-videofluoroscopic swallow study)

Esophageal Speech

Esophageal speech is produced by insufflating the esophagus with air and then allowing this air to be released through the UES where vibration creates sound.[56,57] As opposed to tracheoesophageal speech, which occurs when pulmonary air is shunted through a prosthesis, esophageal speech relies on active air insufflation from the mouth. Air can enter the esophagus only when there is higher pressure above the UES than below. Thus, air insufflation occurs either when patients produce high intra-oral pressure or when they create low pressure at the level of the UES by relaxing the cricopharyngeus muscle. The primary advantage of esophageal speech is that it does not rely on any device. Thus, once mastered, the patient no longer will rely on the SLP for long-term care. Unfortunately, esophageal speech is challenging for patients to learn with acquisition rates as low as 40% despite extensive speech therapy.[58,59] Additionally, as esophageal speech depends on smaller air "charges," phrase length may be negatively impacted and natural speech may be judged as inferior than other options.[60,61] Thus, esophageal speech is not as commonly used as tracheoesophageal speech.

Esophageal speech training includes strategies to accomplish air insufflation as well as treatment of distracting secondary behaviors. Positive pressure injection methods rely on using the articulators to force high-pressure air through the cricopharyngeus, while the inhalation method relies on chest expansion and dropping of UES pressures to pull air into the esophagus.[62] In both cases, the patient will need to redirect the air through the UES to create voice, which is then articulated in the normal fashion. Unfortunately, some patients may develop distracting behaviors during air insufflation such as grimacing or tensing the neck/shoulders. The SLP can use mirrors and video biofeedback to help patients extinguish such distractions.

- Esophageal speech is produced by insufflating the esophagus with air that is allowed to be released through the UES, where vibration creates sound.
- The primary advantage of esophageal speech is that it does not rely on any device.
- Esophageal speech is challenging for patients to learn with acquisition rates as low as 40%.

Augmentative/Alternative Communication

While most patients are able to successfully acquire alaryngeal communication techniques, there are some patients who require alternative options. In particular, patients who undergo extensive surgeries involving the majority of the tongue require other options. Augmentative and alternative communication options should be sought to meet the unique communication needs of each patient. Fortunately, there are a number of high- and low-tech options that can be explored by the SLP, including writing, specialized medical communication augmentative and alternative communication (AAC) devices, as well as text to speech apps available on many smartphones and tablets. The SLP should work with the patient to ensure communication needs are met through whatever method necessary.

Pulmonary Rehabilitation

In addition to communication rehabilitation, the SLP has an active role in the pulmonary rehabilitation of patients following laryngectomy. Prior to laryngectomy, the nose and mouth serve to filter, moisten, and warm the air before it reaches the lungs.[63] As this function is disrupted after laryngectomy, rehabilitation efforts should focus on compensating for these changes. The heat and moisture exchange unit (HME) (**Figure 9.11**) is designed to replicate the typical functions of the upper airway.[64] One important function of the HME is humidification. Humidity in the trachea is important for the ciliary activity, which assists in clearance of materials out of the lungs and airway. Ciliary activity becomes impaired when relative humidity in the trachea drops below 70%. Studies of tracheal humidity reveal ~50% relative humidity following laryngectomy compared to ~99% in nose/mouth breathers. Use of an HME increases relative humidity back to ~70% thereby protecting ciliary function for airway clearance.[64.65] Additionally, HME use thins tracheal secretions leading to improved airway clearance.[66] From a patient perspective, this leads to improved cough efficiency, reduced cough frequency, improved sleep, and enriched quality of life.[67] Benefits extend not only to acute symptoms but also to long-term lung function.[65,68]

Figure 9.11 Atos HME

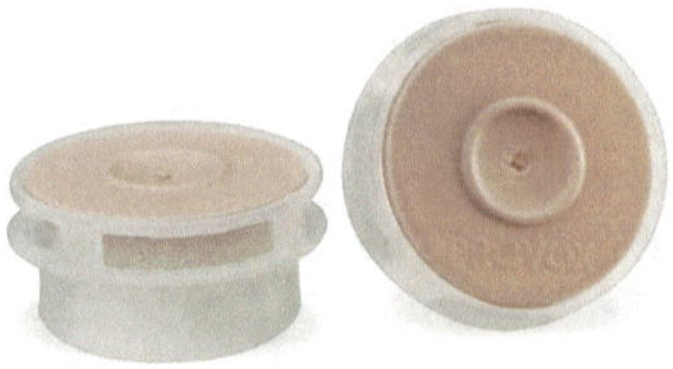

Image © Atos Medical AB and Chris Edghill

The HME is not directly attached to the stoma; therefore, an interface is required to keep the HME in place. Patients may opt for either adhesive peristomal attachments (**Figure 9.12**) or intraluminal devices such as laryngectomy tubes (**Figure 9.13**) and buttons (**Figure 9.14**). Adhesive peristomal attachments work best for patients with flat neck topography or large and irregular stomas.[69] Laryngectomy tubes and buttons are preferred for patients with deep-set stomas, irregular neck topography, and/or smaller, round stomas.[70]

Figure 9.12 Atos Adhesive Baseplate

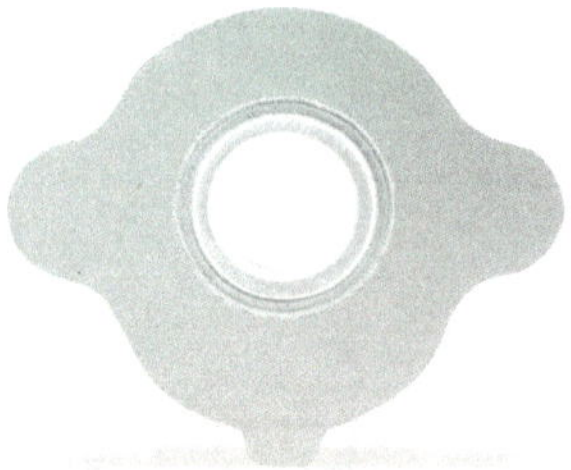

Image © Atos Medical AB and Chris Edghill

Figure 9.13 Atos Larytube

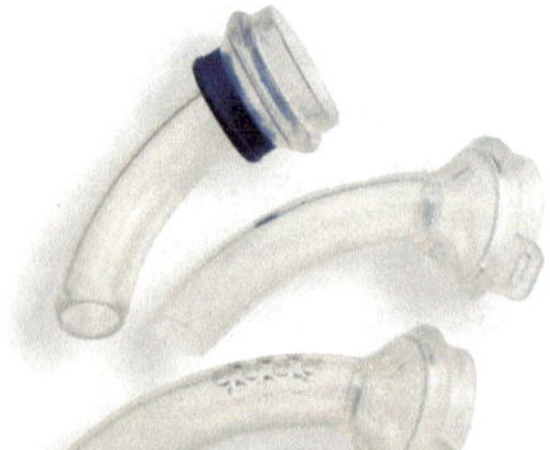

Image © Atos Medical AB and Chris Edghill

Figure 9.14 Atos Laryngectomy Button

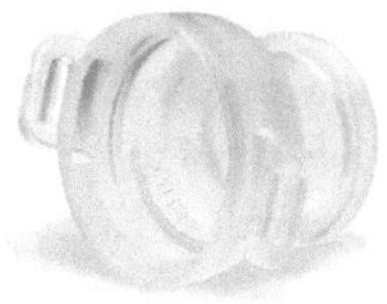

Image © Atos Medical AB and Chris Edghill

For patients who opt not to use HME filters, it remains important to keep the stoma covered to protect the airway from matter such as dust, pollen, insects, and other airborne particulates. It is important, however, to recognize that stoma covers function only to filter and not to moisten or warm the air. Stoma covers may also serve a cosmetic function to minimize visibility of the stoma. Stoma covers range from small foam squares that stick to the neck above the stoma to "dickie" mock t-shirts. Patients are often creative in using items like scarves and jewelry to "mask" the stoma as well.

Stoma Care

The patient will need to learn to care for the stoma in order to facilitate effortless breathing. If the stoma is not cleaned regularly, thick mucus may accumulate and eventually block the airway.[71] While stoma cleaning is required frequently immediately after surgery, patients will have a lower burden for stoma care over time. Patients should be reminded of the need to minimize the risk of contamination and infection; therefore, hands and instruments used during cleaning should be kept free of contamination. Saline can be used around the stoma to help loosen crusts that may accumulate. If accumulated crusts are difficult to clear, a mixture of equal parts water and hydrogen peroxide can be used to loosen for easy removal. Tweezers can be used to clean softened crusts. Water based lubricants can be used if the stoma is dry; however, petroleum-based products such as Vaseline should never be used around the airway.

Tracheal suctioning will be necessary for the majority of patients immediately after surgery. Fortunately, over time, most patients are able to produce adequate cough strength to expel secretions without the need for a suction device. However, for the first 3-4 months, many patients will require tracheal suctioning as an adjunct to coughing for airway clearance. Patients and their caregivers should be trained in sterile suctioning during the hospital stay.

In addition to cleaning the stoma and the surrounding skin, patients also need to regularly clean the laryngectomy tube/button to prevent clogging from secretions. If the laryngectomy tube becomes clogged with secretions, it may restrict air passage to the point where the patient is unable to breathe. In general, the tube will need to be cleaned at least twice daily immediately after surgery and less frequently over time. The laryngectomy is typically cleaned with soft brushes, saline, and hydrogen peroxide. However, peroxide should not be used with tubes made of silicone, nylon, or metal, so specific recommendations for cleaning are available from the manufacturer of each device.

SWALLOWING

Total laryngectomy results in the surgical division of the trachea and the esophagus; therefore, aspiration is typically not a concern. By contrast, swallowing efficiency may be significantly altered, leading to a predominant patient perception of dysphagia, up to 71% in one study.[72] It is particularly important for the SLP to note that swallowing difficulties associated with surgery may be further compounded by side effects of radiation. Swallowing difficulty after laryngectomy may be anatomic or physiologic in nature and is best assessed with videofluoroscopy.

There are a number of reasons why patients may experience dysphagia following laryngectomy. Typically, opening of the UES is facilitated by the anterior-superior excursion of the hyoid and larynx.[73] As these structures are removed during laryngectomy, there may be an impact on bolus propulsion into the esophagus. In addition, removal or denervation of the pharyngeal constrictors may lead to reduced pharyngeal clearing forces.[74] Another potential cause of post-laryngectomy dysphagia is formation of a pseudoepiglottis and pseudovallecula where food or liquid may become entrapped.[75] This is typically due to scar formation when the surgical defect is closed horizontally. Finally, patients undergoing laryngectomy may experience stricture either due to surgery or radiation therapy.[76,77] A stricture is a narrow region in the pharynx or upper esophagus that limits bolus passage, particularly with solid foods.

Treatment of post-laryngectomy dysphagia depends on the underlying etiology. When dysphagia is the result of reduced pharyngeal driving forces, the SLP can provide exercises to strengthen the base of the tongue. Additionally, patients may be provided with strategies such as soft food preparation and liquid wash to facilitate pharyngeal clearance. In cases where the UES does not open adequately or there is stricture, surgical procedures may be employed to reduce obstruction. These procedures include myotomy (division of muscle fibers), dilation (stretching), or Botox (denervation).[78] In cases where a pseudovallecula is causing problematic residue, laser resection of the scar band may be offered.[79]

CLINICAL SCENARIO CONT'D.

Mr. Jones requires radiation after his laryngectomy. About six months after radiation, he reports an increase in swallowing difficulty to his SLP. He also notes an increase in strain when trying to voice and difficulty using his hands-free valve. She performs a videofluoroscopic swallowing evaluation that reveals a stricture at the upper esophageal sphincter. He is referred for dilation, which resolves his concerns.

In addition to the anatomic and physiologic changes associated with laryngectomy, patients may also experience sensory changes that may impact eating. Following laryngectomy, lack of airflow through the nose and mouth may result in diminished smell and taste.[80] This is particularly problematic when patients have also been exposed to radiation therapy. The SLP can train the patient in techniques to draw air in through the nose to improve sense of smell/taste. The "polite yawn" is a technique where patients can use rapid lowering of the jaw and soft palate to draw air in through the nose. This simple technique may offer a substantial positive impact on quality of life.[81]

Additional Medical Issues After Laryngectomy

Lymphedema

Lymphedema is an abnormal accumulation of protein-rich fluid in the space between cells. The fluid accumulation causes chronic inflammation and reactive fibrosis of the affected tissues. It is a common complication of radiation and surgery for head and neck cancer. Radiation creates scarring, which interferes with the function of the lymphatic system. Additionally, surgical removal of lymph nodes may result in swelling as the lymphatic fluid cannot re-enter the systemic circulation and accumulates in the tissues. There are two types of lymphedema that can develop in patients with head and neck cancer: an external visible swelling of the skin or soft tissue and an internal swelling of the mucosa of the pharynx and larynx.[82] Lymphedema generally starts slowly and is progressive. While rarely painful, lymphedema causes discomfort in the form of a sensation of heaviness and achiness, and may lead to skin changes.

Lymphedema has several stages:

Stage 0: Latency stage – No visible/palpable edema.

Stage 1: Accumulation of protein-rich pitting edema that can be reduced with elevation.

Stage 2: Progressive pitting, proliferation of connective tissue (fibrosis).

Stage 3: No pitting, presence of fibrosis, sclerosis, and skin changes.

Lymphedema of the head and neck can cause several functional impairments. These include:

- Difficulty in breathing
- Impairment in vision
- Motor limitations (reduced neck motion, jaw tightness or trismus and chest tightness)
- Sensory limitations
- Speech, voice and swallowing problems (inability to use an electrolarynx, difficulty in articulation, drooling, and loss of food from mouth)
- Emotional issues (depression, frustration, and embarrassment)

Over time, the lymphatic system may establish an alternative way of drainage leading to reduced edema. Neck tightness and swelling due to lymphedema generally improve over time, particularly if treated in the early stages. Lymphedema therapy may be provided by specialty-trained physical, occupational, or speech therapists. Complete decongestive therapy to treat lymphedema includes:[83]

- Manual lymph drainage (a hands-on manual massage to move fluid)
- Compressive bandages and garments
- Remedial exercises
- Skin care
- Elastic therapeutic tape (Kinesiotape)
- Oncology rehabilitation
- Elevation of the head when sleeping

Diuretics, surgical removal (debulking), liposuction, compression pumps, and elevation of the head alone are ineffective treatments.

Hypothyroidism

Most laryngectomees develop hypothyroidism. This is due to the effects of radiation and/or the removal of part or all of the thyroid gland during laryngectomy surgery.[84] The symptoms of hypothyroidism vary: Some individuals have no symptoms, while others have dramatic or, rarely, life-threatening symptoms. Thyroid deficiency can be corrected by taking synthetic thyroid hormones. The symptoms of hypothyroidism are nonspecific and mimic many normal changes of aging:

- General symptoms - The thyroid hormone stimulates the body's metabolism. Most symptoms of hypothyroidism are due to the slowing of metabolic processes. Systemic symptoms include fatigue, sluggishness, weight gain, and intolerance to cold temperatures.
- Skin - Decreased sweating, dry and thick skin, coarse or thin hair, disappearance of eyebrows, and brittle nails.
- Eyes - Mild swelling around the eyes.
- Cardiovascular system - Slowing of the heart rate and weakening of cardiac contractions, decreasing its overall function. Thus, these can cause fatigue and shortness of breath with exercise. Hypothyroidism can also cause mild hypertension and raise cholesterol levels.
- Respiratory system - Respiratory muscles may weaken and lung function can decrease. Symptoms include fatigue, shortness of breath with exercise, and decreased ability to exercise.
- Gastrointestinal system - Slowing of the digestive tract motility, causing constipation.
- Reproductive system - Menstrual cycle irregularities, ranging from absent or infrequent periods to very frequent and heavy.

Thyroid deficiency can be corrected by taking a synthetic thyroid hormone (Thyroxine) which is best taken on an empty stomach with a full glass of water 30 minutes before eating, preferably before breakfast or at a similar time of day. This is because food containing high fat (e.g., eggs, bacon, toast, hash brown potatoes, and milk) can decrease thyroxine absorption by 40 percent.[85]

Several formulations of synthetic thyroxine are available, but there has been considerable controversy over their relative efficacy. In 2004, the US FDA approved a generic substitute for branded levothyroxine products. The American Thyroid Association, Endocrine Society, and the American Association of Clinical Endocrinologists objected to this decision, recommending that patients remain on the same brand.[86] If patients must switch brands or use a generic substitute, serum thyroid stimulating hormone (TSH) should be checked six weeks later. Because there may be subtle differences between synthetic thyroxine formulations, it is better to stay with one formulation when possible. If the preparation must be changed, follow-up monitoring of TSH and sometimes thyroxine (T4) serum levels should be done to determine if dose adjustments are necessary.

After starting therapy, the patient should be reevaluated and serum TSH should be measured in three to six weeks, and the dose adjusted if needed. Symptoms of hypothyroidism generally begin to resolve after two to three weeks of replacement therapy and may take at least six weeks to dissipate. A thyroxine dose can be increased in three weeks in patients who continue to have symptoms and who have a high serum TSH concentration. It takes about six weeks before a steady hormone state is achieved after therapy is initiated or the dose is changed.

The process of increasing the dose of hormone every three to six weeks is continued, based upon periodic measurements of TSH until it returns to normal (from approximately 0.5 to 5.0 mU/L).

Once this is achieved, periodic monitoring is needed. After identification of the proper maintenance dose, the patient should be examined and serum TSH measured once a year (or more often if there is an abnormal result or a change in the patient's condition). Dose adjustment may be needed as patients age or have a weight change.

Pain

The degree of pain experienced after laryngectomy is subjective, but as a general rule, the more extensive the surgery, the more likely the patient will experience pain. Certain types of reconstructive procedures where tissue is transferred as a flap from the chest muscles, forearm, thigh, jejunum, or a stomach pull up are more likely to be associated with increased or prolonged pain.[87] For individuals who experience chronic pain as a result of laryngectomy or any other head and neck surgery, evaluation by a pain management specialist is usually helpful. Treatments may include oral medication, nerve blocks, acupuncture, acupressure, massage, physical therapy, meditation, relaxation, and even humor. Specialists in pain management can offer these treatments.[88]

Patients who require a radical neck dissection as part of the surgery may experience additional pain. At present, most patients undergo a "modified radical neck dissection" when the spinal accessory nerve is not removed.[89] If the spinal accessory nerve is cut or removed during surgery, the patient is more likely to have shoulder discomfort, stiffness, and long-term loss of range of motion and strength. Some of the associated discomfort of this procedure can be prevented by exercise and physical therapy.

Treating pain can both increase patients' well-being and ease the hardship imposed on their caregivers. As chronic pain may interfere with rehabilitation efforts, pain management is an important aspect of rehabilitation. Patients should be encouraged to talk to their health care providers about their pain and seek treatment. Clinicians should remain vigilant regarding patient pain and initiate appropriate referrals when necessary.

Clinical Scenario Cont'd.

Mr. Jones continues to have pain in the months following his surgery and radiation. He notes stiffness and reduced mobility of his neck. He is referred to the pain management team who recommends a combination of medication, physical therapy, and massage. After three months of treatment, he reports reduction in his neck pain as well as improvement in function and quality of life.

Psychological Issues

Head and neck cancer survivors, including laryngectomees, face many psychological, social, and personal challenges. Head and neck cancer and its treatment affect some of the most basic human functions, such as breathing, eating, communication, and social interaction.[90] Understanding and treating these issues are no less important than dealing with medical concerns. Post-traumatic stress disorder is one of the psychological results of laryngectomy and is more common in females.[91]

Individuals diagnosed with cancer experience numerous feelings and emotions which can change from day to day, hour to hour, or even minute to minute and can generate a heavy psychological burden. Some of the feelings include, anger, mood swings, fear, stress, anxiety, depression, sadness, guilt, and loneliness. Some of the psychological and social challenges faced by laryngectomees include depression, anxiety and fear of recurrence, social isolation, substance abuse, body image concerns, sexuality issues, return to work matters, economic impact, and changes in interaction with spouses, family, friends, and co-workers.

Depression

Many people with cancer feel sad or depressed. This is a normal response to any serious illness. Depression is one of the most difficult issues faced by a patient with cancer,[92] and yet the social stigma associated with admitting depression makes it difficult to reach out and seek therapy. The challenges of life as a laryngectomee in the shadow of cancer means it is even more difficult to deal with depression. The inability to speak or difficulties with speech make it harder to express emotions and can lead to isolation. Surgical and medical care is often not sufficient to address such issues, and more emphasis should be placed on mental well-being after laryngectomy.

Coping with and overcoming depression are important for the well-being of the patient. Managing depression may facilitate recovery and increase one's chance for a longer survival and ultimately a cure. There is growing scientific evidence of a connection between mind and body. Although many of these connections are not yet understood, it is well recognized that individuals who are motivated to get better and exhibit a positive attitude recover faster from serious illnesses, live longer, and sometimes overcome immense odds. It has been shown that this effect may be mediated by alterations in the cellular immune responses and a decrease in natural killer cell activity. [93]

Naturally, there are many reasons to feel depressed after learning one's cancer diagnosis, and then, living with it.[94] It is a devastating illness for patients and their families, particularly because of the lack of a cure for most types of cancer. By the time the disease has been discovered, it is too late for prevention, and, if the cancer has been discovered at an advanced stage, the risk of dissemination is high and the chance of an ultimate cure is significantly decreased. Hopefully, the patient can find the strength within to fight depression. Immediately after a laryngectomy, individuals may be overwhelmed by new daily tasks and realities. They often experience a mourning period for their many losses, including their voice and prior state of health. They also have to accept many permanent deficits, including not being able to speak "normally." Some may feel they have a choice between succumbing to a creeping depression or becoming proactive and returning to life. A desire to get better and overcome a handicap can be the driving force to reversing the downhill trend. Depression may recur, requiring a continuous struggle to overcome it.

Support from family members and friends is important. Continuous involvement and contribution to others' lives can be invigorating. One can draw strength from enjoying, interacting and impacting the lives of their children and grandchildren. Setting an example to one's children and grandchildren not to give up in the face of adversity can be the driving force to be proactive and resist depression.[95] Getting involved in activities that one liked before the surgery can provide a continuous purpose for life. Participating in the activities of a local laryngectomee club can be a new source of support, advice, and friendship.

Seeking the help of a mental health professional such as a social worker, psychologist or psychiatrist can also be helpful. There are many treatment options available to treat depression. These include psychotherapy, medications, and transcranial magnetic stimulation. Having a caring and competent physician and a speech and language pathologist who can provide continuous follow-up is vital. Their involvement can help patients deal with emerging medical and speech problems and can contribute to their sense of well-being.

Suicide

Patients with head and neck cancer have more than three times the incidence of suicide compared with the general population. A recent investigation cited a nearly 12-fold higher incidence of suicide in patients with hypopharyngeal cancer and a five-fold higher incidence in those with laryngeal cancer.[96] The higher rate of suicide in these patients could be attributed to prolonged dysphagia and dependence tracheostomy and gastrostomy tubes. These factors clearly point to the urgent need to recognize and treat psychiatric problems such as depression and suicidal ideation in laryngectomees.

Most studies have reported a high incidence of major and minor depressive mood disorders associated with suicide among cancer patients.[97] Elderly cancer patients suffer less severe depression, which is sometimes not recognized and often undertreated. Approximately half of all suicides among people with cancer were preceded by major depression and other contributing factors, including anxiety, lack of social support systems, and demoralization.[98]

Screening cancer patients for depression, hopelessness, distress, severe pain, coping problems, and suicidal ideation is a useful way to identify those at risk. Counseling and referral to mental health specialists, when appropriate, may prevent suicide in at-risk cancer patients.[99] This approach also involves speaking with patients at heightened risk for suicide (and their families) about reducing access to the most common methods used to commit suicide.

Coping with Uncertain Future

Once cancer had been diagnosed, and despite successful treatment, it is difficult to completely free oneself from the fear that it may return. Some people are better than others at living with this uncertainty. Those who adjust well become happier and more able to go on with their lives than those who do not.[100]

One of the difficult challenges is waiting for the results of an important test or scans. Many individuals feel anxiety and are worried during the waiting period. What makes predicting the future difficult is that the scans used to detect cancer (positron emission tomography or PET, magnetic resonance imaging or MRI, and computed tomography or CT) only detect with certainty cancer lesions that are larger than one centimeter; thus, physicians may miss a small lesion located at a site that is difficult to detect. Patients, therefore, have to accept the reality that the cancer may return and that physical examination and vigilance are the best ways of monitoring their condition. Hopefully, over time, one strikes a balance between fear and acceptance as coping with, and learning to accept, an uncertain future improves.

Coping and Adjusting to One's Disfigurement

Dealing with disfigurement of the face and neck as a result of surgery and radiation is one of the greatest challenges for laryngectomees. It may influence their self-image and self-identity.[101] Cancer and its treatment can cause significant changes to how one looks, feels, and functions. For many whose appearance changed significantly after treatment, adjusting to their new looks, as well as impaired ability to communicate and eat, is difficult. Unlike many other types of cancer, the deformities and scars from head and neck cancer are often visible and cannot be hidden. This may make one feel self-conscious and less confident, wondering if these visible disfigurements will influence relationships. It may push some to social isolation and depression. Hopefully, over time, the patient can adjust to their disfigurements. These adjustments require dealing with physical, emotional, and social issues. Physical adjustments include dealing with difficulties in drinking, chewing, swallowing, breathing, speaking, hearing, and head and neck movements. These issues may affect one's social adjustment, as they can limit one's ability to eat out or enjoy other social interactions, leading to isolation. The need to find new ways to communicate can be frustrating and difficult. Overcoming one's functional challenges and fears about how others may react to them is an important step in adjustment. Maintaining an active social life can facilitate adjustment by preventing or even reversing depression, anxiety, and isolation.

Some individuals struggle more with changes in their appearance than how they function. Adjusting to changes in both appearance and function may be even more challenging.[102] The visibility of emotions on the face can exacerbate patients' self-consciousness and fear of social interactions, creating uncertainty about how people will react to them.

Even though it is difficult to control how others will react, there are coping strategies that can help one interact more confidently and avoid negative encounters. Clinical research showed that individuals with facial disfigurements who approach others with confidence and the belief that they will accept their appearance are more likely to be successful socially and emotionally than those who are not confident or expect rejection. Most people will respond positively and adapt quickly to one's appearance and will react better to those who are confident and positive. A potentially positive and uplifting consequence of openly displaying their deformities reveals the patients' medical history, and the fact they are cancer survivors who go on with their lives despite their handicap.

SURVIVORSHIP

Continual medical follow-up by specialists, including the otolaryngologist, radiation oncologist, and medical oncologist is important. As time passes from the initial diagnosis and surgery, follow-up occurs with less frequency.[103] Most otolaryngologists recommend monthly follow-up examinations in the first year after diagnosis, and less often afterwards, depending on the patient's condition. Patients should be encouraged to contact their physician whenever new symptoms arise.

Most major cancer medical centers in the US follow the National Comprehensive Cancer Network (NCCN) guidelines and recommendations[104] for follow-up of head and neck cancer patients. These guidelines are based on the potential risk of relapse and second primary cancers, treatment sequelae and toxicities resulting from treatment. The guidelines recommend a complete head and neck exam every 1-3 months for the first year after treatment and/or surgery, every 2-6 months for the second year, every 4-8 months for the third through fifth years, and then every 12 months thereafter. However, each patient's head and neck surgeon, medical oncologist, and radiation oncologist generally determines the frequency of follow-up visits based on the relative risk of recurrence. Recurrence generally depends on the site of the original tumor, the stage of the disease when first detected, and whether the disease spread to lymph nodes in the neck or other organs in the body.

The NCCN also recommends baseline imaging of the tumor site and neck within six months of treatment. Follow-up imaging is based on concerning signs and symptoms, smoking history, and areas that could not be seen on clinical exam. Chest imaging is recommended for individuals with a smoking history based on the guidelines for lung cancer screening. Thyroid checkup is recommended if the neck has been irradiated or the thyroid has been removed. Regular follow-up includes smoking cessation; alcohol counseling, if needed; dental, nutritional, and swallowing evaluation; speech and hearing assessments; and ongoing surveillance for depression.

It is critical that patients and their care providers are vigilant to identify cancer recurrence or emergence of a second primary tumor. There is a higher probability of cancer recurrence or a new cancer occurring in the first few years after diagnosis. Early identification of recurrence increases survival, which can reach 90% when the cancer is in stage I, and only 70% in stage ll.[105] It is also important to be followed by an internist or family physician, as well as a dentist, to address other medical and dental issues.

Smoking and excessive alcohol consumption are known risk factors for developing many types of head and neck cancer, in addition to several other types of cancer. Individuals with head and neck cancer should receive counseling about the importance of smoking cessation[106] because continued smoking can worsen cancer prognosis. Patients with laryngeal cancer who continue to smoke and drink are less likely to be cured and are more likely to develop a second tumor.[107] Continued smoking, either during or after radiation therapy, can increase the severity and duration of mucosal reactions, worsen dry mouth (xerostomia), and compromise patient outcome.

Urgent Care

Laryngectomees and other neck breathers are at great risk of receiving inadequate acute care when they experience breathing difficulties or when they need cardiopulmonary resuscitation (CPR).[100] Emergency departments and emergency medical response personnel often do not recognize a patient who is a neck breather, do not know how to administer oxygen properly, and may erroneously give mouth-to-mouth or bag-valve-mask ventilation when mouth-to-stoma or bag-valve/mask to stoma ventilation is indicated. Many medical personnel are also not familiar with the care of laryngectomees because a laryngectomy is a relatively rare procedure. This can lead to devastating consequences, with potential anoxia. As such, care providers working with patients following laryngectomy should be aware of altered approaches of providing rescue care.

It is important for medical personnel to differentiate partial neck breathers from total neck breathers (total laryngectomees) because the management of each group is different. The trachea is not connected to the upper airway following total laryngectomy, and all breathing is accomplished through the tracheal stoma. By contrast, partial neck breathers retain a connection between the trachea and upper airway, even though there is a tracheal stoma. Thus, partial neck breathers are also able to breathe through their mouth and nose. However, the extent of breathing through the upper airway in those individuals varies and failure to recognize a partial neck breather may lead to inappropriate treatment.

The most common cause of sudden breathing difficulty in total laryngectomees is airway blockage due to aspiration of a foreign body or a mucous plug. Laryngectomees may also suffer from other medical conditions including heart, lung, and vascular problems. It may be difficult to detect a carotid artery pulse in the neck of some laryngectomees because of post-radiation fibrosis. Some patients may not have a radial artery pulse in one of their arms if tissue from that arm was used as a free flap to reconstruct the upper airway.

Preparation for Rescue Breathing

Resuscitation of a patient following total laryngectomy is different than a patient with a tracheostomy tube). Resuscitation of a total neck breather (after total laryngectomy) is different from a partial neck breather (after partial laryngectomy or tracheostomy). A total neck breather may or may not have a tube in place. The steps to rescue a total neck breather are:

1. Determine the patient's responsiveness.
2. Activate the emergency medical services.
3. Position the person supine when possible and extend shoulders to expose the chest and neck.
4. Remove anything covering the stoma (such as filter or cloth that may prevent access to the airway).
5. Clear any mucus from the stoma.
    - Secure an airway in the stoma (such as a laryngectomy, tracheostomy, or endotracheal tube). Remove anything blocking the airway, such as a filter or an HME.

The stoma of a total neck-breather may have within it a tube, a button, or a housing, supporting structures such as an HME (**Figures 9.11-9.14**). For total neck-breathers, all resuscitation efforts should focus on the stoma. It is not necessary to remove the stoma's housing unless it blocks the airway. If a tube is present, saline lavage may be performed through instillation of 2-5 cc of sterile saline to clear any mucous plugs.[108] Otherwise, the tube can be removed (outer and inner cannulas).

Laryngectomy tubes or stoma buttons should be carefully removed. The voice prosthesis should not be removed, unless it is blocking the airway, breathing, or suctioning. If the prosthesis is dislodged, it should be removed and replaced with a catheter to prevent aspiration and fistula closure. Next, the stoma should be wiped and suctioned and breath sounds should be heard over the stoma. If breath sounds are present, then ventilation can be supported by placing a tube within the airway or manually ventilating with a pediatric face mask. Care should be used in inserting the tube so that it does not dislodge the voice prosthesis, which may necessitate inserting a tube with a smaller diameter. If a tube is inserted to facilitate ventilation, the resuscitator should ensure the distal tip is above the carina and that bilateral breath sounds can be auscultated and both sides of the chest rise.

If the tracheostomy tube is blocked, the chest may fail to rise. Another basic rescue maneuver would be to administer direct mouth-to-stoma ventilation. It is useless to try to perform mouth-to-mouth ventilation on a neck breather, and doing so would waste precious time.

Even if the patient has a normal breathing pattern, he or she should be treated like any unconscious patient. If prolonged administration of oxygen is required, it should be humidified.

Care of Laryngectomees During Anesthesia or Procedures

Undergoing a procedure (e.g., colonoscopy) under sedation, or surgery with either local or general anesthesia can be challenging for laryngectomees.[109] Unfortunately, most medical personnel who care for laryngectomees before, during, and after surgery are not familiar with their unique anatomy, how they speak, and how to manage their airway during and after the procedure or operation. These include nurses, medical technicians, surgeons and even anesthesia personnel. It is advisable that laryngectomees explain their unique needs and anatomy before the surgery to those who will be treating them. Using illustrations or pictures is helpful. Anesthetists should view the stoma in order to understand the function of the voice prosthesis and its position in the airway and be cautioned not to remove it unless it is dislodged. It is important to discuss the patient's special requirements with the surgical and anesthesia teams during the pre-surgical evaluation and on the day of surgery. The patient should inform the caring teams how they will notify them of pain or the need to be suctioned.

SUMMARY

Total laryngectomy is a distinct procedure which shares common features with tracheostomy, but also has marked differences. The rehabilitation of individuals following laryngectomy is complex and should include consideration of communication needs, swallowing, respiration, and psychological adaptation. Care providers must be cognizant of the complexity of post-laryngectomy rehabilitation and vigilant for a multitude of factors that may arise. Though complex, rehabilitation of patients following laryngectomy can be highly rewarding and lead to long-term benefits for both the patient and the provider. All care providers should be familiar with the unique resuscitation needs of a laryngectomee.

KEY POINTS:

- Unlike patients with a tracheostomy, patients are completely unable to breathe through their nose and mouth following laryngectomy.
- Total laryngectomy results in removal of the entire larynx, not merely a bypass of the larynx as seen in tracheostomy.
- Rehabilitation of communication following laryngectomy revolves around establishment of an alternative sound source.
- Rehabilitation following laryngectomy should not stop at restoration of communication, but should also encompass swallowing, pulmonary, and olfactory rehabilitation.
- There is great complexity to consider in patients following laryngectomy, including medical and mental health issues.

REVIEW QUESTIONS

1. What is the primary difference between patients undergoing tracheostomy and patients undergoing total laryngectomy?
    a. Patients are able to breathe through the nose and mouth following laryngectomy.
    b. The entire larynx is removed during a total laryngectomy leading to total neck breathing.
    c. Patients are unable to use their vocal folds to create voice following tracheostomy.
    d. After tracheostomy, patients must receive all oxygen only through the tracheostomy site.

    ANSWER: B. The primary difference between tracheostomy and laryngectomy is the presence/absence of the larynx. After total laryngectomy, the patient is a total neck breather as the nose and mouth are structurally separated from the trachea/lungs. Choice A is incorrect as the nose and mouth are surgically separated from the trachea/lungs during total laryngectomy. Choice C is incorrect because patients undergoing tracheostomy can redirect air through the larynx by digital tracheostomy occlusion, use of a speaking valve, or plugging the tracheostomy tube. Choice D is incorrect as tracheostomy does not separate the upper and lower airways. Thus, while applying oxygen to the tracheostomy site is more efficient, oxygen may be delivered to the upper airway in some patients following tracheostomy.

2. What is the source of vibration for tracheoesophageal speech?
    a. Pharyngoesophageal segment
    b. The voice prosthesis
    c. The vocal folds
    d. The tracheal wall

    ANSWER: A. Following laryngectomy, the pharyngeoesophageal segment (also called neoglottis) is put into vibration when exhaled air passes through the voice prosthesis into the esophagus. This vibration is the foundation for tracheoesophageal speech. Choice B is incorrect as the prosthesis serves as a conduit for airflow but does not actually vibrate. Choice C is incorrect as the vocal folds are removed during total laryngectomy. Choice D is incorrect as the tracheal wall does not vibrate in response to egressive airflow.

3. Which communication option following total laryngectomy is typically judged as most natural and acceptable to listeners?
    a. Electrolaryngeal speech
    b. Tracheoesophageal speech
    c. Esophageal speech
    d. Augmentative/alternative communication

    ANSWER: B. Tracheoesophageal speech uses exhaled air to drive pharyngoesophageal vibration. This provides the most fluent speech using natural anatomy. Choice A is incorrect as the mechanical vocal quality is often considered unacceptable or difficult to understand. Choice C is incorrect because phrase length is shorter since exhaled air is not the driving force. Additionally, behaviors during air charging may be distracting to the listener. Choice D is incorrect as it often prevents natural, fluent conversation and relies on technological devices.

4. What is the most common cause of leakage around a tracheoesophageal voice prosthesis?
    a. Biofilm accumulation
    b. Cancer recurrence
    c. Inadequate prosthesis size
    d. Esophageal stricture

ANSWER: C. Excessive length of a voice prosthesis can lead to pistoning in and dilation of the puncture tract, allowing fluids to seep around the prosthesis. Presentation with leakage around the voice prosthesis is often due to excessive length. Choice A is incorrect as biofilm is more commonly associated with leakage through a voice prosthesis. Choice B is incorrect since recurrent disease is much less common than inappropriate prosthesis size. Similarly, esophageal stricture is a less common problem that may contribute to leakage around a prosthesis.

5. Why is it important for a patient to wear a heat moisture exchange unit following total laryngectomy?
    a. To detract attention from the stoma.
    b. Because ciliary clearance is reduced with changes in temperature and humidity associated with neck breathing.
    c. Because it is the only way laryngectomees can speak after surgery.
    d. Because it can prevent drowning.

ANSWER: B. The nose and mouth play an important role in preparing the air for the trachea and lungs. Neck breathing is associated with reduction in temperature and humidity in the airway and leads to reduction in ciliary function. Lack of ciliary function may lead to increased accumulation of airway secretions and coughing. Thus, the HME plays an important role in restoring normal airway function. Choice A is incorrect because other strategies can be employed to mask the stoma, such as foam or cloth stoma covers. Choice C is incorrect since the HME does not produce voice. It may be used to help occlude the stoma for tracheoesophageal speech; however, patients are able to communicate using esophageal or electrolaryngeal speech. Choice D is incorrect because the HME is not designed to create a water-tight seal at the stoma. Thus, a patient wearing an HME is still at risk for drowning if submerged in water.

References

1. Cocek A. The history and current status of surgery in the treatment of laryngeal cancer. *Acta Medica.* 2008;51(3):157-63.
2. National Cancer Institute, Surveillance, Epidemiology, and End Results (SEER) Program; Cancer Stat Facts: Larynx Cancer 2017. https://seer.cancer.gov/statfacts/html/laryn.html. Accessed July 25, 2020.
3. American Cancer Society; Cancer Facts and Figures 2017; Special section – Rare Cancers in Adults. http://www.cancer.net/cancer-types/laryngeal-and-hypopharyngeal-cancer/statistics Accessed July 25, 2020.
4. Underwood JM, Richards TB, Henley SJ, et al. Decreasing trend in tobacco-related cancer incidence, United States 2005-2009. *J Community Health.* 2015;40(3):414-18.
5. Gupta B, Johnson NW, Kumar N. Global epidemiology of head and neck cancers: A continuing challenge. *Oncology.* 2016;13-23.
6. Siegel RL, Miller KD, Jemal A. Cancer Statistics. *CA Cancer J Clin.* 2016;66:7-30.
7. Scheich, L. Looking at laryngeal cancer. *Nursing.* 2007;37(5):50-55.
8. Machado RA, Moubayed SP, Hernandez-Prera JC, Urken ML. Influence of previous treatment of oral squamous cell carcinoma on the geographic distribution of recurrent neck metastases: A case series of unusual level 4 metastases. *Am J Otolaryngol.* 2016;37:459-462.
9. Nachalon Y, Cohen O, Alkan U, Shvero J, Popovtzer A. Characteristics and outcome of laryngeal squamous cell carcinoma in young adults. *Oncol Lett.* 2017;13:1393-1397.
10. Mortuaire G, Chevalier D, Mouawad F. Open partial laryngectomy after failure of (chemo) radiation: Indications, oncologic and functional outcomes. *Curr Opin Otolaryngol Head Neck Surg.* 2017;25:159-162.
11. Succo G, Peretti G, Piazza C, et al. Open partial horizontal laryngectomies: S proposal for classification by the working committee on nomenclature of the European Laryngological Society. *Eur Arch Otorhinolaryngol.* 2014;271:2489-2496.
12. Piazza C, Barbieri D, Del Bon F, et al. Functional outcomes after different types of transoral supraglottic laryngectomy. *Laryngoscope.* 2016;126:1131-1135.
13. Lörincz BB1, Knecht R. Transoral robotic total laryngectomy and neck dissection: The concept of robotic combo surgery. *Laryngorhinootologie.* 2013;92:585-588.
14. Leone CA, Capasso P, Topazio D, Russo G. Supracricoid laryngectomy for recurrent laryngeal cancer after chemoradiotherapy: a systematic review and meta-analysis. *Acta Otorhinolaryngol Ital.* 2016;36:439-449.
15. Mardini S, Salgado CJ, Kim Evans KF, Chen HC. Reconstruction of the esophagus and voice. *Plast Reconstr Surg.* 2010;126:471-485.
16. Hellstadius Y, Lagergren J, Zylstra J, et al. Prevalence and predictors of anxiety and depression among esophageal cancer patients prior to surgery. *Dis Esophagus.* 2016;29(8):1128-1134.
17. Aarstad HJ, Aarstad AK, Heimdal JH, Olofsson J. Mood, anxiety, and sense of humor in head and neck cancer patients in relation to disease stage, prognosis, and quality of life. *Acta Otolaryngol.* 2005;125(5):557-565.
18. Almonacid CI, Ramos AJ, Rodriguez-Borrego MA. Level of anxiety versus self-care in the preoperative and postoperative periods of total laryngectomy patients. *Rev Lat Am Enfermagem.* 2016;24.
19. Zeine L, Larson M. Pre- and post-operative counseling for laryngectomees and their spouses: an update. *J Commun Disord.* 1999;32:51-61.

20. Fitzgerald E, Perry A. Pre-operative counseling for laryngectomy patients: a systematic review. *J Laryngol Otol.* 2016;130(1):15-20.
21. Shenson JA, Craig JN, Rohde SL. Effect of preoperative counseling on hospital length of stay and readmissions after total laryngectomy. *Otolaryngol Head Neck Surg.* 2017;156(2):289-298.
22. Lauder E. Self-help for the laryngectomee. San Antonio, TX: Lauder Publishing; 1994.
23. Brook I. The Laryngectomee Guide. Washington D.C. CreateSpace Independent Publishing; 2013.
24. Gress CD. Preoperative evaluation for tracheoesophageal voice restoration. *Otolaryngol Clin North Amer.* 2004;37(3):519-530.
25. Ackerstaff AH, Hilgers FJ, Aaronson NK, et al. Heat and moisture exchangers as a treatment option in the post-operative rehabilitation of laryngectomized patients. *Clin Otolaryng Allied Sci.* 1995;20(6):504-509.
26. Brook I. Urgent care of neck breathers. *J Emerg Nurs.* 2011;37:163-4.
27. de Maddalena H. The influence of early speech rehabilitation with voice prostheses on the psychological state of laryngectomized patients. *Eur Arch Otorhinolaryngol.* 2002;259(1):48-52.
28. McCombe AW, Jones AS. Radiotherapy and complications of laryngectomy. *J Laryngol Otol.* 1993;107(2):130-132.
29. Ganly I, Patel S, Matsuo J, et al. Postoperative complications of salvage total laryngectomy. *Cancer.* 2005;103(10):2073-2081.
30. Xi S. Effectiveness of voice rehabilitation on vocalization in postlaryngectomy patients: a systematic review. *Int J Evid Based Healthcare.* 2010;8:256-258.
31. Doyle P.C. Foundations of voice and speech rehabilitation following laryngeal cancer. San Diego, CA. Singular Publishing. 1994.
32. Wood BG, Rusnov MG, Tucker HM, Levine HL. Tracheoesophageal puncture for alaryngeal voice restoration. *Ann Otol Rhinol Laryngol.* 1981;90:492-4.
33. Merwin GE, Goldstein LP, Rothman HB. A comparison of speech using artificial larynx and tracheoesophageal puncture with valve in the same speaker. *Laryngoscope.* 1985;95(6):730-734.
34. Sedory SE, Hamlet SL, Connor NP. Comparisons of perceptual and acoustic characteristics of tracheoesophageal and excellent esophageal speech. *J Speech Hear Disord.* 1989;54(2):209-214.
35. Saurajen AS, Chee NW, Siow JK, Lim F, Mok PK, Earnest A. Tracheoesophageal puncture outcomes and predictors of success in laryngectomized patients. *Ann Acad Med Singap.* 2000;29(4):452-456.
36. Lewin JS, Baumgart LM, Barrow MP, Hutcheson KA. Device life of tracheoesophageal voice prosthesis revisited. *JAMA Otolaryngol Head Neck Surg.* 2017;143(1):65-71.
37. van Weissenbruch R, Kunnen M, Albers FW, van Cauwenberge PB, Sulter AM. Cineradiography of the pharyngoesophageal segment in postlaryngectomy patients. *Ann Otol Rhinol Laryngol.* 2000;109(3):311-319.
38. Blom ED, Singer MI, Hamaker RC. A prospective study of tracheoesophageal speech. *Arch Otolaryngol Head Neck Surg.* 1986;112:440-447.
39. Lavertu P, Scott SE, Finnegan EM, Levine HL, Tucker HM, Wood BG. Secondary tracheoesophageal puncture for voice rehabilitation after laryngectomy. *Arch Otolaryngol Head Neck Surg.* 1989;115(3):350-355.

40. Blom ED, Singer MI, Hamaker RC. An improved esophageal insufflation test. *Arch Otolaryngol.* 1985;111:211-212.
41. Lewin JS, Baugh RF, Baker SR. An objective method for prediction of tracheoesophageal speech production. *J Speech Hear Disord.* 1987;52(3):212-217.
42. Singer S, Wollbruck D, Cook S, Fuchs M, Meuret S. Speech rehabilitation during the first year after total laryngectomy. *Head Neck.* 2013;35(11):1583-1590.
43. van As CJ, Op de Coul BM, van den Hoogen FJ, Koopmans-van Beinum FJ, Hilgers FJ. Quantitative videofluoroscopy: A new evaluation tool for tracheoesophageal voice production. *Arch Otolaryngol Head Neck Surg.* 2001;127(2):161-169.
44. Op de Coul BM, Ackerstaff AH, van as Brooks CJ, et al. Compliance, quality of life, and quantitative voice quality aspects of hands-free speech. *Acta Otolaryngol.* 2005;125(6):625-637.
45. Roxburgh J, Perry A. Use of a "hands-free" tracheostoma valve in patients with laryngectomy and tracheoesophageal puncture. *Ann Otol Rhinol Laryngol.* 2004;113(7):565-570.
46. Gerwin JM, Culton GL. Prosthetic voice restoration with the tracheostomal valve: A clinical experience. *Am J Otolaryngol.* 1993;14(6):432-439.
47. Graville D, Gross N, Andersen P, Everts E, Cohen J. The long-term indwelling tracheoesophageal prosthesis for alaryngeal voice rehabilitation. *Arch Otolaryngol Head Neck Surg.* 1999;125(3):288-292.
48. Laccourreye O, Menard M, Crevier-Buchman L, Couloigner V, Brasnu D. In situ lifetime, causes for replacement, and complications of the Provox voice prosthesis. *Laryngoscope.* 1997;107(4):527-530.
49. Yenigun A, Eren SB, Ozkul MH, Tugrul S, Meric A. Factors influencing the longevity and replacement frequency of Provox voice prostheses. *Singapore Med J.* 2015;56:632-636.
50. Talpaert MJ, Balfour A, Stevens S, Baker M, Muhlschlegel FA, Gourlay CW. Candida biofilm formation on voice prostheses. *J Med Microbiol.* 2015;64(Pt 3):199-208.
51. Bunting GW. Voice following laryngeal cancer surgery: Troubleshooting common problems after tracheoesophageal voice restoration. *Otolaryngol Clin North Am.* 2004;37(3):597-612.
52. Op de Coul BM, Hilgers FJ, Balm AJ, Tan IB, van den Hoogen FJ, van Tinteren H. A decade of postlaryngectomy vocal rehabilitation in 318 patients: A single institution's experience with consistent application of Provox indwelling voice prostheses. *Arch Otolaryngol Head Neck Surg.* 2000;126(11):1320-1328.
53. Jacobs K, Delaere PR, Vander Poorten VL. Submucosal purse-string suture as a treatment of leakage around the indwelling voice prosthesis. *Head Neck.* 2008;30(4):485-491.
54. Lewin JS, Hutcheson KA, Barringer DA, Croegaert LE, Lisec A, Chambers MS. Customization of the voice prosthesis to prevent leakage from the enlarged tracheoesophageal puncture: Results of a prospective trial. *Laryngoscope.* 2012;122(8):1767-1772.
55. Seshamani M, Ruiz C, Kasper Schwartz S, Mirza N. Cymetra injections to treat leakage around a tracheoesophageal puncture. *ORL J Otorhinolaryngol Relat Spec.* 2006;68(3):146-148.
56. Diedrich WM. The mechanism of esophageal speech. *Ann New York Acad Sci.* 1968;155:303-317.
57. Kearney A. Nontracheoesophageal speech rehabilitation. *Otolaryngol Clin North Am.* 2004;37(3):613-625.

58. Gates GA, Ryan W, Cooper JC, et al. Current status of laryngectomee rehabilitation: I. Results of therapy. *Am J Otolaryngol.* 1982;3:1-7.
59. King PS, Lowlles ES, Peirson GA. Rehabilitation and adaptation of laryngectomy patients. *Am J Phys Med.* 1968;97:192-303.
60. Pindzola RH, Cain BH. Acceptability ratings of tracheoesophageal speech. *Laryngoscope.* 1988;98(4):394-397.
61. Williams SE, Watson JB. Speaking proficiency variations according to method of alaryngeal voicing. *Laryngoscope.* 1987;97:737-739.
62. Salmon SJ, Keith RL, Darley FL. Methods of air intake for esophageal speech and their associated problems. In Keith RL & Darley FL, eds. *Laryngectomy Rehabilitation.* San Diego, CA; College Hill Press, 1979:55-69..
63. Ackerstaff AH, Hilgers FJ, Meeuwis CA, Knegt PP, Weenink C. Pulmonary function pre- and post- total laryngectomy. *Clin Otolaryngol Allied Sci.* 1999;24(6):491-494.
64. Zuur JK, Muller SH, de Jongh FH, van Zandwijk N, Hilgers FJ. The physiological rationale of heat and moisture exchangers in post-laryngectomy pulmonary rehabilitation: A review. *Eur Arch Otorhinolaryngol.* 2006;263:1-8.
65. van den Boer C, Muller SH, van der Noort V, et al. Effects of heat and moisture exchangers on tracheal mucociliary clearance in laryngectomized patients: A multi-center case control study. *Eur Arch Otorhinolaryngol.* 2015;272(11):3439-3450.
66. Ackerstaff AH, Hilgers FJ, Aaronson NK, Balm AJ, van Zandwijk N. Improvements in respiratory and psychosocial functioning following total laryngectomy by the use of a heat and moisture exchanger. *Ann Otol Rhinol Laryngol.* 1993;102(11):878-883.
67. Bien S, Okta S, van As-Brooks CJ, Ackerstaff AH. The effect of a head and moisture exchanger (Provox HME) on pulmonary protection after total laryngectomy: A randomized controlled study. *Eur Arch Otorhinolaryngol.* 2010;267:429-435.
68. Icuspit P, Yarlagadda B, Garg S, Johnson T, Deschler D. Heat and moisture exchange devices for patients undergoing total laryngectomy. *ORL Head Neck Nurs.* 2014;32(1):20-23.
69. van der Houwen EB, van Kalkeren TA, Post WJ, Hilgers FJ, van der Laan BF, Verkerke GJ. Does the patch fit the stoma? A study on peristoma geometry and patch use in laryngectomized patients. *Clin Otolaryngol.* 2011;36:235-241.
70. Lewin JS, Lemon J, Bishop-Leone JK, Leyk S, Martin JW, Gillenwater AM. Experience with Barton button and peristomal breathing valve attachments for hands-free tracheoesophageal speech. *Head Neck.* 2000;22(2):142-148.
71. Hilgers FJ, Ackerstaff AH, Aaronson NK, Schouwenburg PF, van Zandwijk N. Physical and psychosocial consequences of total laryngectomy. *Clin Otolaryngol Allied Sci.* 1990;15(5):421-425.
72. Maclean J, Cotton S, Perry A. Dysphagia following total laryngectomy: The effect on quality of life, functioning, and psychological well-being. *Dysphagia.* 2009;24(3):314-321.
73. Lang IM, Shaker R. An overview of the upper esophageal sphincter. *Curr Gastroenterol Rep.* 2000;2(3):185-190.
74. Lippert D, Hoffman MR, Britt CJ, et al. Preliminary evaluation of functional swallow after total laryngectomy using high-resolution manometry. *Ann Otol Rhinol Laryngol.* 2016;125(7):541-549
75. Davis RK, Vincent ME, Shapshay SM, Strong MS. The anatomy and complications of "T" versus vertical closure of the hypopharynx after laryngectomy. *Laryngoscope.* 1982;92(1):16-22.

76. Hutcheson KA, Alvarez CP, Barringer DA, Kupferman ME, Lapine PR, Lewin JS. Outcomes of elective total laryngectomy for laryngopharyngeal dysfunction in disease-free head and neck cancer survivors. *Otolaryngol Head Neck Surg.* 2012;146(4):585-590.
77. Vu KN, Day TA, Gillespie MB, et al. Proximal esophageal stenosis in head and neck cancer patients after total laryngectomy and radiation. *ORL J Otorhinolaryngol Relat Spec.* 2008;70:229-225.
78. Sweeny L, Golden JB, White HN, Magnuson JS, Carroll WR, Rosenthal EL. Incidence and outcomes of stricture formation postlaryngectomy. *Otolaryngol Head Neck Surg.* 2012;146(3):395-402.
79. van der Molen L, Kornman AF, Latenstein MN, van den Brekel MW, Hilgers FJ. Practice of laryngectomy rehabilitation interventions: A perspective from Europe/the Netherlands. *Curr Opin Otolaryngol Head Neck Surg.* 2013;21:230-238.
80. Riva G, Sensini M, Corvino A, Pecorari G, Garzaro M. Smell and taste impairment after total laryngectomy. *Ann Otol Rhinol Laryngol.* 2017;126(7):548-554.
81. Hilgers FJ, Jansen HA, Van As CJ, Polak MF, Muller MJ, Van Dam FS. Long-term results of olfaction rehabilitation using the nasal airflow inducing ("polite yawning") maneuver after total laryngectomy. *Arch Otolaryngol Head Neck Surg.* 2002;128(6):648-654.
82. Smith BG, Hutcheson KA, Little LG, et al. Lymphedema outcomes in patients with head and neck cancer. *Otolaryngol Head Neck Surg.* 2015;152:284-291.
83. Shaitelman SF, Cromwell KD, Rasmussen JC, et al. Recent progress in the treatment and prevention of cancer-related lymphedema. *CA Cancer J Clin.* 2015;65:55-81.
84. Dutta S, Biswas KD, Ghatak S, Haldar D, Sen I, Sinha R. Postoperative hypofunctioning of the thyroid gland after total laryngectomy. *Ear Nose Throat J.* 2016;95:E23-7.
85. Mourad M, Saman M, Sawhney R, Ducic Y. Management of the thyroid gland during total laryngectomy in patients with laryngeal squamous cell carcinoma. *Laryngoscope.* 2015;125:1835-1838.
86. American Association of Clinical Endocrinologists, the Endocrine Society, and the American Thyroid Association Joint Position Statement on the Use and Interchangeability of Thyroxine Products, 2004. www.thyroid.org/thyroxine-products-joint-position-statement/. Accessed Jully 25, 2020.
87. Gane EM, Michaleff ZA, Cottrell MA, et al. Prevalence, incidence, and risk factors for shoulder and neck dysfunction after neck dissection: A systematic review. *Eur J Surg Oncol.* 2017;43:1199-1218.
88. Pattison N, Brown MR, Gubbay A, et al. Towards a pain free hospital: An in-depth qualitative analysis of the pain experiences of head and neck cancer patients undergoing radiotherapy. *Br J Pain.* 2016;10:29-37.
89. Stubblefield MD. Clinical evaluation and management of radiation fibrosis syndrome. *Phys Med Rehabil Clin N Am.* 2017;28:89-100.
90. Terro W, Crean SJ. Prospective, longitudinal assessment of quality of life in patients with cancer of the head and neck and their primary carers. *Br J Oral Maxillofac Surg.* 2017;55:613-617.
91. Keszte J, Danker H, Dietz A, et al. Mental disorders and psychosocial support during the first year after total laryngectomy: A prospective cohort study. *Clin Otolaryngol.* 2013; 38: 494-501.
92. Offerman MP, Pruyn JF, de Boer MF, Busschbach JJ, Baatenburg de Jong RJ. Psychosocial consequences for partners of patients after total laryngectomy and for the relationship between patients and partners. *Oral Oncol.* 2015; 51: 389-398.

93. Manceaux P, Zdanowicz N. Immunity, coping and depression. *Psychiatr Danub.* 2016; 28(Suppl-1):165-169.
94. Brook I. A physician as a cancer of the neck patient: Overcoming depression after laryngectomy. *Palliative and Supportive Care.* 2012; 10: 63-64.
95. Perry A, Casey E, Cotton S. Quality of life after total laryngectomy: Functioning, psychological well-being and self-efficacy. *Int J Lang Commun Disord.* 2015; 50: 467-75.
96. Kam D, Salib A, Gorgy G, et al. Incidence of suicide in patients with head and neck cancer. *JAMA Otolaryngol Head Neck Surg.* 2015; 141: 1075-1081.
97. Jayakrishnan TT, Sekigami Y, Rajeev R, Gamblin TC, Turaga KK. Morbidity of curative cancer surgery and suicide risk. *Psychooncology.* 2016;Jul 16. doi: 10.1002/pon.4221 (epub ahead of print).
98. Anguiano L, Mayer DK, Piven ML, Rosenstein D. A literature review of suicide in cancer patients. *Cancer Nurs.* 2012;35:E14-26.
99. K Hughes M. Suicide screening in the oncology population. *J Adv Pract Oncol.* 2016;7:101-104.
100. Brook I. A physician as a cancer of the neck patient: Am I cured. *Palliative and Supportive Care.* 2011;9:213-214.
101. Brook I. A physician's personal experience as a cancer of the neck patient. *Otolaryngol Head Neck Surg.* 2010;143:324-326.
102. Dooks P, McQuestion M, Goldstein D, Molassiotis A. Experiences of patients with laryngectomies as they reintegrate into their community. *Support Care Cancer.* 2012;20:489-498.
103. Cohen EE, LaMonte SJ, Erb NL, et al. American cancer society head and neck cancer survivorship care guideline. *CA Cancer J Clin.* 2016;66:203-239.
104. National Comprehensive Cancer Network Guidelines. https://nccn.org. Accessed July 25, 2020.
105. Kao SS, Ooi EH. Survival outcomes following salvage surgery for oropharyngeal squamous cell carcinoma: Systematic review. *J Laryngol Otol.* 2017;15:1-15.
106. Maasland DH, van den Brandt PA, Kremer B, Goldbohm RA, Schouten LJ. Alcohol consumption, cigarette smoking and the risk of subtypes of head-neck cancer: Results from the Netherlands Cohort Study. *BMC Cancer.* 2014;14:187.
107. Peterson LA, Bellile EL, Wolf GT, et al. Cigarette use, comorbidities, and prognosis in a prospective head and neck squamous cell carcinoma population. *Head Neck.* 2016;38:1810-1820.
108. Walsh EM. New use of a tracheal tube for rescue breathing in laryngectomees in the community. *Resuscitation.* 2006;69:335-338.
109. Brook I. Ventilation of neck breathers undergoing a diagnostic procedure or surgery. *Anesth Analg.* 2012;114:1318-1322.

10

Complications of Tracheostomy

Samuel D. Racette, Michiel J. Bové,
M. Sherif Afifi, Linda L. Morris

Clinical Scenario

The patient is a 36-year-old male with a history of tracheotomy performed two weeks ago following head trauma sustained in a motor vehicle accident. Earlier today, the patient was reported to have bright red blood in his tracheal secretions, but this has subsided. On exam, the patient is alert and appropriately oriented. Suddenly, the patient coughs, and pulsatile bright red bleeding projects from the tracheostomy tube.

Objectives

- Discuss immediate, early, and late complications related to tracheotomy
- List the steps necessary in evaluation, prevention, and management of each complication
- Develop a structured approach for managing respiratory distress in a patient with a tracheostomy tube
- Highlight incidence and emergency management of potentially lethal complications, including tracheo-innominate fistula, tube dislodgement/false passage, intraoperative fire, and tube obstruction

Introduction

There is a myriad of complications that can arise following tracheotomy. These complications are often classified into immediate, early, and late subgroups (**Table 10.1**). Immediate complications of the procedure include hemorrhage and pneumothorax. Early complications (within 7 days) include mucous plugging, pneumonia, stomal infection, pneumomediastinum, pneumopericardium, tube obstruction, subcutaneous emphysema, and inadvertent decannulation. Later complications include the development of mucous plugs, infection, tracheo-innominate hemorrhage, tracheo-innominate fistula, tracheo-esophageal fistula, tracheo-cutaneous fistula, stomal stenosis, stomal granulation tissue, tracheomalacia, tracheal stenosis, mediastinitis, mediastinal fistula, and tracheocele.[1-10] The time frames for early, intermediate, and late complications can overlap.

Table 10.1 Complications of Tracheostomy

Immediate	Early	Late
Hemorrhage Pneumothorax Intra-operative fire Air embolism	Pneumonia Stoma infection Pneumomediastinum Pneumopericardium Obstruction Subcutaneous emphysema (crepitus) Inadvertent decannulation, loss of airway False passage Mucous plugs	Mucous plugs Pneumonia Stomal infection Tracheitis Tracheomalacia Tracheoinnominate fistula Tracheoesophageal fistula (persistent stoma) Stomal stenosis Stomal granulation tissue Tracheal stenosis Mediastinitis Mediastinal fistula Tracheocele

In the clinical case above, it is essential to assess the etiology of the bleeding discovered during routine suctioning. The differential diagnosis for this presentation is wide-ranging, from the innocuous and common "suction related trauma" to the devastating and life-threatening tracheo-innominate (TI) fistula/hemorrhage. Although the rate of devastating complications is quite low (less than 1% for TI fistula). concern for any complication following tracheotomy must be promptly evaluated.[11]

Overview of Tracheotomy Complications

In a landmark retrospective review,[12] the rate of complications was found to be significantly elevated in specific patient populations, including pediatric, post-head trauma, obese, burn, or seriously debilitated patients. Furthermore, the overall complication rate was low, the most common being tracheal stenosis. The investigators concluded that the majority of these cases were attributed to prolonged intubation, and that careful surgical planning and post-operative care may prevent many complications. Other published rates of tracheotomy-related complications varied significantly (5%–65%), due to differences in study design, length of follow-up, and definition of complications.[13,14]

The first study to prospectively quantify complications from tracheotomy observed 40 patients and did not include intraoperative complications.[15] In regard to early complications, 5% (two patients) had significant bleeding from the wound and another 5% had bleeding from stomal granulation tissue. One patient bled upon decannulation, while another bled endotracheally as a result of granulation tissue extending from the stoma to the tracheal lumen. It is noted that these two patients later developed stomal stenosis. One patient developed tube obstruction, two developed bilateral tension pneumothorax during the first tube change, and four developed severe necrotizing pneumonia. The investigators followed up all patients with a bronchoscopic exam. Fifteen patients died while still receiving mechanical ventilation, all of whom were found to have severe tracheitis. All 25 patients who were successfully decannulated survived. Of these survivors, 60% had minimal deformity of the trachea, 32% had moderate deformity, and 8% had symptomatic tracheal stenosis.

A recently published study by Spataro[16] sought to prospectively determine inpatient and outpatient complications which can occur following tracheotomy. Their study included patients receiving tracheotomies by any service at a single academic institution. They excluded patients who received total laryngectomies, were under the age of 18, or those who had a tracheotomy performed at an outside institution prior to arrival. They quantified their demographics and found that patients undergoing tracheotomy at their institution were more likely to be male, obese, and Caucasian. The most common primary diagnosis listed for patients was cardiorespiratory failure, followed by head and neck cancer. The vast majority (94%) were planned procedures: 50% open tracheotomies and 50% percutaneous dilatational tracheotomies. Of the open procedures, 40% were completed using the Björk flap technique. Regarding decannulation, 54% of patients were successfully decannulated prior to discharge, while 11% of their cohort were decannulated as outpatients.

Their study found that 47% of patients experienced an inpatient complication following their procedure. From most commonly occurring to least, these complications included mucous plugging, bleeding from the stoma, infection, accidental decannulation, stoma breakdown, false passage, tracheal or subglottic stenosis, tracheo-innominate fistula, trachea-esophageal fistula, pneumothorax, and death. Tracheostomy-related death was reported to be 1%, while overall mortality was reported at 11%, indicating the high comorbidities related to this patient population.[16]

It should be noted that the only death related to tracheostomy in this study was attributed to accidental decannulation and subsequent respiratory arrest at post-operative day 96. Although there is significant chance of complication immediately following tracheotomy, clinician and caregivers should always be vigilant.

Intraoperative Complications

Intraoperative complications include hemorrhage (usually from the anterior jugular veins, the thyroid isthmus, or vascular variants such as the thyroid ima artery), creation of a false passage, electrocautery-induced airway fire, and surgical injury to adjacent structures.

Recognition of False Passage

Evaluation

The inability to ventilate immediately after placement of the tracheostomy tube suggests that the tube may have entered a false passage, usually anterior to the tracheal wall or, rarely, posterior to the trachea into the esophagus.

Prevention

The best way to avoid a false passage is to exercise meticulous attention, always having a high index of suspicion, and confirm successful tracheal cannulation.

Management

The inability to pass a soft suction catheter into the newly placed tracheostomy tube suggests placement in a false passage. In addition, all retractors and cricoid hooks should be kept in place until successful cannulation is confirmed to allow for an immediate re-attempt at cannulation should difficulties arise. Confirmation of successful tracheal cannulation is confirmed with the return of end-tidal CO_2 and/or direct visualization of the tracheal lumen with a bronchoscope.

Hemorrhage

Evaluation

Hemorrhage can occur as a result of the laceration of blood vessels in the neck during the procedure. Low tracheotomies, below the fourth tracheal ring, have a higher incidence of damage to the innominate artery. Minor bleeding from another source is far more common and is estimated to occur in up to 40% of cases.

Minor intraoperative bleeding commonly results from injury to the anterior jugular veins early in the dissection (especially during emergent procedures), or to the thyroid isthmus during attempts to mobilize it from the anterior tracheal wall or during attempts to divide and ligate it. High-riding innominate arteries present a significant risk of severe hemorrhage when the dissection is carried out inferiorly.

Prevention

Finger palpation in the substernal region should always precede instrumentation to rule out prominent pulses in this region. Bleeding can be minimized by carefully identifying and staying in the midline, cautiously dissecting layer by layer, and maintaining excellent lighting and retraction of the soft tissues in the operative field. Patient position and neck extension should be optimized. If local anesthesia is used, the procedure should not be started until the vasoconstrictive agent in the local anesthetic has taken effect. Structures such as the anterior jugular vein and the thyroid isthmus should be carefully identified in order to avoid inadvertent trauma and bleeding. An aberrant innominate artery may traverse anterior to the trachea in the field of dissection, making it vulnerable to laceration and potentially, life-threatening hemorrhage.[11]

Management

After the insertion of the tracheostomy tube, the surgical wound should be carefully inspected for any bleeding sources. A Valsalva maneuver is commonly used to identify bleeding vessels. If necessary, the tracheostomy tube should be removed to allow for better inspection of the surgical field, and to locate any source of bleeding. Superficial sources of bleeding can be addressed by slightly lifting the flange of the tracheostomy tube, while leaving the cannula in the trachea. Placement of hemostatic agents may be helpful in patients with coagulopathies; however, any packing should be removed prior to tracheostomy tube change to reduce risk of aspiration.

Pneumothorax

Evaluation

Pneumothorax is usually the result of a traumatic puncture of the pleura. It is more common during pediatric tracheotomy, where the pulmonary apices are relatively more elevated within the lower neck. In adults, this complication usually involves the rupture of a pulmonary bleb in a patient struggling to breathe during an awake, emergency tracheotomy. Pneumothorax can also result from damage to the posterior tracheal wall during the tracheal incision, access to the tracheal lumen during PDT, or during insertion of the tracheostomy tube. More commonly, the tracheostomy tube can be inadvertently inserted between the anterior tracheal wall and the anterior mediastinum. The insertion of the tube into this false passage results in worsening respiratory status and can be confirmed by the inability to pass a flexible suction catheter into the tracheal lumen. While some suggest obtaining postoperative radiographs for all tracheotomy patients, published data suggests this is unnecessary in routine, uncomplicated, elective cases. The detection rate of pneumothorax in one systematic review was 2.2% following surgical tracheostomies, and 3.2% for percutaneous dilatational tracheotomies. Those cases requiring intervention was even lower at 0.7% and 1.8%, respectively. The authors suggest restricting chest radiographs to emergency procedures, difficult procedures, or patients exhibiting signs or symptoms of pneumothorax.[17]

Prevention

Pneumothorax is best prevented by controlled and careful midline dissection. The tracheostomy tube should be inserted under direct visualization and good illumination. The ability to suction the trachea with a flexible suction catheter and the presence of end tidal CO_2 should be immediately confirmed after placement of the tracheostomy tube. Positive pressure through the tracheostomy tube should be delayed until these confirmatory measures are performed to avoid insufflating the mediastinum. If there remains any doubt about the placement of the tube, retractors can be placed within the stoma to maintain its patency while the tracheostomy tube is removed and replaced under direct visualization. Confirmation in difficult cases may, at times, necessitate use of flexible bronchoscopy.

Management

When pneumothorax is significant, it should be treated by the insertion of a chest tube.

Intraoperative Fire

Evaluation

The incidence of airway fire during tracheotomy is exceedingly low, but reports do exist of this devastating complication. In fact, by 2014 only 25 cases had been reported in the literature.[18] The majority of cases were a consequence of unipolar electrocautery.[19,20] The tracheotomy procedure involves significant risk due to the inclusion of the three elements necessary to initiate a fire: heat, fuel, and an oxidizer.

A number of different objects and fluids used in the operating room are flammable and can serve as a fuel source.[21] Tincture of benzoin has ignited with the use of cautery during wound closure.[22] Similarly, skin preparations that include alcohol provide highly flammable residue.[21,23] Gauze sponges have acted as fuel in many reported fires.[22,24] Draping material[25] and tape[26] can also ignite if the oxygen tension is high. Although surgical drapes must be flame-retardant, many other materials are flammable and serve as a fuel source if a sufficiently high oxygen tension exists. Endotracheal tubes are generally made of polyvinyl chloride (PVC) because of its low implant toxicity and pliability. PVC endotracheal tubes are known to ignite in oxygen-rich environments, but have been shown to be flammable in oxygen concentrations as low as 25%.[27,28]

Prevention

Prevention of intra-operative fires is the responsibility of each member of the surgical team. Communication between the surgeon and anesthesiologist is essential. Extreme care should be taken not to use cautery close to the trachea after entering it. Concentrations of oxygen in excess of 50% FiO_2 (fraction of inspired oxygen) have been shown to support airway fires.[29] The FiO2 should, therefore, be kept as low as possible during tracheotomy. Additionally, it is essential that only cuffed endotracheal tubes be used during tracheotomy in order to limit oxygen from leaking into the zone where the trachea is entered.[30-32]

All personnel should be aware that an airway fire can occur during tracheotomy, whether at the bedside or in the operating room. Saline should be available at all times to help extinguish a fire. A fire extinguisher should also be available within reach.[33] Other recommended guidelines for the prevention of surgical fires during tracheotomy include the following:

- Keep the cautery unit in the holster when not in use.
- Use a nonconductive plastic clamp to attach cautery to the surgical field.
- Adjust cautery settings to prevent sparks.
- Disconnect power to high-intensity light sources when not in use.
- Never allow fiber-optic cables to come into contact with flammable materials.
- Advance the endotracheal tube close to the carina and further distal to the surgical incision (24–25 cm from the teeth in the average male).
- Use saline to inflate the endotracheal tube cuff. Ensure there is no leak of anesthetic gas past the cuff.
- Never use cautery to enter the trachea.
- Avoid nitrous oxide or any flammable anesthetic agents.
- Avoid tenting surgical drapes to prevent the accumulation of oxygen.
- Avoid alcohol-based skin preparations and petroleum-based eye products.
- Stop supplemental oxygen at least one minute before using cautery.
- If bleeding occurs upon tracheal incision, ensure the airway is secured and then use diathermy while suctioning to clear oxygen from the wound.
- Use an incise drape to isolate head and neck incisions from flammable vapors underneath.
- Use fire-retardant surgical drapes.
- Wet all gauze sponges and cotton pledgets.
- Use suction to scavenge gases from the mouth.

Prevention of fire consists of the removal of one of the elements of the fire triangle. This includes shaving the entire neck and shoulders of a patient with excess body hair, adequate drying of the prep solution, and, if tolerated, decreasing high oxygen delivery.[19]

Management

In the event of an airway fire, the following steps should be taken immediately:

- Stop the flow of oxygen to the endotracheal tube.
- Remove the endotracheal tube.
- Flood the field with fluids, if appropriate. Consider flushing saline down the endotracheal tube to extinguish any intraluminal fire.[34]
- Re-intubate the patient as soon as possible.
- Consider adding PEEP, maintaining ventilator support, and administering high-dose steroids.
- Urgently consult an otolaryngologist to evaluate the extent of the airway burn.

Air Embolism

Evaluation

Air embolism results from aspiration of a volume of air through any tear in venous circulation. Deep inspiratory chest movements produce markedly negative venous pressure in the neck veins that cause air to enter the venous system during neck surgery. Air that enters the neck veins is transported through the pulmonary venous drainage to the right atrium and ventricle and can continue to the pulmonary arteries. Gas embolism in the pulmonary arteries may cause interference with gas exchange, cardiac arrhythmias, pulmonary hypertension, and even cardiac failure and arrest. A large bolus of air entering the venous system can cause an air-lock in the right side of the heart, leading to decreased pulmonary venous return, and subsequent decreased left ventricular preload and cardiac output. Intermediate amounts of air collect in the pulmonary circulation and produce a pulmonary vascular injury manifested by pre- and post-capillary pulmonary vasoconstriction, pulmonary hypertension, endothelial injury, and subsequently, pulmonary edema. Resultant ventilation-perfusion mismatch can cause right-to-left circulation shunting and increased arterial hypoxemia. Small amounts of air do not produce symptoms because the air is broken up into small particles absorbed in the circulation. Shock and cardiac arrest can occur after introduction of as little as 10–20 ml of air in the venous system. Furthermore, 0.5 ml of air in the left anterior descending coronary artery has been shown to lead to ventricular fibrillation.[35,36]

Death from air embolism after tracheostomy is extremely rare. One early case report described a postoperative death from air embolism in an 18-month-old child who died suddenly a few hours after tracheotomy. The procedure had been performed under general anesthesia. The neck veins were notably engorged, and there was profuse hemorrhage. The patient coughed immediately after extubation, and the venous hemorrhage from the lower aspect of the wound was controlled by gauze packing. The patient left the operating room in stable condition and was breathing spontaneously, but coughing occasionally. Four hours postoperatively, the patient died suddenly and without warning. Upon autopsy, the right heart was shown to be filled with air and the cerebral arteries contained air bubbles.[37]

Prevention

To avoid this potentially lethal complication, all venous hemorrhage should be completely controlled with non-slipping ligature (e.g., silk). Immediate and careful assessment should be performed for early postoperative excessive coughing, hemostasis, and unexplained circulatory collapse.

Management

Once air embolism is suspected, the procedure in progress should be terminated immediately.

- Administer 100% oxygen and intubate for significant respiratory distress or refractory hypoxemia. Oxygen may reduce bubble size by increasing the gradient for nitrogen to dissolve.
- Promptly place the patient in Trendelenburg (head-down) position and rotate toward the left lateral decubitus position. This maneuver helps trap air in the apex of the ventricle, prevents its ejection into the pulmonary arterial system, and maintains right ventricular output.
- Maintain systemic arterial pressure with fluid resuscitation and vasopressors and beta-adrenergic agents, if necessary.
- Immediate imaging with echocardiography may assist in detecting residual air in the central circulation, and subsequent direction of its aspiration through a central venous catheter.
- Temporary support of the circulation may be required with institution of extracorporeal membrane oxygenation (ECMO).
- Consider transferring the patient to a hyperbaric chamber. Potential benefits of this therapy include (a) compression of existing air bubbles, (b) establishment of a high diffusion gradient to speed the dissolution of existing bubbles, and (c) improve oxygenation of ischemic tissues and lower intracranial pressure.

Early Postoperative Complications

Tracheostomy Tube Displacement and Loss of Airway

Evaluation

The tracheostomy patient requires vigilant care to prevent complications, especially in the first several days post-operatively. One study showed that health care professionals lack knowledge of what to do in the event of inadvertent decannulation.[38] One of the most hazardous complications of a tracheostomy is inadvertent decannulation occurring before the tract between the skin and the trachea has matured, which occurs approximately 3 to 6 days after the procedure. If the stoma has not yet matured, the tissue planes collapse upon each other when the tracheostomy tube is removed. Inadvertent decannulation before a stable tract has formed can, therefore, result in a loss of airway. Several factors can predispose a patient to tube dislodgement, including (a) loose tracheostomy tube ties and sutures securing the tracheostomy tube in place (as may occur after edema or subcutaneous emphysema resolves); (b) use of adjustable-length tracheostomy tubes; (c) excessive coughing; (d) excessive movements of an agitated, uncooperative, confused, or under-sedated patient; (e) an overweight patient with an elongated tract from skin to trachea that causes relative shortening of the tracheostomy tube; and (f) an improperly fitted tracheostomy tube that may be affected by positioning or circuit attachments.

Tracheostomy tube displacement may not always be immediately evident, especially if the patient's airway obstruction was incomplete and the patient is not dependent on positive-pressure ventilation. In these situations, displacement may present with respiratory distress and the inability to pass a suction catheter. It is important to have heightened urgency to identify partial dislodgement, as subtle presentations can potentially lead to respiratory arrest and death.

Prevention

While the incidence of tube displacement is low, it has a high mortality rate. Care should be taken to secure the tracheostomy tube with sutures placed through the neck flange and with snug-fitting tracheostomy ties. Tube security should be regularly checked, and transporting the patient should be minimized as much as possible in the early postoperative period. Tube security should also be checked prior to moving the patient in any way, and care should be taken to relieve any added weight or traction from the ventilator circuit.

Management

When the airway is lost due to tube displacement in the early postoperative period, a mature stoma has not yet developed. Tissue planes collapse, and emergency efforts to replace the tube are not advised because of the likely development of a false passage. Rather, the immediate management of a lost airway in a patient with an immature stoma should include mask ventilation until an oral endotracheal airway can be established. The tracheotomy can then be revised under more controlled conditions, including adequate lighting, personnel, and equipment. If stay sutures were placed, traction on these sutures will spread the skin edges and bring the stoma up to the level of the opening in the skin.[39-41].

Tube Obstruction

Evaluation

In a patient with a tracheostomy tube, the most frequent cause of respiratory or cardiac arrest is tube obstruction. Tube obstruction secondary to mucous plugs, blood clots, or tube displacement can occur in the early postoperative period. Mucous plugs are one of the most frequent complications of tracheostomies. Because the upper airway is bypassed, patients are at risk for drying of secretions, which can lead to mucous plugs. Adequate measures to mobilize secretions are of the utmost concern in managing the patient with a tracheostomy.

Prevention

Tube obstruction may be minimized by attentive nursing care that includes frequent suctioning, adequate hydration, and the use of humidified oxygen. The prevention of obstruction is markedly facilitated by the use of tracheostomy tubes with inner cannulas, which allows regular inspection and cleaning. The two primary interventions to prevent the development of mucous plugs are adequate hydration and promoting mobility of secretions. Adequate hydration is necessary to keep secretions thin and mobile so they can be easily coughed or suctioned. This can be a challenge in a patient whose fluid intake may be restricted for other reasons. Heat moisture exchangers (HMEs) can be effective in helping humidify secretions; however, these devices can become easily clogged with secretions themselves, and may need to be changed periodically. Recent Cochrane reviews have not delineated a difference between high humidity tracheostomy collars and HMEs in decreasing the risk and incidence of artificial airway obstruction.[42]

Management

Mucous plugs are most often a respiratory emergency and usually present as acute dyspnea. **Figure 10.1** is an algorithm for the management of airway obstruction. Immediate treatment measures include checking the inner cannula for obstruction. If the inner cannula is clear, the obstruction may be further into the airway; in which case, deep suctioning is necessary. This can be accompanied by vigorous use of the manual resuscitation bag in order to promote productive coughing and oxygenate a patient in distress. If there is difficulty passing a suction catheter or the manual resuscitation bag meets resistance, the clinician should be highly suspicious of secretions narrowing the diameter of the tracheostomy tube. If the aforementioned measures have not relieved the obstruction, the entire tracheostomy tube should be changed. Frequently, a large mucous plug will be removed with the tracheostomy tube. If this does not relieve the obstruction, the clinician should remove the tracheostomy tube and suction directly into the mature stoma. Bronchoscopy can be used to identify and remove mucous plugs that are deep in the tracheobronchial tree. In patients for whom it is not contraindicated, the Heimlich maneuver can be considered to "bring a mucous plug up the airway" to facilitate its removal.

Figure 10.1 Obstruction Algorithm

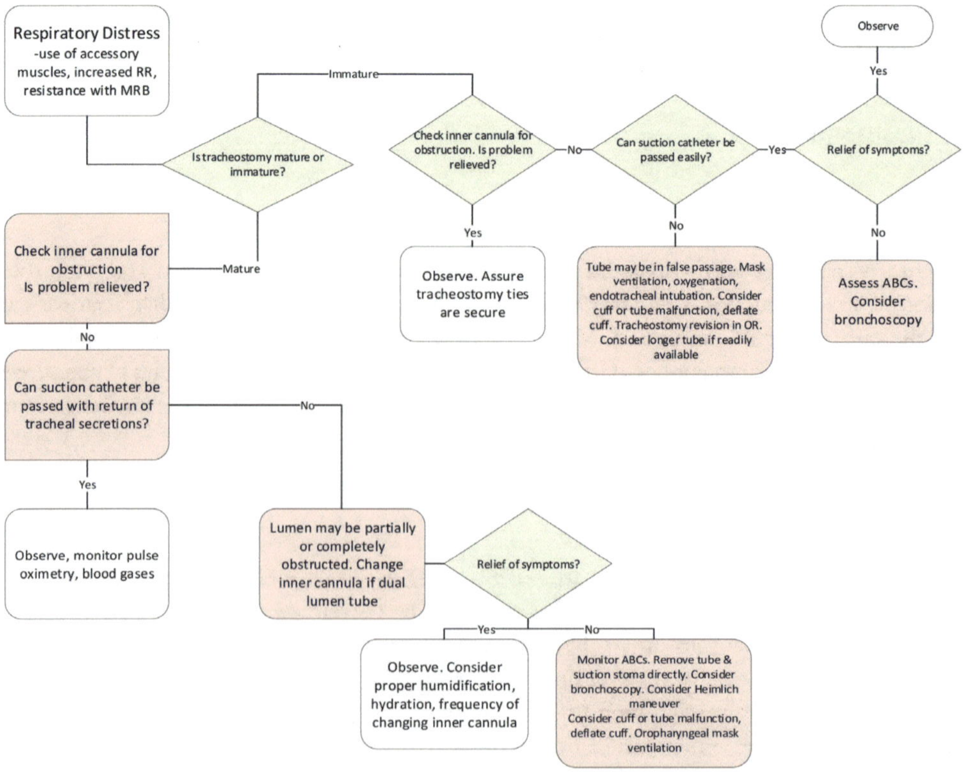

Internal Stomal Erosion

Evaluation

Internal stomal erosion results from undue force creating outward pull or torque on the tracheostomy tube, most often due to traction from the ventilator circuit. These traction forces are magnified when more weight is added to the circuit, including closed suction systems and in-line humidifiers. Excessive traction can enlarge the stoma to the extent that the entire shaft of the tracheostomy tube as well as the cuff is visible within the stoma.

Prevention

Excessive force against the stoma must be minimized by adequately supporting the ventilator circuit and removing unneeded attachments. Unless the patient is hemodynamically unstable, a closed suction system should be removed. Unnecessary in-line features should also be removed, relocated, or minimized. When moving the patient in any way, the ventilator circuit should always be checked for excessive traction. To minimize traction when providing care, patients should always be first turned toward the ventilator and then turned away. When patients are positioned facing away from the ventilator, extra care must be taken to minimize traction forces.

Management

A longer tracheostomy tube may be required to avoid further trauma to the stoma. The wound can then granulate and heal from within. If the integrity of the cartilaginous framework of the trachea has been compromised, the patient may require stenting or resection of the affected portion of the trachea in order to allow decannulation.

External Stomal Erosion

Evaluation

External stomal erosion occurs as a result of inward pressure from the tube flange digging into the tissues of the neck. It can be exacerbated by flexion of the neck or added weight from in-line attachments to the ventilator circuit.

Prevention

In the case of external stomal erosion, prevention and treatment are the same. The neck should be maintained in a neutral position, and any added weight that creates inward pressure should be eliminated. In some cases, the erosion is so deep that packing may be required to eliminate drainage and allow the tissues to heal.

Management

Local wound care is important to avoid infection. Necrotic tissue should be carefully debrided with regular wet to dry dressings. Semi-permeable dressings can be used to retain moisture and encourage cell growth. Dressings also provide a barrier between the tracheostomy tube flange and the peristomal skin.

Bleeding

Evaluation

Bleeding can result from ligated thyroid isthmus, erosion into nearby blood vessels, or aggressive suctioning against granulation tissue or the tracheal wall. Postoperative bleeding can occur after the vasoconstrictive effect of epinephrine added to local anesthesia has worn off, or from elevated blood pressure in a previously hypotensive patient. One study reported a 5.7% incidence of clinically relevant bleeding, with similar rates seen in both open and percutaneous tracheotomy.[43]

Prevention

Bleeding after a tracheotomy may be prevented by careful dissection and attention to details, adequate blood pressure control immediately after tracheotomy, and selection of softer suction catheters when needed.

Management

Brisk bleeding can arise from veins of thyroid tissue lacerated during surgery and should be managed by a return to the operative setting for wound exploration. Prolonged oozing should make the surgeon suspect a coagulopathy. If oozing is limited and the patient has a cuffed tracheostomy tube, the wound can be lightly packed.

Infection

Evaluation

A tracheostomy is considered a clean contaminated wound. The reported incidence of infection is highly dependent upon the definition of infection in individual studies. The incidence of cellulitis and purulence has generally been reported at 3% to 8%.[43] Stomal infection usually manifests as an indolent infection, mild cellulitis, or granulation tissue. Serious infections such as mediastinitis, fasciitis, abscess, and clavicular osteomyelitis are rare. When they do occur, they present with greater fluctuations in the patient's vital signs.

Prevention

The peristomal region is quickly colonized with multiple species of organisms. Over 85% of tracheostomies have been shown to be colonized with *Pseudomonas*.[44] Thus, the role of antibiotic prophylaxis has been highly controversial. One animal study demonstrated that perioperative prophylaxis with systemic antibiotics and povidone-iodine reduced bacterial growth and laryngeal damage.[45] Other studies concluded that perioperative antibiotics merely selected for resistant pathogenic organisms, such as beta-hemolytic streptococcus and Staphylococcus *epidermidis*, and decreased the numbers of normal skin flora. Others have suggested that the use of gauze induces secondary wound injury and prevents wound healing.[46] The use of fibrous wound dressings such as Aquacel (carboxymethylcellulose natrium sheet) and antimicrobial drain sponges (polyhexamethylene biguanide) can be used as adjuncts in controlling peristomal wound infections.[46,47]

The indwelling tracheostomy tube accumulates debris and serves as a source of device-related infection, similar to urinary and central venous catheters. It has been found that the tracheostomy tube has a biofilm greater than 80% of the time six days after placement.[48] Biofilm plays an important role in the pathogenicity of the infecting organism by protecting the embedded microbes and reducing the efficacy of host defenses and antimicrobial killing. Although most biofilms do not harbor pathogenic organisms, it is still possible for the tracheostomy tube to be a reservoir for infection.[49,50]

Avoiding colonization is impossible. Meticulous hygiene involving careful suctioning, care of the stoma, cleaning the inner cannula, and regular changes of the stomal dressing, tracheostomy tube holder, and tracheostomy tube is necessary to decrease the burden of crust and debris, thereby reducing bacterial loads. Traction sutures should be removed with the first tracheostomy tube change after the tract has matured (3–5 days).

Management

True necrotizing wound infections with purulence and surrounding cellulitis should be treated with culture-specific antibiotic regimen, frequent debridement, and dressing changes..

Subcutaneous Emphysema

Evaluation

The incidence of subcutaneous emphysema after tracheotomy ranges from 1% to 4%.[51] Air can be forced into a subcutaneous tissue plane during tube placement, especially if the patient frequently coughs intra- or postoperatively. This complication is more likely if an uncuffed tracheostomy tube is used, if the tracheotomy wound is closed with sutures, or if it is packed. An uncuffed tracheostomy tube causes air to pass from the airway into the subcutaneous peristomal tissues.

Subcutaneous emphysema is usually mild and manifests as an area of crepitus in the region of the skin surrounding the tracheostomy site. Rarely, it may present more extensively with swelling of the entire body, which can occur with forceful use of the manual resuscitation bag within an immature stoma.

Prevention

There are several methods to avoid subcutaneous emphysema from tracheostomy placement. Securing the airway with endotracheal intubation prior to tube placement allows the administration of general anesthesia and prevents coughing in the awake patient. Another measure is to avoid excessive dissection in the pretracheal plane or lateral to the trachea. Finally, the clinician should avoid closing the skin incision when a tracheotomy wound is packed to allow air to escape the trachea.

Management

Most cases of subcutaneous emphysema can be managed expectantly as the trapped air is usually resorbed spontaneously in the body over a few days. If the wound is sutured closed, the sutures should be removed; and if the wound is packed, the packing should be removed. An uncuffed tracheostomy tube should be replaced with a cuffed tube.

Pneumomediastinum

Evaluation

Pneumomediastinum is the accumulation of air within the thoracic cavity, potentially resulting in decreased cardiac output, cardiovascular collapse, and difficult ventilation. Symptoms include coughing, shortness of breath, and chest pain that is often pleuritic and occasionally radiates to the neck, back, or shoulders. It is a well-recognized complication following tracheotomy, especially in children where it is reported to occur in up to 43% of those patients older than 12 months, and 28% of those younger than 12 months.[52] The accepted mechanism describes forceful inspiratory movements resulting from respiratory obstruction, when high negative intrathoracic pressures have developed. The incision through the skin and cervical fascia creates an initial pathway for the aspiration of air through the wound edges into the mediastinum.

Prevention

The development of pneumomediastinum seems related to the extent of peritracheal dissection during the procedure.[53] Dissection along the anterior wall of the trachea should, therefore, be minimized. As with pneumothorax, prevention depends on establishing an airway prior to performing the tracheotomy, either through endotracheal intubation or rigid bronchoscopy.

Management

The treatment of pneumomediastinum depends on the amount of air present. A small amount of air noted on a postoperative chest x-ray in an asymptomatic patient will be reabsorbed spontaneously and warrants no specific treatment. For larger volumes of air or in the symptomatic patient, chest tube placement may be required.

Post-Obstructive Pulmonary Edema

Evaluation

Post-obstructive pulmonary edema, also referred to as negative pressure pulmonary edema, occurs in a variety of circumstances. Although the cause is not clear, the common denominator for its development is hypoxia associated with airway obstruction paired with vigorous inspiratory efforts. Negative intrapleural pressure is the primary pathologic event.[54] This negative intrapleural pressure promotes the translocation of blood from the systemic to the pulmonary circulation, which further increases pulmonary microvascular pressures. When the obstruction is relieved, either via surgical airway or endotracheal tube placement, the pulmonary edema becomes evident either immediately or within hours.

Prevention

Although there are no effective means of prevention, knowledge of the risk factors and recognition of the signs and causes are important. Factors that increase the risk for post-obstructive pulmonary edema include obstructive sleep apnea and acute airway obstruction secondary to bronchospasm, croup, epiglottitis, or tumor.

Management

Prompt recognition and treatment are essential and include adequate oxygen delivery, diuretics, and positive pressure ventilation with PEEP as necessary.

LATE POSTOPERATIVE COMPLICATIONS

Late postoperative complications of tracheostomy typically occur after the first postoperative week.[55] They include tracheo-innominate fistula, tracheo-esophageal or tracheo-cutaneous fistula, granulation tissue, tracheomalacia, and tracheal stenosis.

Tracheo-innominate Fistula/Hemorrhage

Evaluation

Tracheo-innominate fistula is a rare complication, with a reported incidence of 0.7%.[56] The peak incidence occurs between one and three weeks after the initial tracheotomy procedure. The clinical case at the beginning of this chapter emphasizes the two hallmark signs of tracheo-innominate fistula. They are a sentinel hemorrhage, followed by massive pulsatile bleeding. Risk factors include low placement of the tracheostomy tube (below the fourth tracheal ring), excessive tube movement, hypotension causing decreased capillary pressure, sepsis, prolonged corticosteroid use, malnutrition, and diabetes.[6,9]

Prevention

The best way to reduce the incidence of tracheo-innominate fistula is to prevent the risk factors. Low placement of the stoma and hypotension should be avoided. The tracheostomy tube should be of optimal size so the cuff can be centralized within the trachea, which will also eliminate excessive angulation and anterior movement of the tube against the trachea. Cuff pressures should be monitored to avoid over-inflation.[9]

Management

Bleeding from a tracheo-innominate fistula is the most feared complication and carries a mortality rate above 80%.[12] The rupture of an innominate artery can present unexpectedly as a sudden fatal hemorrhage from the stoma. Warning signs of pulsatile tracheostomy tubes and sentinel bleeds must be taken seriously.

If massive hemorrhage is the initial presenting sign, the cuff should be immediately overinflated to tamponade the bleeding or digital pressure on the anterior portion of the trachea may be immediately applied and remain until the patient is transported emergently to the operating room. A thoracotomy may be required for repair of the fistula. Alternatively, the placement of a stent by interventional radiology may be performed.

Tracheo-esophageal Fistula

Evaluation

Tracheo-esophageal fistula is another rare complication following tracheotomy, with an estimated incidence of 1%.[55] This complication usually occurs with prolonged excessive cuff pressure or when a malpositioned tracheostomy tube exerts pressure on the posterior wall, especially in the presence of an indwelling nasogastric tube. Tracheo-esophageal fistula can also develop after a penetrating injury to the posterior tracheal wall at the time of tracheotomy. It is suspected when there are copious secretions, recurrent aspiration, a persistent cuff leak, severe gastric distention, or gastric contents presenting through the tracheostomy tube. Diagnosis is made with contrast esophagography or direct visualization with bronchoscopy.[57]

Prevention

Efforts to ensure the proper fit of the tracheostomy tube within the airway are necessary to prevent tracheo-esophageal fistula. Patients with both nasogastric and tracheostomy tubes should be monitored closely to ensure that cuff pressures remain within acceptable limits.

Management

If the mediastinum is involved in a secondary suppurative infection, thoracotomy or CT-guided drainage may be necessary to drain the wound. If the process is isolated within the cervical region, it may be drained through a neck incision. With adequate drainage of the suppurative collection, treatment with antibiotics, and attention to proper nutrition, a fistula may close spontaneously. If conservative measures are unsuccessful, stenting of the esophagus and trachea may alleviate symptoms.

Tracheo-cutaneous Fistula

Evaluation

Tracheo-cutaneous fistula represents the failure of the tracheostomy stoma to close following decannulation. The squamous epithelial surfaces of the peristomal skin and endotracheal mucosa adhere to one another, creating an uninterrupted epithelial tract. The incidence of tracheo-cutaneous fistula ranges from 3.3% to 42%.[58] Clinical presentation consists of continuous drainage of mucus onto the anterior chest wall, especially with coughing, which can cause skin irritation and poor cosmesis. Tracheo-cutaneous fistula also decreases the efficiency of the patient's cough, promoting recurrent aspiration. By tethering the laryngotracheal complex to the overlying skin, tracheo-cutaneous fistula also impairs swallowing, which is dependent on adequate laryngeal elevation. Fistula formation occurs more often after long-term tracheostomy and has a reported rate of 70% in those who have a tracheostomy tube for over 16 weeks.[59]

Stomas generally close by secondary intention within one week of decannulation; however, it has been reported that up to 29% of all decannulated patients develop a persistent stoma. Epithelialization and/or infection of the tract can cause this failure to close. Atrophy and adhesion of the subcutaneous tissue can also occur, resulting in a depressed scar.[60]

Prevention

Tracheo-cutaneous fistula occurs more often in patients with long-term tracheostomy tube placement. Avoiding this complication is, therefore, most often a function of timely decannulation.

Management

The closure of the fistula may be possible via cautery and curettage of the tract. Cases in which the tract fails to close within six months, however, require operative closure (see **Figure 10.2**). Both the scar and fistula are addressed at the same time. The scar is excised via a horizontally oriented elliptical incision encompassing the fistula. The flaps are raised to release adherent scar tissue, and the squamous epithelium of the tract immediately adjacent to the trachea are left intact and inverted with a purse-string suture so the trachea is lined with squamous epithelium. The skin surrounding the tract is widely undermined. The strap muscles, which are frequently involved in the fistulous tract, are released and re-approximated in the midline. Joining the muscle in the midline fills the depressed area of the tract and, more importantly, separates the laryngotracheal complex from the overlying skin, thus enabling the elevation of the complex during swallowing.

Figure 10.2 Repair of tracheocutaneous fistula

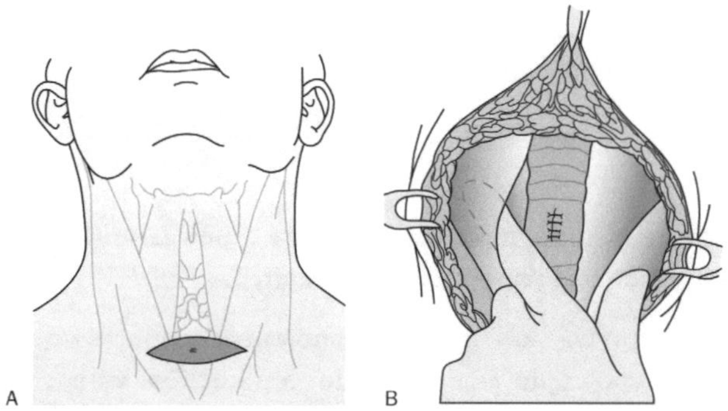

Surgical repair of tracheocutaneous fistula.

A) Scar from tracheostomy is excised down to fistula.

B) Skin flaps superior and inferior to the excision are undermined and strap muscles are dissected.

Complications of tracheo-cutaneous fistula closure include hematoma, infection, keloid formation, and subcutaneous emphysema.[59] Rarely, subcutaneous emphysema develops into a well-defined air pocket located anterior to the trachea. These pockets are referred to as pneumatoceles, pretracheal air cysts, tracheoceles, or aeroceles. Treatment consists of simple drainage and the application of a pressure dressing, and it is performed in an outpatient setting. In cases where the aerocele presents months after the closure of the tracheocele, mucosalization has usually occurred and requires complete excision. Complications of tracheo-cutaneous fistula closures are avoided by minimizing coughing after closure of the fistula as well as by placing a small drain to evacuate any air accumulation under the flaps during the immediate postoperative period.

Stomal Granulation Tissue

Evaluation

Granuloma formation after tracheotomy is common due to the high rate of bacterial colonization of the stoma and the constant mechanical irritation associated with the motion of the tube. The incidence of granulation tissue has been estimated to be 80%, and many times can be attributed to the comorbid presence of gastro-esophageal reflux disease (GERD). The irritation of acidic stomach contents results in inflammation and, at times, ulceration in the traumatized airway.[3,61] Granulation tissue can cause bleeding, difficulty with a tracheostomy tube change, decannulation delay, or obstruction of the tracheostomy tube or trachea itself. The tracheostomy tube can be considered a foreign body that elicits an inflammatory reaction because of its motion due to swallowing and the pistoning effect from positive-pressure mechanical ventilation. At the stoma, a mucocutaneous junction allows contact with the skin and moisture from the tracheal mucosa. The debris that accumulates around the tracheostomy tube can be a source of bacterial colonization and infection. The common problem of granulation tissue is a response to the irritation from indwelling tubes and catheters.

Prevention

Meticulous skin care and antimicrobial and corticosteroid preparations play important roles in decreasing the burden of bacterial contamination as well as the resultant inflammatory reaction that promotes granulation tissue formation. A program of regular tracheostomy tube changes significantly decreased the episodes of granulation tissue requiring operative intervention.[3] One study showed that frequent tube changes also appeared to decrease the likelihood of forming granulation tissue or inflammation at the stoma. However, there was no indication whether more frequent tracheostomy tube changes (every two weeks) would eliminate the problem, or whether a certain subset of patients would require less frequent changes.[3]

Management

Although some granulomas may resolve spontaneously, topical silver nitrate cauterization, inhaled beclomethasone, treatment of GERD, and/or surgical removal may be required.

When granulation tissue becomes obstructive and prevents ventilatory support, surgical intervention is necessary. The use of bronchoscopic equipment in conjunction with sharp dissection has been described as a safe, reliable method for removing suprastomal granulation tissue.[62] Simple eversion of the granulation tissue through the stoma with a skin hook and blind resection may lead to hemorrhage and incomplete excision. Other strategies include endoscopic laser, electrocautery, microdebrider, or coblation. No strategy has been found to be superior in regard to efficacy at this time.[63]

Tracheomalacia

Evaluation

Tracheomalacia, or a weakening of the tracheal wall, results from ischemic injury to the trachea followed by chondritis and the subsequent destruction and necrosis of supporting tracheal cartilage.[57,64] Such injury can result from either direct pressure from the tracheostomy tube itself or from its cuff. When the cuff is overinflated, it places increased pressure on the mucosa leading to ischemic injury. Consequently, when the cuff is inflated, cuff pressure should be maintained between 20-30 cm H_2O.[65]

With the loss of airway support, the compliant tracheal airway collapses during expiration, which may result in expiratory airflow limitation, air trapping, and retained respiratory secretions. In addition, the loss of cartilaginous support may cause the trachea to be compressed by surrounding structures. In the acute setting, tracheomalacia may present as a failure to wean from mechanical ventilation. Alternatively, it may present as dyspnea in a patient with a history of previous tracheotomy. Diagnosis of tracheomalacia depends on a high index of suspicion. Bronchoscopy can reveal excessive expiratory collapse of the trachea in a patient on mechanical ventilation. In the spontaneously breathing patient, a flow-volume loop study shows evidence of variable intrathoracic obstruction. Another approach is dynamic CT scan images of the trachea, which can depict expiratory tracheal collapse.[66]

Prevention

The single most important preventive strategy is to monitor cuff pressure and ensure it remains within acceptable range. If obtaining an adequate seal with normal cuff pressure is not possible, a diagnosis of tracheomalacia should be investigated, rather than continue increasing the cuff pressure. A bronchoscopic examination may confirm the diagnosis.

Management

The treatment of tracheomalacia is first directed at those patients who are symptomatic. Once symptomatic, the initial approach is medical optimization of frequently comorbid conditions including asthma, COPD, and GERD. In mild cases, this conservative approach may be effective. Placement of a longer tracheostomy tube which bypasses the region of expiratory collapse may facilitate ventilation. Additionally, moving the cuff away from the affected area prevents further injury and allows healing. Once optimized, a more thorough assessment using pulmonary function tests (PFT), a six-minute walk test, dyspnea and cough scores may be obtained.[67] In more severe cases, therapeutic options include stenting, tracheal resection, or tracheoplasty.

Tracheal Stenosis

Evaluation

Stenosis of the trachea can occur at the stoma, superior to the stoma, at the level of the cuff, or at the tip of the tube. The primary cause of stenosis is mucosal ischemia. One study found that 89% of patients with subglottic stenosis had a previous tracheostomy for at least 17 days.[68]

Substantial stenosis of the trachea at any location can be treated either surgically or by stenting the stenotic area.[69]

Tracheal and subglottic stenosis are well recognized complications of tracheostomy. Their reported incidence varies and ranges from 0.6% to 21%.[70] Stenosis is categorized into suprastomal, stomal, or infrastomal and is considered clinically relevant when the diameter is reduced by more than 50%.[57] Suprastomal or subglottic stenosis is thought to be caused by damage to the cricoid cartilage followed by cricoiditis and bacterial infection, resulting in cartilage destruction and scar formation. One report revealed that stenosis secondary to PDT occurs earlier and is more commonly subglottic.[71] The mechanism is thought to be due to the tracheal puncture site being more superiorly located than the open tracheotomy site.

Stenosis at the stomal level may be due to infection, peristomal chondritis, or an excessively large tracheostomy tube, or aggressive dilation of the stoma at the time of the procedure. Stomal stenosis is more common in patients who remain ventilator dependent because traction of the ventilator circuit against the tube causes ulceration of the stoma. Infrastomal stenosis most commonly occurs where the cuff comes in contact with the endoluminal tracheal mucosa. Alternatively, it can occur at the tip of the tube as it rubs against the wall of the trachea if the tube lies within it at an abnormal angle.

At the level of the cuff, high pressure leads to ischemia of the mucosa, which, in turn, leads to mucosal edema and ulceration. As ulceration deepens, normal ciliary flow is interrupted, and mucociliary stasis promotes secondary infection and perichondritis. With further infection, chondritis and cartilaginous necrosis develop. Healing occurs by secondary intention with granulation tissue proliferation in the area of ulceration and the deposition of fibrous tissue in the submucosa. Primary intention healing is hindered by poor blood supply to the cartilage, and the constant motion of the laryngotracheal complex associated with swallowing and head movement. Historically, the use of high-volume, low-pressure cuffs markedly decreased the incidence of this type of injury. Placement of a nasogastric tube with a tracheostomy tube can also increase pressure on the mucosa in the posterior trachea and should be avoided when possible.

Tracheal stenosis is caused by the pressure of the cuff, or the tube itself, against the trachea, which leads to commissural scarring and can result in necrosis. One study[70] examined the incidence of tracheal stenosis over a 19-year period, and followed 45 patients with postintubation tracheal stenosis: 38 had tracheal stenosis, and 7 had infraglottic stenosis. Causes and risk factors varied by approach, which was either open surgical tracheotomy or percutaneous dilatational tracheotomy. Risk factors for stenosis after open tracheotomy included infection at the stoma site (10 patients), cervical soft tissue trauma (6), urgent tracheotomy (4), pediatric age group (2), and hypotension (3). Risk factors for stenosis after the percutaneous approach included high tracheotomy (5 patients), tracheal or cartilage damage (1), infection at the stoma site (2), and hypotension (1).[70]

The leading complication in a 10-year sample of 1,130 patients was tracheal stenosis, which was attributed to the presence of an endotracheal tube in situ for at least 12 days prior to tracheotomy.[12]

Previous studies have reported that the most common site of tracheal stenosis is at the level of the cuff; however, Sarper and others[70] found only a 31% rate of stenosis at the level of the cuff and a 64% rate of stenosis at the stoma. Two patients in their study had double stenosis at both the stoma and cuff. Stenosis can be a fixed scar, or it can manifest as functional stenosis due to tracheomalacia, which can narrow the tracheal wall during coughing or forced expiration.[6]

An undersized tracheostomy tube can contribute to overinflation of the cuff in order to provide an adequate seal. Symptoms of stenosis are often unrecognizable until the narrowing approaches 5 mm, when the patient may develop stridor. If patients fail to be liberated from mechanical ventilation, they should be evaluated for tracheal stenosis. It takes an 80% narrowing of the trachea before spirometry can detect evidence of tracheal stenosis.[6]

Prevention

Damaged cartilage is the most common cause for stenosis at the stoma site. The stoma should not be made too large, nor should there be too much force exerted when inserting the tube. Excessive movement of the tube within an overly large stoma can produce damage to the tissue around the stoma.[6] Wound sepsis and trauma to the tracheal area also affect wound healing. Sarper and others[70] found that 42% of their cases of stomal stenosis following open tracheotomy were due to wound sepsis.

Keeping the cuff pressure less than 20 cm H_2O can help prevent stenosis at the level of the cuff, [69] although it should be noted that the recommended cuff pressure to prevent aspiration or a cuff leak is 20-30 cm H_2O. Subglottic stenosis can be prevented with early discontinuation from mechanical ventilation and aggressive efforts toward expeditious decannulation.

High tracheotomy should be avoided, and careful placement of the stoma should be guided by bronchoscopy. Other preventive measures include use of large-volume, low-pressure cuffs, avoidance of large stomal apertures, elimination of heavy equipment connected to the tube, and meticulous nursing care.[70]

Management

Resection of the trachea may be necessary (see **Figure 10.3**), especially in those who have multiple stenoses. Complications are low for tracheal lesions but are significantly higher for larygotracheal resections. In one study, the most common late complication of tracheal resection was granulation tissue at the suture line.[70]

Figure 10.3 Repair of tracheal stenosis

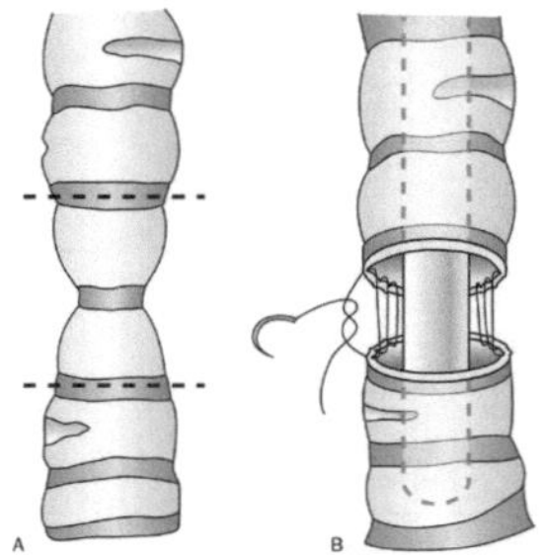

Surgical repair of tracheal stenosis.

A) Area of tracheal stenosis is identified.

B) Portion of trachea has been resected and closure is begun. Note insertion of anode endotracheal tube through the anastomosis.

Summary

Numerous complications can result from the placement of a tracheostomy. Although there is an overlap, complications are typically categorized as immediate/intraoperative, early (during the first postoperative week), or late. Many complications can be prevented by attention to detail and meticulous care. Good intraoperative communication between the surgeon and anesthesiologist is essential. During the first postoperative week, tube security is a priority to prevent inadvertent decannulation. Many of the later complications can be prevented by minimizing cuff pressure to avoid sequelae including stenosis, tracheomalacia, and granulation tissue. Knowledge of potential complications promotes quick action in the event of an emergency.

Key Points

- Potentially dangerous complications can occur in the immediate, early, or late periods after tracheotomy. Prompt recognition and knowledge of management steps are integral to successful patient outcomes. Particular attention should include surveillance for severe hemorrhage, false passage, air collection in the chest, intraoperative fires, post-obstructive pulmonary edema, and fistulous tracts leading to the trachea.
- Tube displacement and loss of airway can occur before the stoma has matured (prior to the fifth postoperative day). Signs of tube displacement include resistance with use of a manual resuscitation bag, inability to pass a suction catheter, subcutaneous emphysema, and the inability to obtain an end-tidal CO_2 measurement.
- Mucous plugs are common and potentially catastrophic. Their incidence can be lessened by adequate hydration and effective mobilization of secretions.
- Maintaining optimal cuff pressures can decrease the high incidence of tracheal stenosis and tracheomalacia.

REVIEW QUESTIONS

1. A patient who underwent tracheotomy one week prior is found to have massive hemorrhage from the tracheostomy tube. Appropriate interventions to control the bleeding and stabilize the patient are attempted unsuccessfully and the patient expires. What preventive measure significantly decreases the risk of tracheo-innominate fistula development?
    a. Use of electrocautery during tracheotomy
    b. Placement of the tracheal incision above the fourth tracheal ring
    c. Over-inflation of the tracheostomy cuff in the peri-operative period
    d. Use of corticosteroid post-operatively

    AMSWER: B. The risk of tracheo-innominate fistula decreases with increasing space between the tracheal opening and the innominate artery. Entering the trachea below the fourth tracheal ring has been associated with a higher risk of developing a tracheo-innominate fistula. Overinflation of the cuff has been associated with tracheal stenosis as well as an increased risk of tracheo-innominate fistula if the trachea is damaged at the same level as the innominate artery. The use of electrocautery is not associated with tracheo-innominate fistula, and the use of corticosteroids is detrimental to wound healing.[6,9]

2. At what percentage of tracheal stenosis does it become clinically relevant in adults?
    a. 25%
    b. 50%
    c. 75%
    d. 90%

    ANSWER: B. Patients will typically not have clinically apparent signs of stenosis until 50% of their airway is narrowed. Pulmonary function testing will not reveal a stenosis until it is above 75%.[57] The rate of significant stenosis (75% or greater) has been reported at 0.6% to 21% of patients.[70]

3. A 62-year-old male is undergoing awake tracheotomy due to tumor obstruction of the airway. The procedure is complicated by intra-operative hemorrhage secondary to injury to the internal jugular vein. During the repair of the injured vessel, the patient's blood pressure and oxygen saturation suddenly collapse, despite 100% FiO2. What is the likely etiology?
    a. Acute blood loss anemia
    b. Myocardial infarction
    c. Venous air embolism
    d. Mucous plugging

    ANSWER: C. Although all answers may lead to clinically relevant hemodynamic collapse, the most likely cause in this scenario is venous air embolism. Forceful inspiration during an awake tracheotomy in the presence of venous injury above the level of the heart creates a negative force which entrains air. The entrance of air into the venous system, typically greater than 5 ml/kg, leads to decreased gas exchange in the lung, cardiac arrhythmias, pulmonary hypertension, and even cardiac failure and arrest.[35,36]

4. What factor is associated with an increased risk of tracheal stenosis following tracheotomy?
    a. Performing tracheotomy greater than 10 days after intubation for respiratory failure
    b. Treatment with prophylactic perioperative antibiotics
    c. Placement of a nasogastric tube at the time of tracheotomy
    d. Low placed tracheostomy

    ANSWER: C. The risk factors that may increase the likelihood of developing a clinically relevant tracheal stenosis include placement of a nasogastric tube at the time of tracheotomy which increases pressure on the tracheal wall, inflation of the cuff above 20 mm Hg, improperly sized tracheostomy tube, and excessive rubbing of the tracheostomy tube on the tracheal wall.[70]

5. A 40-year-old morbidly obese male with a history of tracheotomy two days prior is found unresponsive. Positive pressure ventilation is initiated, and movement of air is found to be difficult with no return of end tidal CO_2. The patient expires and on post-mortem examination, the tracheostomy tube is found to be outside the airway within a false passage. What may have prevented this complication from occurring?
    a. Placement of a tracheostomy tube of appropriate size and length
    b. Use of stay sutures at the time of tracheotomy
    c. Minimize sedation in the post-operative period
    d. More frequent suctioning of the tracheostomy tube

    ANSWER: A. The loss of end-tidal CO_2 and the inability to pass air is indicative of tracheostomy tube displacement and loss of the airway. The risk of this complication is increased with loosened straps holding the tracheostomy tube in place, excessive coughing, under-sedation, obesity, and improper tracheostomy tube length and/or size. This patient with morbid obesity likely had an improperly sized tracheostomy tube for his body habitus, and movement led to tube displacement, creating a false passage. Stay (traction) sutures may be helpful in management of this devastating complication, but it would not prevent it from occurring.[39-41]

REFERENCES

1. Watanakunakorn C. Successful novel drainage treatment of mediastinal abscess complicating tracheostomy. *Chest.* 1989;96(4):946-948.
2. Henderson CG, Harrington RL, Izenberg S, Dyess DL, Silver FM. Tracheocele after routine tracheostomy. *Otolaryngol Head Neck Surg.* 1995;113:489-490.
3. Yaremchuk K. Regular tracheostomy tube changes to prevent formation of granulation tissue. *Laryngoscope.* 2003;113:1-10.
4. Wright SE, Van Dahm K. Long-term care of the tracheostomy patient. *Clin Chest Med.* 2003;24:473-487.
5. St. John RE, Malen JF. Contemporary issues in adult tracheostomy management. *Crit Care Nurs Clin N Amer.* 2004;16(3):413-430.
6. Heffner JE. Management of the chronically ventilated patient with a tracheostomy. *Chron Respir Dis.* 2005;2:151-161.
7. Neema PK, Manikandan S. Tracheostomy and its variants. *Ind J Anaesth.* 2005;49(4):323-327.
8. DeLeyn P, Bedert L, Delcroix M, Depuydt P, Lauwers G, Sokolov Y, et al. Tracheotomy: Clinical review and guidelines. *Eur J Cardiothorac Surg.* 2007;32:412-421.
9. Singh N, Fung A, Cole IE. Innominate artery hemorrhage following tracheostomy. *Otolaryngol Head Neck Surg.* 2007;136(4):S68-S72.
10. Fernandez-Bussy S, Mahajan B, Folch E, Caviedes I, Guerrero J, Majid A. Tracheostomy tube placement: Early and late complications. *J Bronchol Intl Pulmonol.* 2015;22(4):357-364.
11. Grant CA, Dempsey G, Harrison J, Jones T. Tracheo-innominate artery fistula after percutaneous tracheostomy: Three case reports and a clinical review. *Brit J Anaesth.* 2006;96:127-131.
12. Goldenberg D, Ari EG, Golz A, Danino J, Netzer, A, Joachims HZ. Tracheotomy complications: A retrospective study of 1130 cases. *Otololaryngol Head Neck Surg.* 2000;123(4):495-500.
13. Waldron J, Padgham ND, Hurley SE. Complications of emergency and elective tracheostomy: A retrospective study of 150 consecutive cases. *Ann Royal Coll Surg Engl.* 1990;72(4):218-220.
14. Francois B, Clavel M, Desachy A, Puyraud S, Roustan J, Vignon P. Complications of tracheostomy performed in the ICU: Subthyroid tracheostomy vs. surgical cricothyroidotomy. *Chest.* 2003;123(1):151-158.
15. Dane TE, King EG. A prospective study of complications after tracheostomy for assisted ventilation. *Chest.* 1975;67(4):398-404.
16. Spataro E, Durakovic N, Kallogjeri D, Nussenbaum B. Complications and 30-day hospital readmission rates of patients undergoing tracheostomy: A prospective analysis. *Laryngoscope.* 2017;127:2746-2753.
17. Yeo WWX, Phua CQ, Lo S. Is routine chest X-ray after surgical and percutaneous tracheostomy necessary in adults: A systemic review of the current literature. *Clin Otolaryngol.* 2014;39(2):79-88.
18. Gorphe P, Sarfati B, Janot F. Airway fire during tracheostomy. *Eur Ann Otorhinolaryngol Head Neck Dis.* 2014;131:197-199.
19. Weber SM, Hargunani CA, Wax MK. Duraprep and the risk of fire during tracheostomy. *Head and Neck.* 2006;28:649-652.

20. Rinder CS. Fire safety in the operating room. *Curr Op Anaesthesiol.* 2008;21(6):790-795.
21. Institute for Safe Medication Practices (ISMP). Surgical fires caused by skin preps and ointments: Rare but dangerous and preventable. *Nurse AdviseERR.* 2018;16(4):1-4.
22. Axelrod EH, Kusnetz AB, Rosenberg MK Operating room fires initiated by hot wire cautery. *Anesthesiol.* 1993;79:1123-1126.
23. Plumlee JE. Operating-room flash fire from use of cautery after aerosol spray: A case report. *Anesth Analg.* 1973;52:202-203.
24. Blanchard DL. Fire in surgery. *Ophthal Plas Reconstr Surg.* 1987;3:59.
25. Stouffer DL. Fires during surgery: Two fatal incidents in Los Angeles. *J Burn Care Rehabil.* 1992;13,114-117.
26. Nicholson MJ. Case history number 82: "Nonflammable" fires in the operating room. *Anesth Analg.* 1974;54:152-153.
27. Wolf GL, Simpson JI. Flammability of endotracheal tubes in oxygen and nitrous oxide enriched atmosphere. *Anesthesiol.* 1987;67:236-239.
28. deRichmond AL, Bruley ME. Head and neck surgical fires. In Eisele DW ed., *Complications in head and neck surgery.* St. Louis, MO: Mosby-Year Book, 1993.
29. Thompson JW, Colin W, Snowden T, Hengesteg A, Stocks RM, Watson SP. Fire in the operating room during tracheostomy. *S Med J.* 1998;91(3):243-247.
30. Marsh B, Riley RH. Double-lumen tube fire during tracheostomy. *Anesthesiol.* 1992;76(3):480-481.
31. Michels AM, Stott S. Explosion of tracheal tube during tracheostomy. *Anaesthesia.* 1994;49(12):1104.
32. Wilson PT, Igbaseimokumo U, Martin J. Ignition of the tracheal tube during tracheostomy. *Anaesthesia.* 1994;49(8):734-735.
33. Daane SP, Toth BA. Fire in the operating room: Principles and prevention. *Plast Reconstruc Surg.* 2005;115(5):73e-75e.
34. Wolf GL, Sidebotham GW, Stern JB. Intraluminal flame spread in tracheal tubes. *Laryngoscope.* 1994;104:874-879.
35. Hartveit F, Lystad H, Minken A. The pathology of venous air embolism. *Brit J Exp Pathol.* 1968;49(1):81-86.
36. Agarwal SS, Kumar L, Chavali KH, Mestri SC. Fatal venous air embolism following intravenous infusion. *J Forens Sci.* 2009;54(3):628-684.
37. Asherson N Tracheostomy: Sudden death from delayed air embolism. *J Laryngol Otol.* 1958;72:743-745.
38. Casserly P, Lang E, Fenton JE, Walsh M. Assessment of healthcare professionals' knowledge of managing emergency complications in patients with a tracheostomy. *Brit J Anaesth.* 2007;99:380-383.
39. Walvekar RR, Myers EN. Technique and complications of tracheostomy in adults. In Myers EN, Johnson JR eds., *Tracheotomy: Airway management, communication, and swallowing.* 2nd ed.,San Diego, CA: Plural Publishing, 2008:35-67.
40. Parnes SM, Myers EN. Traction sutures in a tracheostomy using a ligature passer. *Transac Amer Acad Ophthalmol Otolaryngol.* 1997;82(41):479-485.
41. Lee YC, Kim TH, Lee J, Oh IH, Eun YG. Comparison of complications in stroke subjects undergoing early versus standard tracheostomy. *Respir Care.* 2015;60(5):651-657.
42. Gillies D, Todd DA, Foster JP, Batuwitage BT. Heat and moisture exchangers versus heated humidifiers for mechanically ventilated adults and children. *Cochrane Database Syst Rev.* 2017;14(9).

43. Delaney A, Bagshaw SM, Nalos M. Percutaneous dilatational tracheostomy versus surgical tracheostomy in critically ill patients: A systematic review and meta-analysis. *Crit Care.* 2006;10(2):R55.
44. Myers EN, Stool SE, Johnson JT. Technique of tracheotomy. In Myers EN, Stool, SE, Johnson, JT, eds. *Tracheotomy.* New York: Churchill Livingstone, 1985.
45. Sasaki CT, Horiuchi M, Koss N. Tracheostomy-related subglottic stenosis: Bacteriologic pathogenesis. *Laryngoscope.* 1979;89(6):857-865.
46. Tsunezuka Y, Suzuki M, Nitta K, Oda M. The use of fibrous wound dressing sheets made of carboxymethylcellulose natrium in the postoperative management of tracheostomy. *Kyobu Geka.* 2005;58(12):1063-1067.
47. Motta GJ, Trigilia D. The effect of an antimicrobial drain sponge dressing on specific bacterial isolates at tracheostomy sites. *Ostomy Wound Management.* 2005;51(1):60-62,64-66.
48. Lee JM, Hashmi N, Bloom JD, Tamashiro E, Doghramji L, Sarani B, Palmer JN, Cohen NA, Mirza, N. Biofilm accumulation on endotracheal tubes following prolonged intubation. *J Laryngol Otol.* 2012;126:267-270.
49. Mack C. Molecular mechanisms of Staphylococcus epidermidis biofilm formation. *J Hosp Infec.* 1999;43:S113–S125.
50. Kinnari TJ. The role of biofilm in chronic laryngitis and in head and neck cancer. *Curr Opin Otolaryngol Head Neck Surg.* 2015;23(6):448-453.
51. Durbin CG. Early complications of tracheostomy. *Respiratory Care.* 2005;50(4):511-515.
52. Kremer B, Botos-Kremer AI, Eckel HE, Schlöndorff G. Indications, complications, and surgical techniques for pediatric tracheostomies—An update. *J Pediatr Surg.* 2002;37(11):1556-1562.
53. Rabuzzi DD, Reed GF. Intrathoracic complications following tracheotomy in children. *Laryngoscope.* 1971;81(6):939-946.
54. Weymuller EA. Acute airway management. In Cummings CW ed., *Otolaryngology Head and Neck Surgery,* 3rd ed., St. Louis, MO: Mosby-Year Book, 1998.
55. Epstein, SK. Late complications of tracheostomy. *Respir Care.* 2005; 50(4): 542-549.
56. Scalise P, Prunk SR, Healy D, Votto J. The incidence of tracheoarterial fistula in patients with chronic tracheostomy tubes: A retrospective study of 544 patients in a long-term care facility. *Chest.* 2005;128(6):3906-3909.
57. Sue RD, Susanto I. Long-term complications of artificial airways. *Clin Chest Med.* 2003;24(3):457-471.
58. Mohan VK, Kashyap L, Verma S. Life threatening subcutaneous emphysema following surgical repair of tracheo-cutaneous fistula. *Paediatr Anaesth.* 2003;13(4):339-341.
59. Bent JP, Smith RJ. Aerocele after tracheo-cutaneous fistula closure. *Intl J Pediatr Otorhinolaryngol.* 1998;42(3):257-261.
60. Stanton DC, Kademani D, Patel C, Foote JW. Management of post-tracheotomy scars and persistent tracheo-cutaneous fistulas with dermal interpositional fat graft. *J Oral Maxillofac Surg.* 2004;62:514-517.
61. Roh J, Yoon Y. Effect of acid and pepsin on glottic wound healing a simulated reflux model. *Arch Otolaryngol Head Neck Surg.* 2006;132(9):995-1000.
62. Fang TJ, Lee LI, Li HY. Powered instrumentation in the treatment of tracheal granulation tissue for decannulation. *Otolaryngol Head Neck Surg.* 2005;133(4):520-524.

63. Rasband-Lindquist A, Sale K. A novel approach to excision of distal tracheal granulation tissue in tracheostomy patients with difficult anatomy. *Ear Nose Throat J.* 2016;95(10-11):454-456.
64. Feist JH, Johnson TH, Wilson RJ. Acquired tracheomalacia: Etiology and differential diagnosis. *Chest.* 1975;68(3):340-345.
65. Sengupta P, Sessler DI, Maglinger P, Wells S, Vogt A, Durrani J, Wadhwa A. Endotracheal tube cuff pressure in three hospitals, and the volume required to produce an appropriate cuff pressure. *BMC Anesthesiol.* 2004;4:8.
66. Aquino SL, Shepard JA, Ginns LC, Moore RH, Halpern E, Grillo HC, et al. Acquired tracheomalacia: Detection by expiratory CT scan. *J Computer Assis Tomogr.* 2001;25(3):394-399.
67. Carden KA, Boiselle PM, Waltz DA, Ernst A. Tracheomalacia and tracheobronchomalacia in children and adults: An in-depth review. *Chest.* 2005;127:984.
68. Pena J, Cicero R, Marin J, Ramirez M, Cruz S, Navarro F. Laryngotracheal reconstruction in subglottic stenosis: An ancient problem still present. *Otolaryngol Head Neck Surg.* 2001;125(4):397-400.
69. Rana S, Pendem S, Pogodzinski MS, Hubmayr RD, Gajic O. Tracheostomy in critically ill patients. *Mayo Clin Proc.* 2005;80(12):1632-1638.
70. Sarper A, Ayten A, Eser I, Ozbudak O, Demircan A. Tracheal stenosis after tracheostomy or intubation: Review with special regard to cause and management. *Texas Heart Inst J.* 2005;32(2):154-158.

11

Downsizing and Decannulation

By Linda L. Morris

Objectives

- Identify patient, ventilator, and tube factors that predict successful decannulation
- Outline a protocol for successful decannulation
- Provide investigative approach to causes of decannulation failure
- Promote a multidisciplinary approach to manage patients with tracheostomies

Introduction

Unless a tracheostomy is placed for irreversible conditions, the clinician must always consider the goal of decannulation. The decannulation process does have some risk, but there are several benefits. Not only is the tube itself a foreign object irritating the airway, but it also interferes with swallowing, coughing, taste, olfaction, defecation, and phonation. There are psychosocial issues associated with the presence of a tracheostomy tube, including loss of control, anxiety, inability to communicate, reduced quality of life, and body image concerns,[1,2,3] all of which can create frustration at best and severe depression at worst.

Planning for downsizing and decannulation should begin as soon as the patient has recovered from the immediate postoperative period and is looking toward the first tracheostomy tube change. Downsizing is the gradual process of decreasing the size of the tracheostomy tube, usually with the eventual goal of decannulation. Downsizing has several advantages, including decreasing long-term complications such as tracheal stenosis and tracheomalacia as well as improving swallow and decreasing the risk of aspiration. Another theoretical advantage to the downsizing process is minimizing scarring; however, the literature relating scarring and downsizing is sparse.

CLINICAL SCENARIO

Bill P. suffered a large hemorrhagic stroke, and a tracheostomy was placed in the ICU because of inability to wean from mechanical ventilation. A size 8 Shiley DCT (dual-cannula, cuffed) tube was placed at the bedside by open surgical technique. Two days later, the patient was liberated from mechanical ventilation, and the cuff remained inflated. On post-operative day seven, the surgeon returned, assessed the airway, and changed the tracheostomy tube to another 8 Shiley cuffed DCT.

Assessment for downsizing should begin with a thorough review of the medical record and discussion with the primary care practitioner and the surgeon who placed the tracheostomy. When the medical condition has stabilized and there are no factors that necessitate continued cannulation, planning for decannulation should take place. Decannulation should be considered when the reason for tracheostomy placement is resolved, when airway secretions have abated, when mechanical ventilation is no longer required, and the patient demonstrates sustained spontaneous unlabored breathing.[1]

Two systematic reviews address tracheostomy decannulation. Santus and colleagues[4] reviewed 10 studies and found that cough effectiveness and ability to tolerate capping were the most important parameters to progress to decannulation. In addition, they also proposed a decannulation score to assist clinicians in choosing the optimal timing for decannulation. However, this score has not yet been tested in clinical practice. Singh and others[5] conducted a systematic review of 18 studies. Their main findings were that there were no randomized controlled trials that study decannulation, and there is no standard accepted method of decannulation. Perhaps this is because different populations have special considerations, which will be discussed later in this chapter.

FACTORS TO CONSIDER PRIOR TO DECANNULATION

It is important to consider the reason for placement of the tracheostomy in the plan for downsizing and decannulation. Decannulation of patients who have had a prolonged period of mechanical ventilation is markedly different from decannulation in those who have had a resolution of an upper airway obstruction.[1] Patients who have had a prolonged period of mechanical ventilation have other comorbidities to consider, poor respiratory reserve, are also likely to be deconditioned, and may also have limited ability to protect their airway. Morris and colleagues[6] proposed a tracheostomy progression checklist for patients in the ICU (**Table 11.1**). When each question can be answered with Yes, the patient is ready for decannulation.

Table 11.1 Tracheostomy Progression Checklist

Questions	Circle a Response		Date Completed
1. Is the patient free from ventilator support?	Yes	No	
2. Can the cuff be deflated?	Yes	No	
3. Can the tracheostomy be changed to cuffless or TTS?	Yes	No	
4. Does the patient tolerate prolonged capping of the cuffless (or TTS) tracheostomy?	Yes	No	
5. Is the vital capacity at least 1 liter (15 ml/kg)?	Yes	No	
6. Can the patient manage his/her own secretions?	Yes	No	
7. Has the initial need for the tracheostomy been resolved, with no further need for the tracheostomy?	Yes	No	

After tracheostomy placement, the clinician must always consider the initial reason for placement. Once the initial reason for tracheostomy has been resolved, the patient can enter along the pathway toward decannulation. In the case of Bill P., once he was weaned from mechanical ventilation, the process can begin.

Clinical Scenario Cont'd.

A tracheostomy specialist evaluated Mr. P. and deflated the cuff on his tracheostomy tube. The patient remained stable, with no change in respiratory rate and oxygen saturation.

The decannulation process is likely to be different in acute care hospitals versus inpatient rehabilitation and long-term care hospitals. A retrospective study by the National Association of Long-Term Hospitals (NALTH) found that 54% of patients were able to discontinue mechanical ventilation support after a prolonged period, but only 59% of those weaned were ultimately decannulated.[7] O'Connor and colleagues[8] studied the process of decannulation in patients who had received prolonged mechanical ventilation in 23 long-term-care hospitals. They found that within a median of 45 days after tracheostomy placement, decannulation was successful in 35% of patients. The patients who were decannulated successfully had tracheostomy tubes placed earlier and had shorter stays in the acute care hospital. Three years later, 35% of all patients were alive, including 62% of those who were decannulated.

Several studies have proposed that decannulation may be (and perhaps, should be) different in selected populations. Shrestha and others[9] compared a gradual versus an abrupt decannulation technique in a group of severe head trauma patients. They found that, of the variables assessed, the significant factors for abrupt decannulation were cough reflex, suction requirements, X-rays, and antibiotics for more than seven days. Kang and colleagues[10] used an external glottic control device for decannulation in patients with neuromuscular diseases and cervical spine injuries and found that the device was beneficial in substituting for innate glottic function in order to determine readiness for tracheostomy decannulation. Wirtz and investigators[11] reported 10 years of pediatric outcomes with decannulation. After undergoing operative laryngoscopy and bronchoscopy, all 35 children with long-term tracheostomies were decannulated and discharged within two days, without capping, downsizing, or polysomnography, and without complications. Thomas and colleagues[12] studied time to decannulation and associated risk factors in patients with ICU-acquired weakness. In their sample of 122 patients, successful decannulation was achieved after a median of 89 days from onset of primary illness. In a population of neuromuscular patients with tracheostomy, Chadda[13] found that decannulation resulted in increased dead space and a 30% increase in work of breathing. Because each specialized population of patients may have individual concerns, they may benefit from a structured approach toward decannulation based on specific needs.

Resistance and Work of Breathing

The prolonged placement of an endotracheal tube and subsequent tracheostomy interferes with the normal airway-protective mechanisms of cough and swallow. The disadvantages of tracheostomy include loss of the upper airway for ventilation, loss of laryngeal function, and imposed resistance of the artificial airway.[14] The presence of a tracheostomy tube interferes with the normal swallowing mechanism. The vocal cords in the larynx are bypassed by the tracheostomy tube, which interferes with effective coughing and partial regulation of breathing. When the vocal cords are partially closed, subglottic pressure is maintained, and physiologic PEEP maintains airway patency. Subglottic pressure also contributes to effective swallowing and reduction of the risk of aspiration. Intrinsic PEEP is lost with a tracheostomy tube.[1] Furthermore, the laryngeal blast that produces an effective cough is lost.

Compared to endotracheal tubes, tracheostomy tubes have been associated with significant reductions in airflow resistance, work of breathing, and intrinsic PEEP.[15,16] Diehl and colleagues[15] demonstrated a decrease in these measures comparing tracheostomy to mechanical ventilation through an endotracheal tube. Moscovici da Cruz and colleagues[14] showed this difference by comparing spontaneously breathing non-intubated patients to patients with tracheostomies. Presumably, this difference is due to decreases in airflow resistance.[16]

The primary factors involved in resistance and work of breathing are the following:[17]

1. The larger the diameter, the lower the resistance.
2. The shorter the tube, the lower the resistance.
3. Secretions within the walls of the tube increase resistance.
4. The sharper the curve of the tube, the greater the resistance.
5. Higher gas flows require increased pressure.

The small radius and curvature of a tracheostomy tube increase turbulence and airway resistance. However, when compared to endotracheal tubes, these effects are offset by the tracheostomy tube's shorter length, which results in an overall lowering of airway resistance and muscle loading. In addition, secretions within the lumen of the tracheostomy tube also increase resistance, but the ease of suctioning and removable inner cannulas mitigate this effect.[18]

CLINICAL SCENARIO CONT'D.

Because Mr. P. remained stable with cuff deflation over the next two days, the tracheostomy specialist returned to assess the airway and progress the tracheostomy. With the cuff fully deflated, she performed brief digital occlusion of the tube and found that the patient was unable to breathe comfortably around the tube. She then changed the tube to a Shiley 6 CFS cuffless tube, and again performed digital occlusion of the tube. This time, the patient was able to breathe comfortably, so she applied a cap. The patient was able to breathe comfortably and phonate with strong voice quality. Oxygen saturation was 98% on room air.

Downsizing allows more air to pass around the outside of the tracheostomy tube rather than through the tube. A progressively smaller size promotes this gradual increase in airflow around the tube (see **Figure 11.1**). The patient gradually becomes reacquainted with air passing through the upper airway. The general principle during downsizing is that, as the tube gets smaller, it is more difficult to breathe through it but easier to breathe around it. With each change in tube size comes a change in airway dynamics. If the patient is breathing *through* a smaller tube, airway resistance increases. If the patient is breathing *around* a smaller tube, airway resistance decreases. The caveat here is that the tube itself creates an increasingly hindering obstruction as the ratio of tube size to airway diameter increases. This explains why some patients who do not tolerate capping can be successfully decannulated.[19]

Figure 11.1 Airflow larger vs. smaller tube

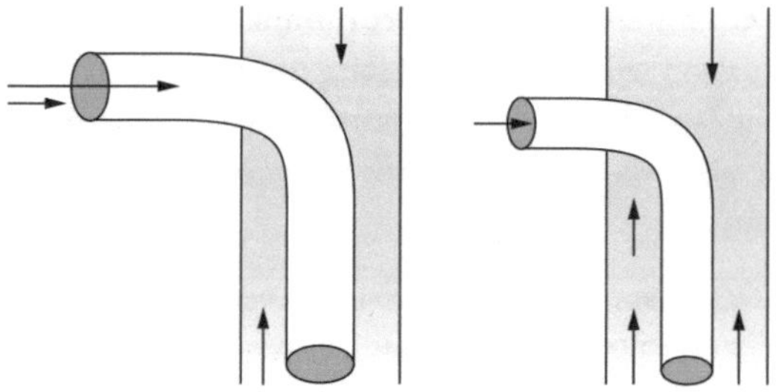

Airflow through a smaller tube compared to a larger one. Note less resistance with breathing through a larger tube. As the tube gets smaller, resistance (and hence, work of breathing) increases.

It is estimated that 10%[20-22] to 16.9%[23,24] of all mechanically ventilated patients receives a tracheostomy, and this trend appears to be increasing. A more recent study[25] reported that up to 24% of ICU patients receives a tracheostomy. Cox and co-investigators[23] reviewed a 10-year database comprising 144,875 patients requiring mechanical ventilation. Approximately one-third of these mechanically ventilated patients (49,872) required longer ventilator support (greater than or equal to four days). Approximately one-fifth of these patients who required prolonged mechanical ventilation (9,794) underwent a tracheostomy. Of interest is that the incidence of tracheostomy placement increased 200% over the 10-year duration of their study.

Aerodynamics not only change during the downsizing process but also after decannulation. Chadda and others[13] found that tidal volume increased without any change in respiratory rate, inspiratory time, or arterial pCO_2. A return to mouth breathing resulted in a 17.5% increase in tidal volume. These changes were due to a significant increase in physiologic dead space and were associated with a significant increase in work of breathing. Similarly, Villalba and others[26] found that work of breathing is higher when breathing through the upper airway than when breathing through a tracheostomy tube with an inflated cuff. Dellweg and investigators[27] found that decannulation resulted in increased or decreased respiratory burden depending on upper airway morphology and pathology. Upper airway morphology was shaped by anatomy, position, muscle tone, secretions, infection, edema, or the presence of an artificial airway. Moscovici da Cruz and investigators[14] studied seven patients with head and neck cancer and also found that upper airway resistance changed with individual differences in airway morphology. Thus, following decannulation, the changes in airway dynamics necessitate continued observation.

Cannulation Times

The course and outcome following tracheostomy varies with the reason for intubation. One Australian group[28] retrospectively studied all patients in their ICU over one year. Of 100 patients who had tracheostomies during that time, 35 were admitted for respiratory causes, 35 for neurologic conditions, 17 due to trauma, and the remaining 13 for cardiovascular, gastrointestinal, sepsis, and metabolic complications. The authors found that 47 patients required tracheostomies because of prolonged mechanical ventilation, 45 for bronchial hygiene or the risk of aspiration, and eight for an unstable or obstructed airway. During the study period, 37 patients died, 30 of whom had the tracheostomy tube in place. Seventy patients were successfully decannulated; 63 survived, and seven died after being decannulated for at least one week. Total cannulation times varied with the reasons for tracheostomy tube placement. As expected, the authors noted that cannulation times were shorter for respiratory than neurologic diagnosis, and even shorter for trauma. Median cannulation time was 25 days, but three patients had cannulation times longer than six months.

Leung and coauthors[28] noted that patients with unstable airways were cannulated for a mean of 13 days. Those with prolonged mechanical ventilation were cannulated for a mean of 25 days, and those with aspiration were cannulated for a mean of 33 days. Comparatively, Dellweg and colleagues[27] reported an average cannulation time of 37 days, and Rumbak and coauthors[16] reported an average intubation/cannulation time of 2.4 weeks.

O'Connor and co-investigators[29] studied patients on prolonged mechanical ventilation. In their study of 135 patients, 58 (43%) were successfully liberated from mechanical ventilation and 81% (47/58) of those weaned were ultimately decannulated. Mean time to decannulation was 45 days. Of those who were weaned, 23% were not decannulated because of an ongoing need for airway protection. In their study, the most common diagnoses were pneumonia, COPD, and septic shock. The median time to placement of a tracheostomy was 18 days after trans-laryngeal intubation. A survival analysis found that 35% of patients were alive 3.5 years later. Those who were decannulated had improved survival compared with those who remained on mechanical ventilation. A more recent study[30] reported median time to tracheostomy at 22 days after intubation, and one-year mortality was 52.4%. After ICU discharge, mortality rate was 29.8% and was higher in non-decannulated patients.

Cannulation times in children tend to be even longer. Kontzoglou and colleagues[31] reported an average cannulation time of 26.4 months. Other studies reported a mean cannulation time of 21.6 months.[32,33] Furthermore, the duration of the decannulation process is also longer in children. Waddell and colleagues[34] described a detailed protocol for decannulation in children that took up to 11 days. This prolonged decannulation schedule could be due to the much longer cannulation times. This study involved children with tracheostomy tubes in place for a mean of 3.5 years who had more complex airway issues. Nonetheless, it is important to consider several factors when planning for decannulation in children. More detailed discussion on decannulation in children can be found in chapter 8.

REASON FOR INITIAL PLACEMENT OF TRACHEOSTOMY

The most important factor when considering decannulation is the initial reason for tracheostomy placement. If the primary issues are not resolved, attempts to downsize and decannulate will not be successful. Factors affecting the decision to place a tracheostomy are the same factors affecting the decision to decannulate. An easy way to remember the indications for the placement of an artificial airway is the acronym *VOPS*: ventilation, obstruction, protection, and secretions.[35]

Ventilation

Patients who continue to require any form of positive-pressure ventilation will benefit from continued use of the tracheostomy. Noninvasive means of positive-pressure ventilation are often met with other complications—such as gastric insufflation, discomfort, and air leak—which can contribute to less than optimal delivery of volume. If the tracheostomy was placed because of the need for prolonged mechanical ventilation, it is usually safe to consider downsizing and decannulation as soon as the patient has been liberated from *continuous* positive-pressure ventilation for at least 24 hours.

Obstruction

Depending on the nature of the obstruction, the tracheostomy tube can usually be decannulated after the obstruction is relieved. A direct view of the trachea is often indicated if obstruction is suspected or documented.

Causes of obstruction include vocal cord paralysis, head or neck masses, edema after prolonged surgery, granulation tissue, stenosis, tracheomalacia, and obstructive sleep apnea.

Protection

The two primary mechanisms that contribute to airway protection are an adequate cough and an adequate swallow. Patients who cannot protect their airway require a cuffed tracheostomy tube, but even an inflated cuff provides imperfect protection.

Cough effectiveness should be evaluated during the downsizing and decannulation process. Failure to produce an adequate cough can result in atelectasis, inspissation of secretions, or tube obstruction because of the incomplete clearance of secretions. The clinical measure of cough effectiveness is vital capacity, and a normal measurement is considered to be 70 ml/kg ideal body weight.[36] The accepted minimum vital capacity is considered to be 15 ml/kg ideal body weight; below this point, patients are unable to effectively clear secretions. A regression equation has been described for calculating accepted minimum vital capacity based on gender, age, and height;[37] however, a simpler formula to calculate ideal body weight is used most often:

female: 5 feet = 100 pounds; male: 5 feet = 105 pounds

Add five pounds for each inch over five feet. Convert pounds to kilograms by dividing by 2.2 and multiply by 15 ml/kg to find the minimum acceptable vital capacity in milliliters.

It is common for patients to be quite deconditioned after a long stay in the ICU, so a vigorous program of physical mobility is required to provide them with the strength to mobilize secretions themselves. When patients can effectively mobilize secretions on their own, they may no longer require suctioning.

Swallowing Function

Swallowing physiology provides intermittent alimentation and continuous airway protection. The action of swallowing consists of several phases. The oral phase consists of preparing the food for transport. This includes mastication and the addition of saliva to create a bolus. During the pharyngeal stage, the food bolus is pushed downward past the nasopharynx. As it enters the vallecular space, the epiglottis tilts downward. The muscles of the larynx contract, causing it to close tightly, and respiration momentarily ceases. The pharyngeal muscles constrict, and the tongue pushes the bolus posteriorly and downward, propelling it toward the esophagus. The cricopharyngeus muscle relaxes, and the anterior pharyngeal wall is pulled forward. This action allows the bolus to pass into the esophagus. During the esophageal stage, the bolus moves through the esophagus and into the stomach by peristalsis.[38,39]

Prolonged intubation interferes with the glottic mechanism, and it may take some time for normal function to return. This could explain the high incidence of aspiration in patients with tracheostomies, which has been reported by some authors as 69%[40] and 64.8%, with a reported range from 50%–87%.[41] An inflated cuff elevates during the swallow and desensitizes the larynx. In addition, it can bulge posteriorly and compress the esophagus. The tube can also partially interfere with the elevation of the larynx and its anterior movement during swallowing. This tethering effect is magnified with cuff inflation.[38] One study[42] demonstrated that the swallow reflex was progressively more difficult to elicit with increasing cuff pressure. Silent (clinically non-observable) aspiration is a common problem in patients with tracheostomies and has been reported to be 46.2%. Silent aspiration was significantly higher with an inflated cuff compared to a deflated cuff.[41]

Swallow physiology is different with various medical conditions. Patients with neuromuscular disorders show significantly greater frequencies of reduced tongue manipulation, slow oral transit, delayed pharyngeal triggering, and aspiration after the swallow. In contrast, patients with head and neck cancer show significantly higher frequencies of reduced laryngeal closure, aspiration during the swallow, and aspiration after the swallow.[41] Pooled salivary secretions are a predictor of dysphagia.[43,44] Gross and co-investigators[45] found a significantly higher number of inhalations during the swallow in patients with a tracheostomy tube compared to normal controls without a tracheostomy tube. They concluded that this increased tendency to inhale during a swallow places a patient with a tracheostomy at higher risk for aspiration. Finally, while the inflated cuff provides some measure of airway protection, it also interferes with the coughing mechanism. It has been implicated in contributing to aspiration because the larynx is desensitized due to the diversion of airflow through the tracheostomy tube.

Secretions

The failure of patients to manage secretions is a common reason for the continued placement of a tracheostomy tube. The underlying condition may contribute to the production of secretions, but it is often the tracheostomy itself that produces significant secretions.[46] Fortunately, secretions commonly decrease during the capping process. Chapter 7 outlines the management of secretions.

TUBE SIZE

Tube size is an important consideration—both the size of the tube in situ and the size of the tube under consideration. When patients breathe *through* a cuffed tube, the general rule of thumb is to choose a tube with the largest inner diameter in order to minimize resistance and decrease airway pressures. As downsizing is considered, however, it is necessary to choose a tube with a smaller outer diameter in order to allow the patient to breathe more easily *around* the tube.

FUTURE NEED FOR ARTIFICIAL AIRWAY

Before decannulation is performed, there should be an inquiry into any impending need for an artificial airway. If a patient is scheduled for a surgical procedure within the next few days or weeks, it may be beneficial to wait until the recovery is complete.

DETERMINING READINESS FOR DECANNULATION

There is no standard method to determine a patient's readiness for decannulation. Some rely on clinical judgment, some on endoscopy or radiography. Stelfox and others[22] conducted a survey of physicians and respiratory therapists to determine usual practices regarding decannulation. They found that the most important factors influencing readiness for decannulation were the patient's level of consciousness, cough effectiveness, amount of secretions, and ability to tolerate tracheostomy tube capping. Of moderate importance were patient comorbidities, etiology of respiratory failure, swallowing function, respiratory rate, and oxygenation. Compared to respiratory therapists, physicians rated level of consciousness significantly more important, and ability to tolerate tracheostomy tube capping significantly less important. The same investigators[47] found there were differences in decision-making for decannulation between respiratory therapists and physicians. Patients were more likely to be recommended for decannulation if they demonstrated an ability to tolerate capping for 72 hours and had chronic obstructive pulmonary disease.

Capping is also called plugging, corking, or blocking; the principle is the same, but the means may be slightly different. They all involve obstructing the tube. With capping, the *uncuffed* tracheostomy tube is obstructed so the patient breathes around the tube rather than through it. The potential problem is that the blocked tube occupies a significant portion of the airway, depending on its size.

CLINICAL SCENARIO CONT'D.

Mr. P. remained capped continuously for the next 48 hours. Vital signs were stable, oxygen saturation remained over 96%, and vital capacity was 20 ml/kg. The tracheostomy tube was removed and the stoma covered with a gauze dressing.

Gao and others[19] developed a simple device for measuring airflow and subglottal pressure in order to determine a patient's readiness for decannulation. Two groups were compared: a decannulation group (deemed ready based on the usual clinical criteria of capping the tracheostomy tube for 24– 48 hours) and a second group determined unsuitable for decannulation. The researchers took airflow measurements during shallow and deep breathing. A routine examination using a flexible fiberoptic bronchoscope determined the resolution of the initial anatomic reasons for tracheostomy placement as well as assessed any changes in the airway. The decision to decannulate was determined by a surgeon, who made the decision on clinical criteria but was uninformed of the airway resistance measurements. All patients were observed in the hospital for at least 24 hours after decannulation, and all were followed for three months by telephone. All patients in the decannulation group were successfully decannulated without any breathing difficulties during the three-month follow-up period. However, resistance was significantly higher in the group that was not decannulated on all measures of upper airway resistance: inspiratory resistance during shallow breathing, expiratory resistance during shallow breathing, inspiratory resistance during deep breathing, and expiratory resistance during deep breathing. The causes of this increased airway resistance were postoperative scarring, vocal cord paralysis, or neoplasms.[19] Thus, careful clinical examination that determined unsuitability for decannulation correlated well with significant residual airway resistance.

Turbulent airflow requires a greater pressure gradient than laminar flow. The irregular airways noted in the patients who were not decannulated generated more turbulent flow. The investigators found that glottis width was narrower in those patients who failed the protocol. Furthermore, they reported that some patients who could not tolerate plugging or capping were still ready for decannulation. The tube itself created a significant obstruction, and removal of the tube improved breathing. The authors suggested that an objective assessment of airway resistance could lead to quicker decannulation without the need for 24–48-hour capping and potentially decrease costs and length of stay.[19]

There is no accepted definition for decannulation failure; however, Stelfox and colleagues[22,47] found that most clinicians considered decannulation failure to be the reinsertion of an artificial airway between 48 to 96 hours after decannulation. In their study, respiratory therapists considered shorter time frames than physicians for defining decannulation failure: 48 hours versus 96 hours. They also found significant differences in practice between those working in acute care facilities and those working in chronic care facilities.[22,47]

Two studies report decannulation failure in selected populations. One 10-year study of patients with laryngotracheal reconstruction concluded that the certain preoperative and postoperative factors may indicate a higher risk of decannulation failure. These included patients with diabetes, gastroesophageal reflex disease, and grade 4 stenosis.[48] A more recent retrospective study reported factors leading to pediatric decannulation failure. They found that chronic respiratory failure, genetic abnormalities, and feeding dysfunction, as well as the presence of one comorbidity, contributed to decannulation failure. In addition, decannulation based on parental expectations rather than medical readiness was also associated with a higher chance of decannulation failure.[49]

The decision to decannulate is based on clinical judgment and falls within a spectrum of approaches. The more methodical approach requires a host of clinical measures to determine the patient's readiness for decannulation and a very slow downsizing progression from one step to the next before the patient is actually decannulated. A trial-and-error approach is much more rapid and inherently riskier. There are no studies to determine the optimal duration for the process of decannulation. Choate and colleagues[50] studied patients at a tertiary care hospital over a 4.5-year period and recorded a 4.8% decannulation failure rate (40 out of 823 decisions to decannulate). Stomal recannulation was required in 25 cases, whereas 15 cases resulted in reintubation. There was no associated mortality or other adverse events. The most common reason for decannulation failure was sputum retention. The authors advised that nursing staff should closely monitor newly decannulated patients for the initial four hours and for up to 24 hours after decannulation.[50]

Barnes, Barbetti, and Currey[51] studied patients in a rehabilitation facility over 18 months to determine the duration of decannulation. The patients' disorders included spinal cord injury, traumatic brain injury, neuromuscular dysfunction, and ventilator-dependent respiratory failure. A protocol was developed, and an interdisciplinary team was established to implement the decannulation protocol. The team consisted of a respiratory therapist, a nurse practitioner, a primary nurse, and a physician. The study evaluated 93 patients, and 93.5% of them qualified for decannulation; however, 6.5% did not meet criteria because of a prolonged inability to protect their airway and continued ventilator support. All patients who qualified were eventually decannulated within 50 days. The average time for the entire decannulation process in an uncomplicated patient was 10 days, which represented 74% of their population. A more recent study in an acute rehabilitation facility found that successful decannulation was achieved after a median of 40.5 days after study onset and a median of 89 days after onset of primary illness.[12]

Godwin and Heffner[52] recommended several principles to guide the evaluation for decannulation, including adequate ventilatory reserve (spontaneous breathing for 24– 48 hours), adequate nutritional state, patent upper airway, absence of bronchopulmonary infection and impending need for mechanical ventilation, adequate cough without suctioning, minimal aspiration, and medical stability.

Decannulation Protocol

There is currently no recommended protocol for downsizing and decannulation, although many have been proposed.[29,53-56] Some protocols simply recommend cuff deflation and assessment for movement of air around the cuff. Others recommend a fenestrated tracheostomy tube for an added boost of air. Still others recommend capping trials. Downsizing usually begins with cuff deflation, which serves two purposes: to assess airway protection and to assess the movement of air through the upper airway. Cuff deflation involves the admixture of room air, which lowers overall FiO_2 and creates the potential for hypoxemia. If significant hypoxemia results from cuff deflation, the clinician should reinflate the cuff and later reattempt downsizing when the patient can tolerate cuff deflation.

Christopher[1] defined a period of physiologic decannulation as an interim step to evaluate patients with long-term tracheostomy. His study conducted evaluations for cough, secretions, and breathing through the upper airway around an occluded tracheostomy tube, as well as a capping trial period. Kubba and colleagues[57] suggested that tolerating a capped tube during the decannulation process is a test of the patient's reserve and may predict success after decannulation. There are no studies that have tested this notion; however, clinical experience has shown it to be generally true.

The most conservative decannulation protocol was reported by Waddell and colleagues[34] for children. Their protocol began with endoscopic evaluation of the airway. If no anatomical, physiologic, or medical concerns were identified, the child was observed for exercise tolerance for two days. If that evaluation was satisfactory, the tracheostomy tube was replaced by a tube of a smaller size on each consecutive day. When the smallest tracheostomy tube was reached (for children, 3 mm internal diameter), it was left in place for two days and capped for 12 hours on the second morning. If that capping trial was tolerated, a 24-hour capping trial was attempted beginning the following morning. If successful, the tracheostomy would be decannulated and the stoma covered with a dry dressing. Following decannulation, the child was observed on the ward for at least three more days and discharged the fourth day after decannulation. Depending on the number of steps involved in downsizing, the process took up to 11 days.

Some authors have suggested that bronchoscopy should be a routine part of a decannulation protocol; however, Rumbak and colleagues[16] supported their hypothesis that routine bronchoscopy was unnecessary. They studied 75 patients clinically ready to be decannulated. All those patients underwent a tracheostomy occlusion protocol followed by bronchoscopy. They deflated the cuff on a fenestrated tracheostomy tube and occluded it. Patients who developed respiratory distress while the tube was occluded were considered to have failed the protocol. In the study, 84% of patients tolerated the protocol, and 16% failed. Bronchoscopy revealed that all patients had some degree of tracheal injury; however, those who failed the protocol had clinically more significant tracheal obstruction to airflow. The authors concluded that patients who successfully pass the occlusion protocol could be safely decannulated without undergoing bronchoscopy. Conversely, they also suggested that those who fail an occlusion protocol should undergo bronchoscopic evaluation.

Gao and others[19] used a protocol of capping the tracheostomy tube for 24– 48 hours. St. John and Malen[58] reported their decannulation protocol began with a formal swallow evaluation in order to assess for anatomic narrowing or obstruction of the upper airway as well as swallowing function. They recommended endoscopy to assess the function of the vocal cords. When patients could breathe spontaneously and swallow safely, they recommended a low-profile cuffed, metal, or cuffless tube during the transition period. When the patient could tolerate a speaking valve for several days with activity, the patient was downsized to a cuffless tracheostomy tube that was capped. The patient was decannulated when able to tolerate capping for 48 hours with no further need for suctioning or positive-pressure ventilation.

Lewarski[59] and Heffner[60] discussed a rapid "one-step" decannulation protocol that began with assessment for decannulation 48 hours after the patient was liberated from mechanical ventilation. The first step was cuff deflation while assessing for signs of aspiration, at which point the tube was occluded to assess for ease of breathing around the tube. The immediate onset of stridor or the inability to breathe comfortably indicated obstruction or that the tube was too large for the airway, which warranted further bronchoscopic evaluation. If the patient tolerated tube occlusion, it was capped for 30 minutes. If the patient tolerated this brief capping trial, decannulation would be performed, and the patient would be observed for 24–48 hours. However, Heffner[60] acknowledged that most patients benefit from a more systematic approach for downsizing.

One study recommended rapid one-day decannulation in a select group of children during intraoperative laryngoscopy and bronchoscopy. Thirty-five children were decannulated in the OR; however, three patients were re-admitted within 90 days, and two patients ultimately failed decannulation.[11]

Godwin and Heffner[52] began their decannulation protocol with cuff deflation after 24–48 hours of spontaneous ventilation. If there was no immediate evidence of aspiration with cuff deflation, the patient was observed for the next 24 hours with the cuff deflated. At that point, the authors offered several options for decannulation. The tube could be occluded and the patient observed for 12–24 hours. If the patient did not tolerate tube occlusion, a fenestrated tracheostomy tube could be placed. Another option applied progressively smaller cuffless tubes. The smallest tube could be placed and capped for a period of time before decannulation. A third option is a capped tracheal cannula, which offers the advantage of full use of the upper airway, without the resistance of breathing around a capped tube.

Rather than abruptly downsizing the tracheostomy, some practitioners prefer to use progressive capping, sometimes called corking. Corks of different sizes reduce the tube's effective diameter by first blocking one-quarter, then one-half, and then three-quarters of the tube and finally providing total occlusion of the opening as tolerated. However, Gray and others[32] recommended against this practice because one patient aspirated portions of cork.

In a lung model, Hussy and Bishop[61] recommended the use of a fenestrated tracheostomy tube to avoid the significant work of breathing involved with a non-fenestrated tube. Christopher[1] described the use of a small diameter fenestrated or non-fenestrated capped tube with the cuff deflated but also cautioned about the development of granulation tissue. He suggested the interim use of a speaking valve to redirect air to the upper airway but acknowledged that "functional decannulation" would likely not be achieved with this method.

Other practitioners advocate the use of a fenestrated tracheostomy to aid in decannulation; however, this practice may produce granulation tissue within the fenestration if the patient is not properly fitted. Not only would this defeat the purpose of the fenestrated tube, but it might result in a potential complication requiring surgical intervention. For a discussion on proper fitting of a fenestrated tracheostomy tube, see chapter 4.

Still other practitioners use peak cough flow as a predictor of success with decannulation. Bach and Saporito[62] studied patients with neuromuscular ventilatory insufficiency and found the only independent predictor of success was peak cough flow. When peak cough flow was at least 160 liters per minute, patients were more likely to have success with decannulation. Normally, a pre-cough inspiration is approximately 85%–90% of total lung capacity. Then the glottis closes and intrathoracic pressure increases to generate a normal peak cough flow of 360–1,000 liters per minute. Total expiratory volume during normal coughing is approximately 2.3 liters.[62] Patients with neuromuscular disease, however, are often unable to generate sufficient cough effectiveness due to their decreased ability to inflate the lungs, abdominal muscle weakness (weakened expiration), and their inability to adduct the vocal cords and close the glottis in order to generate a deep breath.

Dellweg and others[27] studied patients who had failed at least one attempt at decannulation. Their protocol used a tracheostomy retrainer, a device not available in the United States, that appears similar to a tracheostomy button in that it does not compromise the lumen of the trachea or contribute to airway resistance. These devices provided functional decannulation because the airway was not occluded by a tube. Out of 25 patients, only two did not tolerate this trial. Others had only a slight increase in inspiratory time, but work of breathing, compliance, and resistance were unchanged.

For most adult patients in an inpatient hospital setting, the following methodical approach to decannulation has proven effective and successful to this author. Refer to steps in **Figure 11.2** for a downsizing algorithm.

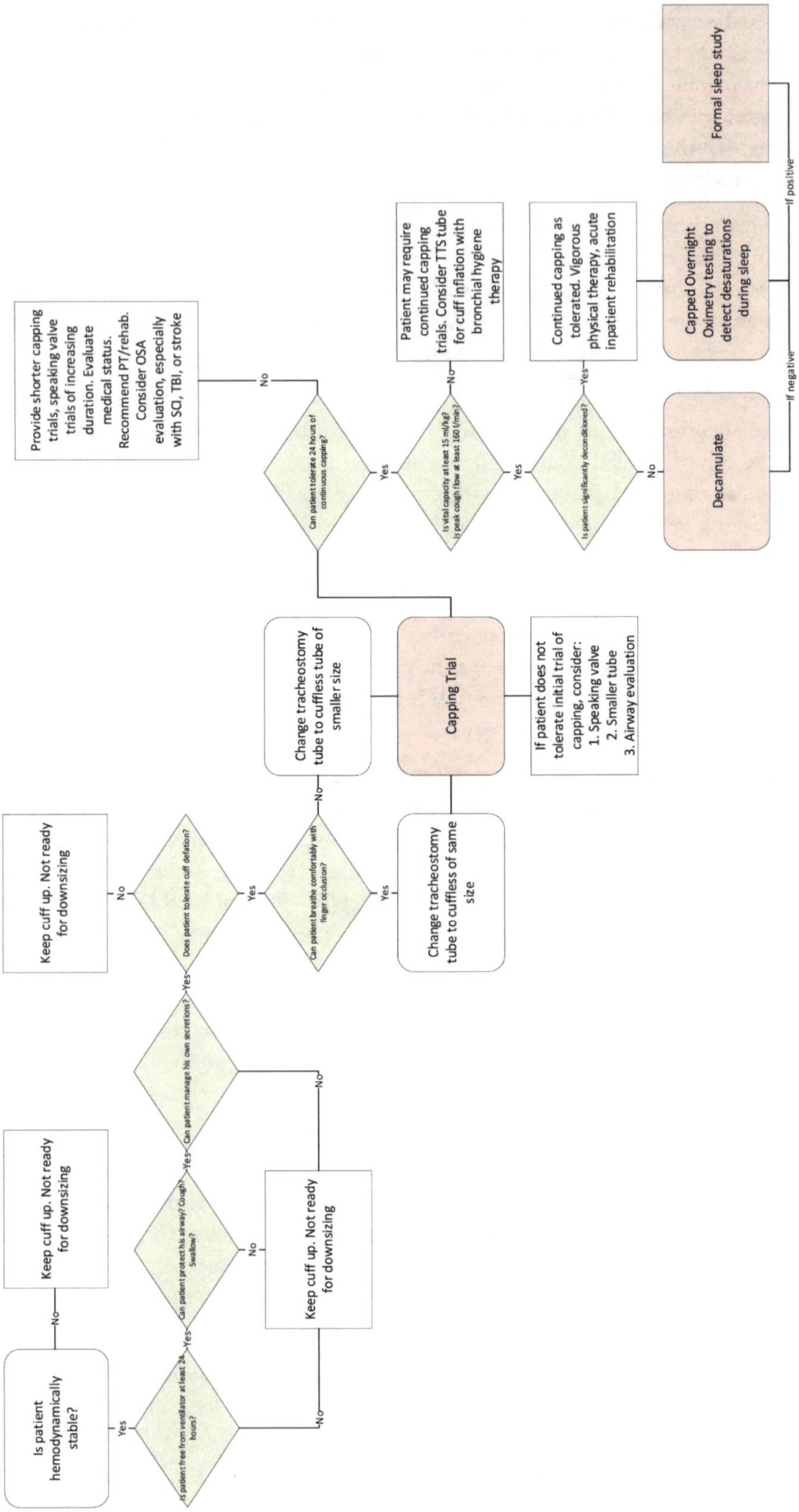

Figure 11.2 Downsizing Algorithm

1. Ensure resolution of the initial reason for tracheostomy tube placement (VOPS: ventilation, obstruction, protection, secretions).
2. Exclude immediate future need of artificial airway. Patients scheduled for a surgical procedure in the near future may benefit from continued cannulation.
3. Determine need for positive-pressure ventilation.
    a. Delivery of positive-pressure breaths during breathing treatments.
    b. Need for intermittent nocturnal positive-pressure ventilation.
4. Examine size and type of tracheostomy tube in situ.
5. Evaluate bedside swallow.
    a. Patients not alert enough to follow commands may be difficult to downsize.
    b. Patients unable to swallow their own saliva are unlikely to be downsized successfully.
    c. Patients with significant central neurological deficits may be challenging to downsize (discussed further in chapter 12).
6. Perform deep subglottic suctioning to remove secretions above the cuff.
7. Deflate the cuff. Instruct patients that the sensation will be unusual because of the unfamiliar feeling of air moving through their upper airway.
8. Occlude the airway with a gloved finger and assess ease of air movement (with cuff deflated). Within two or three breaths, it is usually evident when patients are unable to tolerate digital occlusion. The clinician will observe signs of air hunger and feel pulling against his or her finger as the patient takes a strong inspiratory effort. For this reason, it is important to inform patients prior to this maneuver to gain their cooperation and trust. If patients are able to tolerate finger occlusion, they will be able to breathe easily around the deflated cuff. Patients will have more difficulty when breathing around the cuff of a larger tube.
    a. If the patient is not able to tolerate finger occlusion, the tracheostomy tube may be too large, the folds of the deflated cuff may create too much resistance, or other upper airway factors might be obstructing airflow. See **Figure 11.3**.

Figure 11.3. Deflated cuff compared to cuffless tube of same size

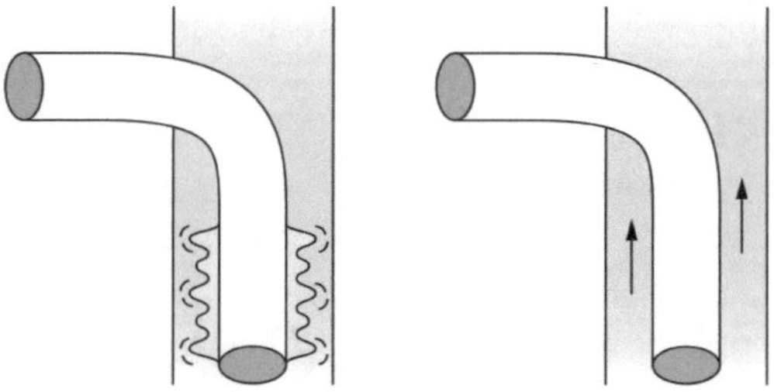

Deflated cuff compared to cuffless tube of the same size. On the left, note turbulent airflow (with increased resistance) around the folds of the deflated cuff. On the right, note laminar airflow around the cuffless tube.

    b. Observe for significant deconditioning. For patients who have been confined to bedrest for long periods of time and are quite weak, Step 7 is generally followed with at least a 24-hour period of cuff deflation. In this way, the patient can be observed for a longer time, and the cuff can be easily reinflated in case of respiratory distress or desaturation. However, if the patient is relatively strong, cooperative, and anxious to proceed, a prolonged cuff deflation is usually unnecessary.

9. Consider formal swallow evaluation by a speech language pathologist.
10. Evaluate amount and thickness of secretions.
    a. Large amounts of thick secretions will require a dual-cannula tube.
    b. Minimal secretions will likely benefit from a single-cannula tube.
11. Test ventilation and phonation without tube.
    a. With the tracheostomy tube removed from the stoma, determine if the tube is a source of obstruction and airway resistance.
    b. Occlude the stoma with a gauze pad and assess for ease of ventilation. If the patient is unable to breathe easily with the stoma occluded, capping will not be tolerated.
    c. Allow the patient to inspire through the stoma, and then occlude upon expiration. This action simulates a speaking valve.
    d. If the patient experiences dyspnea with these maneuvers, endoscopic examination might reveal a source of obstruction.
12. Replace (downsize) the tracheostomy tube with one with a smaller outer diameter.
    a. Steps 1–11 will help determine the type of tube to place.
    b. Generally, a cuffless tube of the same or smaller external diameter is sufficient.
    c. If intermittent positive-pressure ventilation is required, a Bivona TTS tube would be a good choice, especially for the patient who desires to speak.
13. Test readiness to cap.
    a. Digitally occlude the downsized cuffless tube.
    b. If the patient tolerates digital occlusion, cap the tracheostomy tube. *A cuffed tracheostomy tube should never be capped, even when the cuff is completely deflated.* The only exception to this rule is the Bivona TTS tube because its low-profile cuff is designed to be capped when deflated.
    c. If the patient is unable to tolerate digital occlusion, use timed occlusion to simulate a speaking valve. Allow the patient to inspire through the tube, and then occlude it on expiration. The patient's comfort with this intermittent occlusion signals his or her readiness for a speaking valve. Upper airway endoscopic inspection should then exclude any obstructions to airflow.
    d. If the patient tolerates capping, supply oxygen by nasal cannula to guarantee saturation greater than 92%.
    e. If the patient uses a speaking valve, deliver oxygen by high-humidity tracheostomy collar.
14. Cap tracheostomy tube continuously for 24– 48 hours.
    a. If patient is unable to tolerate continuous capping, then cap for progressively increasing lengths of time, especially in patients who received prolonged mechanical ventilation support.
    b. The goal is to keep the tube capped continuously for 24– 48 hours.
    c. Remove cap in case of respiratory distress or desaturation and then suction vigorously and return to high-humidity tracheostomy collar.
    d. Attempt another capping trial later that day or the following day.
    e. Monitor with continuous pulse oximetry.
15. Measure vital capacity.
    a. Vital capacity is an objective measure of cough strength. Vital capacity should be high enough to ensure the patient is able to protect his or her airway.

b. Monitor vital capacity measurements during downsizing and always prior to decannulation.

c. Consider decannulation if vital capacity is greater than 15 ml/kg of (ideal) body weight—approximately 1 liter for most adults. Normal vital capacity is 60–70 ml/kg of body weight.[69]

d. Patients who do not meet minimum vital capacity criteria will benefit from a vigorous exercise program in a rehabilitation center. The patient should remain cannulated during the rehabilitation period and later assessed for decannulation.

e. At the same time, begin a vigorous program of physical therapy to improve cough strength and mobility of secretions.

16. Overnight capped desaturation test.

    a. Patients who cannot be decannulated during their initial hospital stay may require a more conservative approach to decannulation. Frequently, after a prolonged course in the ICU, patients may be too debilitated and require vigorous rehabilitation prior to attempting decannulation. Because the incidence of sleep apnea is quite high in the rehabilitation population, an added overnight desaturation test can provide some insight into possible sleep apnea without a formal sleep study.

    b. For patients who exhibit desaturation episodes during this test, decannulation is postponed until a formal sleep study can be performed. **Figure 11.4** shows a normal overnight oximetry test. **Figure 11.5** shows a pattern of mild obstructive sleep apnea. **Figure 11.6** shows severe complex obstructive sleep apnea.

17. Decannulate.

    a. If the patient tolerates the first 24 hours of continuous capping (without respiratory distress or desaturation) and has a vital capacity greater than 15 ml/kg, remove the tube. Cover the stoma with a gauze dressing.

    b. If patient can tolerate 24 hours of continuous capping but has a vital capacity less than 15 ml/kg, extend continuous capping for another 24 hours.

Figure 11.4 Normal Sleep Oximetry Test

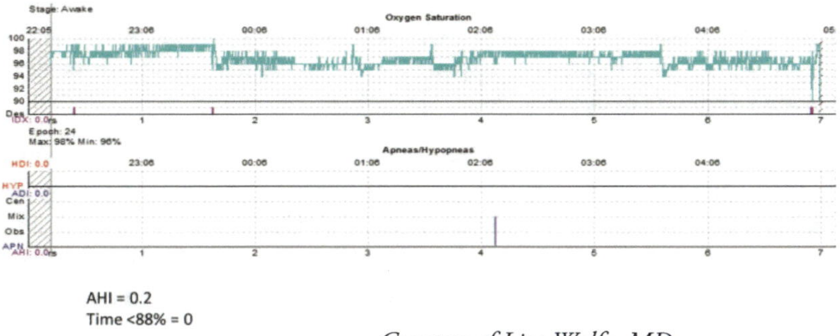

Normal sleep oximetry test. Note that there are no episodes of desaturation less than 88%.

Courtesy of Lisa Wolfe, MD

Figure 11.5 Mild OSA

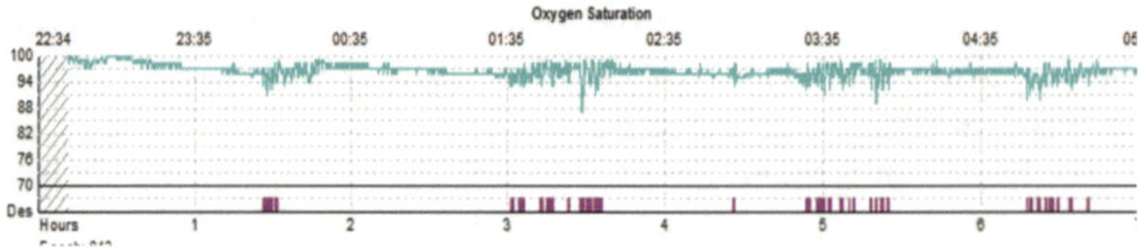

Mild obstructive sleep apnea. Note that there are 0.2 minutes of desaturation less than 88%.

AHI = 7.5
Time <88% = 0.2 min

Courtesy of Lisa Wolfe, MD

Figure 11.6 Severe Complex OSA

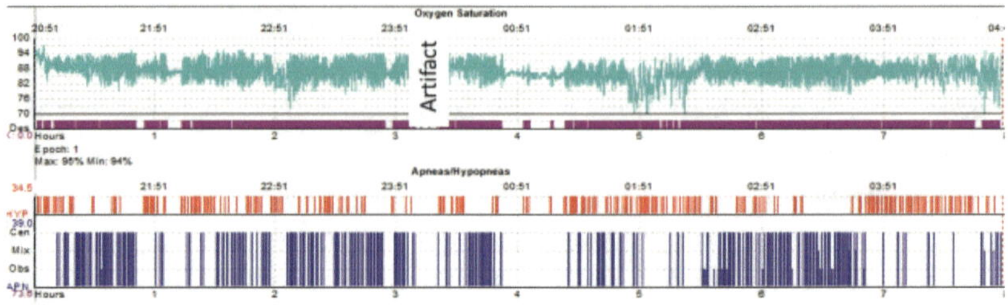

Severe complex obstructive sleep apnea. Note that there are 283 minutes of desaturation less than 88%.

AHI = 73.6
Time<88% = 283 mins

Courtesy of Lisa Wolfe, MD

After Decannulation

It is important to discuss with patients the expected course after decannulation. Patients need to know that they will likely be unable to phonate without digital pressure over the stoma until the stoma heals completely. Phonation without the need for digital pressure can be facilitated by placing a bulky dressing snugly over the stoma. Patients should be instructed to change the dressing twice daily and inspect the stoma for healing and any signs of redness or drainage. Drainage could be a sign of a stomal infection and will often delay complete closure of the stoma. After decannulation, a mature stoma closes slowly. Johnson and colleagues[70] reported that closure of the stoma took an average of 3 to 4 days, with a range of 1 to 26 days. Experience has shown that stomal diameter can shrink by nearly 50% within 12 hours of decannulation.

Occasionally, patients will panic when they realize the tracheostomy tube has been removed and they are unable to speak after decannulation. This is a well-described phenomenon referred to as "decannulation panic" and is most commonly seen in children.[71,72] One author reported that this panic could be attributable to the sudden increase in airway resistance and dead space that occurs after decannulation. Gray and others[32] suggested that more gradual downsizing prior to decannulation does not provoke decannulation panic; however, this author has seen decannulation panic in an adult despite a rather conservative (lengthy) downsizing process. Sherlock and investigators[73] reported that two of eight patients reported panic attacks after decannulation: "Having got rid of [the tracheostomy tube] which was my heart's desire at the time, it just turned out to be my worst nightmare, for a couple of days anyway. But the panic attacks lasted two or three days… I was frightened to go to sleep."

Decannulation in Children

Decannulation appears to have more significance upon speech production in children. A child's age at decannulation may determine whether or not there are delays with speech and language.[75] Simon and colleagues[74] found that children decannulated between birth and three months of age demonstrated normal speech patterns. However, children decannulated between 12 to 47 months developed difficulties with speech and language.[74] It is thought that children decannulated before one year of age may have a better chance at normal speech than those decannulated in their second year.[75]

Decannulation Failure

Occasionally, patients who have been decannulated must be recannulated or reintubated within a relatively short period of time. This situation is called decannulation failure. It is difficult to determine a priori whether or not a patient will require recannulation, but the downsizing process usually identifies patients who may have difficulty.

Multi-Disciplinary Tracheostomy Teams (MDT)

There are several studies reporting the successful outcomes of multi-disciplinary tracheostomy teams (MDT). Tobin and Santamaria[63] reported that the creation of a tracheostomy review team led to shorter decannulation time and length of stay. Patients were decannulated when they could tolerate 24 hours of cuff deflation with the use of either a speaking valve or tube occlusion and could clear secretions without suctioning. Norwood and others[64] reported patient outcomes after the implementation of a tracheostomy team. They found that ICU decannulation rate increased from 14% to 34%, ICU death with tubes in place decreased from 43% down to 16%, and fewer patients were transferred to the wards with their tubes still in situ from 39% down to 18%. Interestingly, time to decannulation did not change between the two groups. They did not describe their decannulation protocol; however, they did report that 25% of the patients were discharged to the wards with a mini-tracheostomy tube in place, which resulted in a significant reduction in complications.

Cameron and colleagues[65] showed the impact of an MDT on patients with spinal cord injury. The team consisted of clinical nurse consultants, physiotherapists, speech pathologists, and physicians who visited patients twice weekly and provided consultation, support, and education on other days as needed. After implementation of the team, they reported a reduced length of stay from 60 to 41.5 days, a decrease in duration of cannulation from 22.5 to 16.5 days, and an eight-fold reduction in cost of care. In addition, time to phonation was decreased from 130 to 10 days. Other studies also reported decreased lengths of stay as a result of MDT. Length of stay was reduced from 50 to 27 days,[66] and ICU length of stay decreased 39.5%.[67]

DeMestral and colleagues[68] also reported the benefits of MDT. They found a decreased incidence of tube blockage from 25% to 5.5%, deceased calls for respiratory distress from 37.5% to 16.7%, increased use of speaking valves from 19.4% to 67.4%, deceased time to downsizing from 26 to 9.4 days, and deceased time to decannulation from 50.4 to 28.4 days. The benefits of MDT seem clear.

SUMMARY

Downsizing and decannulation should be a planned and systematic process with the clinician paying attention to the initial reason for the placement of the tracheostomy tube. For many patients, a simple capping trial is a reasonable test to ensure a safe return to physiologic breathing through the upper airway. However, the tube itself creates an obstruction within the airway, and some patients require a more thoughtful and systematic approach to downsizing and decannulation. Given the shorter length of stay in acute care hospitals, this process is often delayed until the patient has transferred to a less acute level of care. Chapter 12 discusses some specific issues involved in a more long-term approach to downsizing and decannulation in the chronic care and rehabilitation setting.

KEY POINTS

- The issues that led to the placement of the tracheostomy must be resolved before decannulation is considered.
- As a tracheostomy tube gets smaller, it is more difficult to breathe through it and easier to breathe around it.
- A multidisciplinary team approach has demonstrated clear benefits in shortening recovery improving outcomes.
- A planned and systematic approach to downsizing and decannulation usually prevents decannulation failure.
- Deconditioned patients often require a vigorous program of physical exercise prior to decannulation to improve cough strength and ensure airway protection.

REVIEW QUESTIONS

1. When should tracheostomy progression (the downsizing/decannulation process) begin?
   a. When the risk of aspiration has been resolved
   b. When secretions have diminished
   c. When there are no longer factors that necessitate presence of the tube
   c. When the patient is transferred out of the critical care unit

   ANSWER: C. The best answer is C, when the initial reason for placement of the tube has been resolved. For example, if the patient received the tube because of the need for prolonged mechanical ventilation, then tracheostomy progression can begin when the patient is liberated from mechanical ventilation. Choice A is incorrect because the tracheostomy has no effect on the risk of aspiration. Choice B is incorrect because secretions tend to diminish after downsizing/decannulation begins. Choice D is incorrect because tracheostomy progression has no preferred location; it should begin when the patient is ready.

2. Compared to endotracheal tubes, tracheostomy tubes have been associated with all of the following EXCEPT:
   a. Decreased airflow resistance
   b. Increased work of breathing
   c. Reduction in positive end-expiratory pressure (PEEP)
   d. Decreased work of breathing

   ANSWER: B. The answer is B. All of the other choices demonstrate decreased pressure and/or resistance when the patient goes from an endotracheal tube to a tracheostomy tube, and consequently, decrease the work of breathing.

3. A patient is on full ventilator support. Which of the following tracheostomy tubes is the best choice in this situation?
   a. Portex 4 cuffed tube
   b. Shiley 8 cuffed tube
   c. Bivona TTS 8 cuffed tube
   d. TRACOE Comfort 8 uncuffed tube

   ANSWER: B. For a patient on full ventilator support, the priority is effective delivery of tidal volume, so the largest diameter cuffed tube is usually the best. Choice A is incorrect because a size 4 is simply too small to breathe through for an average adult. Choice C is incorrect because the TTS tube is not ideal for continuous cuff inflation due to its high-pressure cuff. Choice D is incorrect because the TRACOE Comfort tube is uncuffed, and therefore, effective accurate delivery of tidal volume is not possible.

4. Reported outcomes of multidisciplinary teams include which of the following?
   a. Increased use of speaking valves
   b. Increased length of stay in ICU
   c. Increased time to decannulation
   d. Increased calls for respiratory distress

ANSWER: A. The correct answer is A. Choices B, C, and D are incorrect because studies have shown a decreased length of stay in ICU, decreased time to decannulation, and decreased calls for respiratory distress.

5. A patient is in the ICU with a Fahl 8 cuffed tracheostomy tube. You deflated the cuff, and the respiratory rate increased 18 to 32 breaths per minute and oxygen saturation decreased from 96 to 88%. Which of the following is the appropriate next step?
   a. Attempt digital occlusion of the tube
   b. Change to Fahl 8 uncuffed tracheostomy tube
   c. Change to Bivona 7 cuffed tracheostomy tube
   d. Re-inflate cuff and attempt cuff deflation at another time

   ANSWER: D. The correct answer is D. Since the patient did not tolerate cuff deflation, the best choice is to re-inflate the cuff and attempt cuff deflation at another time.

REFERENCES

1. Christopher KL. Tracheostomy decannulation. *Respir Care*. 2005;50(4):538-541.
2. Gilony D, Gilboa D, Blumstein T, Murad H, Talmi YP, Kronenberg J, Wolf M. Effects of tracheostomy on well-being and body-image perceptions. *Otolaryngol Head Neck Surg*. 2005;133:366-371.
3. Morris LL, Lupei MI, Afifi MS. Body image perception after tracheostomy. *ORL Head Neck Nurs*. 2017;35(4):13-18.
4. Santus P, Gramegna A, Radovanovic D, Raccanelli R, Valenti V, Rabbiosi D, Vitacca M, Nava S. A systematic review on tracheostomy decannulation: A proposal of a quantitative semiquantitative clinical score. *BMC Pulm Med*. 2014;15(14):201.
5. Singh RK, Saran S, Baronia AK. The practice of tracheostomy decannulation—a systematic review. *J Intens Care*. 2017;5(1):5:38. doi 10.1186/s40560-017-0234-z.
6. Morris LL, McIntosh E, Whitmer A. The importance of tracheostomy progression in the intensive care unit, *Crit Care Nurs*. 2014;34(1):40-50.
7. Scheinhorn DJ, Hassenpflug MS, Votto JJ, Chao DC, Epstein SK, Doig GS, et al. Ventilator Outcomes Study Group. Ventilator-dependent survivors of catastrophic illness transferred to 23 long-term care hospitals for weaning from prolonged mechanical ventilation. *Chest*. 2007;131(1):76-84.
8. O'Connor HH, Kirby KJ, Terrin N, Hill NS, White AC. Decannulation following tracheostomy for prolonged mechanical ventilation. *J Intens Care Med*. 2009;24(3):187-194.
9. Shrestha KK, Mohindra S, Mohindra S. How to decannulate trachestomised severe head trauma patients: A comparison of gradual vs. abrupt technique. *Nepal Med Coll J*. 2012;14(3):207-211.
10. Kang SW, Choi WA, Won YH, Lee JW, Lee HY, Kim DJ. Clinical implications of assisted peak cough flow measured with an external glottic control device for tracheostomy decannulation in patients with neuromuscular diseases and cervical spinal cord injuries: A pilot study. *Arch Phys Med Rehab*. 2016;97:1509-1514.
11. Wirtz N, Tibesar RJ, Lander T, Sidman J. A pediatric decannulation protocol: Outcomes of a 10-year experience. *Otolaryngol Head Neck Surg*. 2016;154(4):731-734.
12. Thomas S, Sauter W, Starrost U, Pohl M, Mehrholz J. Time to decannulation and associated risk factors in the postacute rehabilitation of critically ill patients with intensive care unit-acquired weakness: A cohort study. *Eur J Phys Rehab Med*. 2017;53(4):501-507.
13. Chadda K, Louis B, Benalissa L, Annane D, Gajdos P, Raphael JC, et al. Physiological effects of decannulation in tracheostomized patients. *Intens Care Med*. 2002;28(12):1761-1767.
14. Moscovici da Cruz V, Demarzo SE, Sobrinho JB, Amato MB, Kowalski LP, Deheinzelin D. Effects of tracheotomy on respiratory mechanics in spontaneously breathing patients. *Eur Respir J*. 2002;20:112-117.
15. Diehl JL, El Atrous S, Touchard D, Lemaire F, Brochard L. Changes in the work of breathing induced by tracheotomy in ventilator-dependent patients. *Am J Respir Crit Care Med*. 1999;159:383-388.
16. Rumbak MJ, Graves AE, Scott MP, Sporn GK, Walsh FW, Anderson WM, et al. Tracheostomy occlusion protocol predicts significant obstruction to air flow in patients requiring prolonged mechanical ventilation. *Crit Care Med*. 1997;25(3):413-417.
17. Pierson DJ. Tracheostomy and weaning. *Respir Care*. 2005;50(4):526-533.
18. MacIntyre NR, Cook DJ, Ely EW, Epstein SK, Fink JB, Heffner JE, et al. Evidence-based guidelines for weaning and discontinuing ventilatory support: A collective task force

facilitated by the American College of Chest Physicians; the American Association for Respiratory Care; and the American College of Critical Care Medicine. *Chest.* 2001;120(6, Suppl.):375S-395S.

19. Gao C, Zhou L, Wei C, Hoffman MR, Li C, Jiang JJ. The evaluation of physiologic decannulation readiness according to upper airway resistance measurement. *Otolaryngol Head Neck Surg.* 2008;139(4):535-540.
20. Kollef MH, Ahrens TS, William S. Clinical predictors and outcomes for patients requiring tracheostomy in the intensive care unit. *Crit Care Med.* 1999;27(9):1714-1720.
21. Cox CE, Carson SS, Holmes GM, Howard A, Carey TS. Increase in tracheostomy for prolonged mechanical ventilation in North Carolina, 1993-2002. *Crit Care Med.* 2004;32(11):2219-2226.
22. Frutos-Vivar F, Esteban A, Apeztequia C, Anzueto A, Nightengale P, Gonzalez M, et al. International Mechanical Ventilation Study Group. Outcome of mechanically ventilated patients who require tracheostomy. *Crit Care Med.* 2005;33(2):290-298.
23. Stelfox HT, Crimi S, Berra L, Noto A, Schmidt U, Bigatello LM, Hess D. Determinants of tracheostomy decannulation: An international survey. *Crit Care.* 2008;12(1):R26.
24. Herritt B, Chaudhuri D, Thavorn K, Kubelik D, Kyeremanteng K. Early vs. late tracheostomy in intensive care settings: Impact on ICU and hospital costs. *J Crit Care.* 2018;44:285-288.
25. Adly A, Youssef TA, El-Bergermy MM, Younis HM. Timing of tracheostomy in patients with prolonged endotracheal intubation: A systematic review. *Eur Arch Oto-Rhino-Laryngol.* 2018;275:679-690.
26. Villalba D, Feld V, Leiva V, Scrigna M, Destefano E, Pratto R, Rodriguez M, Collins J, Rocco A, Matesa A, Rossi D, Arcas L, Virgilio S, Golfarini N, Gil-Rosetti G, Diaz-Ballve P, Planells F. Effect of tracheostomy tube on work of breathing: Comparison of pre- and post-decannulation. *Int J Crit Illness Inj Sci.* 2016;6(3):98-102.
27. Dellweg D, Barchfeld T, Haidl P, Appelhans P, Kohler D. Tracheostomy decannulation: Implication on respiratory mechanics. *Head Neck.* 2007;*29*:1121-1127.
28. Leung R, Campbell D, MacGregor L, Berkowitz RG. Decannulation and survival following tracheostomy in an intensive care unit. *Ann Otol Rhinol Laryngol.* 2003;112,853-858.
29. O'Connor HH, White AC. Tracheostomy decannulation. *Respir Care.* 2010;55(8):1076-1081.
30. Martinez L, Demanet J, Mignaux V, Dewavrin F. Tracheostomy performed in ICU: Professional practice assessment and patient outcome. *Rev Mal Respir.* 2018;(1):25-35.
31. Kontzoglou G, Petropoulos I, Noussios G, Skouras A, Benis N, Karagiannidis K. Decannulation in children after long-term tracheostomy. *B-ENT.* 2006;*2*(1),13-15.
32. Gray RF, Todd NW, Jacobs IN. Tracheostomy decannulation in children: Approaches and techniques. *Laryngoscope.* 1998;108:8-12.
33. Zenk J, Fyrmpas G, Zimmerman T, Koch M, Constantinidis J, Iro H. Tracheostomy in young patients: Indications and long-term outcome. *Eur Arch Otorhinolaryngol.* 2008;266(5):705-711.
34. Waddell A, Appleford R, Dunning C, Papsin BC, Bailey CM. The Great Ormond Street protocol for ward decannulation of children with tracheostomy: Increasing safety and decreasing cost. *Int J Ped Otorhinolaryngol.* 1997;39(2):111-118.
35. Shapiro BA, Harrison RA, Kacmarek RM, Cane RD. *Clinical Application of Respiratory Care* (3rd ed.). Chicago: Yearbook Medical Publishers, 1985.

36. Adams AB, Lim S. Monitoring and management of the patient in the intensive care unit. In RL Wilkins, JK Stoller, CL Scanlan (Eds.). *Egan's Fundamentals of Respiratory Care,* 8th ed, St. Louis, MO: Mosby, 2003:1081-1119.
37. Douce FH. Pulmonary function testing. In R. L. Wilkins, J. K. Stoller, & C. L. Scanlan eds. *Egan's Fundamentals of Respiratory Care,* 8th ed., St. Louis, MO: Mosby, 2003:391-425.
38. Tippett DC. Swallowing, tracheostomy, and ventilator dependency. In D. C. Tippett (Ed.), *Tracheostomy and Ventilator Dependency: Management of Breathing, Speaking, and Swallowing.* New York: Thieme, 2000.
39. Sasegbon A, Hamdy S. The anatomy and physiology of normal and abnormal swallowing in oropharyngeal dysphagia. *Neurogastroenterol Motil.* 2017;29(11), doi: 10.1111/nmo.13100.
40. Cameron JL, Reynolds J, Zuidema GD. Aspiration in patients with tracheostomies. *Surgery, Gynecol Obstetrics.* 1973;136(1),68-70.
41. Ding R, Logemann JA. Swallow physiology in patients with trach cuff inflated or deflated: A retrospective study. *Head Neck.* 2005;27:809-813.
42. Amathieu R, Sauvat S, Reynaud P, Slavov V, Luis D, Dinca A, Tual L, Bloc S Dhonneur G. Influence of the cuff pressure on the swallowing reflex in tracheostomized intensive care unit patients. *Brit J Anaesth.* 2012;109(4):578-583.
43. Murray L, Langmore S, Ginsberg S, Dostie A. The significance of accumulated oropharyngeal secretions and swallowing frequency in predicting aspiration. *Dysphagia.* 1996;11:99-103.
44. McGowan SL, Gleason M, Smith M, Hirsch N, Shuldham CM. A pilot study of fiberoptic endoscopic evaluation of swallowing in patients with cuffed tracheostomies in neurological intensive care. *Neurocritical Care.* 2007;6(2):90-93.
45. Gross RD, Tedla M, Ross SB. Breathing-swallowing pattern in tracheostomy vs. controls. *Otolaryngol Head Neck Surg.* 2007;137(2S):P170.
46. Wright SE, Van Dahm K. Long-term care of the tracheostomy patient. *Clin Chest Med.* 2003 *24*:473-487.
47. Stelfox HT, Hess DR, Schmidt UH. A North American survey of respiratory therapist and physician tracheostomy decannulation practices. *Resp Care.* 2009;54(12):1658-1664.
48. Tawfik KO, Houlton JJ, Compton W, Ying J, Khosla SM. Tracheal reconstruction: A ten-year review of risk factors for decannulation failure. *Laryngoscope.* 2014;125:674-679.
49. Bandyopadhyay A, Cristea AI, Davis SD, Ackerman VL, Slaven JE, Jalou HE, Givan DC, Daftary A. Retrospective analysis of actors leading to pediatric tracheostomy decannulation failure: A single-institution experience. *Annals ATS.* 2016;14(4):70-75.
50. Choate K, Barbetti J, Currey J. Tracheostomy decannulation failure rate following critical illness: A prospective descriptive study. *Australian Crit Care.* 2008;22(1):8-15.
51. Barnes WM, Warner RC, Krassen J. Utilization of a tracheostomy weaning protocol in the acute rehabilitation hospital. *Respir Care.* 1999;44(10):1262.
52. Godwin JE, Heffner JE. Special critical care considerations in tracheostomy management. *Clin Chest Med.* 1991;12(3):573-583.
53. Pandian V, Miller CR, Schiavi AJ, Yarmus L, Contractor A, Haut ER, Feller-Kopman DJ, Mirski MA, Morad AH, Carey JP, Hillel AT, Maragos CS, Bhatti NI. Utilization of a standardized tracheostomy capping and decannulation protocol to improve patient safety. *Laryngoscope.* 2014;124:1794-1800.
54. Cohen O, Tzelnick S, Lahav Y, Stavi D, Shoffel-Havakuk H, Hain M, Halperin D, Aki N. Feasibility of a single-stage tracheostomy decannulation protocol with endoscopy in adult patients. *Laryngoscope.* 2015;126:2057-2062.

55. Duro C, Granja C, Castro S, Mestre S. Outcomes of critical patients with tracheostomy: Proposal of a decannuation protocol. *Intens Care Med Exp.* 2015;3(Suppl 1):1-2.
56. Liptzin DR, Connell EA, Marable J, Marks J, Thrasher J, Baker CD. Weaning nocturnal ventilation and decannulation in a pediatric ventilator care program. *Ped Pulmonol.* 2016;51(8):825-829.
57. Kubba H, Cooke J, Hartley B. Can we develop a protocol for the safe decannulation of tracheostomies in children less than 18 months old? *Int J Ped Otorhinolaryngol.* 2004;68(7):935-937.
58. St. John RE, Malen JF. Contemporary issues in adult tracheostomy management. *Crit Care Nurs Clin North Amer.* 2004;16(3):413-430.
59. Lewarski JS. Long-term care of the patient with a tracheostomy. *Respir Care.* 2005;50(4):534–537.
60. Heffner JE. Management of the chronically ventilated patient with a tracheostomy. *Chron Respir Disease.* 2005 2:151-161.
61. Hussey JD, Bishop MJ. Pressures required to move gas through the native airway in the presence of a fenestrated vs. a nonfenestrated tracheostomy tube. *Chest.* 1996;110(2):494-497.
62. Bach JR, Saporito LR. Criteria for extubation and tracheostomy tube removal for patients with ventilatory failure: A different approach to weaning. *Chest.* 1996; 110:1566-1571.
63. Tobin AE, Santamaria JD. An intensivist-led tracheostomy review team is associated with shorter decannulation time and length of stay: A prospective cohort study. *Critical Care.* 2008;12(2):R48.
64. Norwood MG, Spiers P, Bailiss J, Sayers RD. Evaluation of the role of a specialist tracheostomy service: From critical care to outreach and beyond. *Postgraduate Medicine Journal.* 2004;80(946):478-480.
65. Cameron TS, McKinstry A, Burt SK, Howard ME, Bellomo R, Brown DJ, et al. Outcomes of patients with spinal cord injury before and after introduction of an interdisciplinary tracheostomy team. *Critical Care Resuscitation.* 2009;11(1):14-19.
66. Parker V, Giles M, Shylan G, Austin N, Smith K, Morison J, Archer W Tracheostomy management in acute care facilities – a matter of teamwork. *J Clin Nurs.* 2010;19:1275-1283.
67. Pandian V, Miller CR, Mirski MA, Schiavi AJ, Morad AH, Vaswani RS, Kalmar L, Feller-Kopman DJ, Haut ER, Yarmus LB, Bhatti NI. Multidisciplinary team approach in the management of tracheostomy patients. *Otolarygol Head Neck Surg.* 2012;147(4):684-691.
68. deMestral C, Iqbal S, Fong N, LeBlanc J, Fata P, Razek T, Khwaja K. Impact of a specialized multidisciplinary tracheostomy team on tracheostomy care in critically ill patients. *Can J Surg.* 2011;54(3):167-172.
69. Morgan GE, Mikhail MS, Murray MJ. Respiratory physiology: The effects of anesthesia. In G. E. Morgan, Jr., M. S. Mikhail, & M. J. Murray (Eds.), *Clinical anesthesiology* (4th ed.), Retrieved from http://www.accessmedicine.com. 2003.
70. Johnson JT, Wagner RL, Sigler BA. Disposable inner cannula tracheostomy tube: A prospective clinical trial. *Otolaryngology—Head and Neck Surgery.* 1988;99(1):83-84.
71. Black RJ, Baldwin DL, Johns AN. Tracheostomy "decannulation panic" in children: Fact or fiction? *Journal of Laryngology and Otology.* 1984;98(3):297-304.
72. Eber E, Oberwaldner B. Tracheostomy care in the hospital. *Paediatric Respiratory Reviews.* 2006;*7:*175-184.
73. Sherlock ZV, Wilson JA, Exley C. Tracheostomy in the acute setting: Patient experiences and information needs. *Journal of Critical Care.* 2009;24:501-507.

74. Simon BM, Fowler SM, Handler SD. Communication development of young children with long-term tracheostomies. Preliminary report. *International Journal of Pediatric Otolaryngology.* 1983 6:37-50.
75. Kraemer R, Plante E, Green GE. Changes in speech and language development of a young child after decannulation. *Journal of Communication Disorders.* 2005;*38:*349-358.

12

Rehabilitation and Recovery

by John Parson, Lisa Wolfe, Linda L. Morris

Objectives

- Compare patient care between acute care versus a rehabilitation environment
- Provide guidelines for choice of bronchial hygiene therapy
- Outline tracheostomy evaluation in settings of stroke, traumatic brain injury, or airway obstruction
- Chart a management plan for tracheostomy patients in an office or clinic setting

Introduction

Patients who are discharged from the hospital with a tracheostomy have many needs. They need information in order to provide proper care for themselves. They need appropriate supplies. They need support and encouragement. They need confidence in their ability to manage themselves and knowledge of what to do in an emergency. And they often need someone to care for them when they are unable to do it for themselves. This chapter will discuss the issues that face patients and caregivers after discharge from the acute care hospital. The topics will reflect the complexity of issues encountered during rehabilitation. These challenges will be presented during phases of rehabilitation, office visits, and home care, and close with psychosocial concerns and quality of life.

Discharge Disposition of Patients with Tracheostomies

New data on early placement of tracheostomy tubes has been controversial. Early tracheostomy placements are associated with a higher number of tracheostomies placed but are also associated with a reduction in duration of mechanical ventilation, mortality rates, and length of stay in ICU. This paradox notwithstanding, studies have fueled a significant push for ICUs to have early tracheostomy as a standard of care.[1] There is little research that identifies the discharge disposition of tracheostomy patients when they leave the hospital; but, by necessity, this trend will drive a higher number of patients to require Long Term Acute Care (LTAC) and/or Acute Inpatient Rehabilitation (AIR) facilities. At these LTACs and AIRs, choices about tracheostomy care and advancement will be key to the plan of care, influencing many functions of the upper airway, including speech, swallow, cough, etc. There are limited options for patient disposition with a tracheostomy and a multitude of factors to consider when planning for discharge. The usual options are to discharge the patient to home (or to the home of a family member), an extended care facility, a rehabilitation facility, or a skilled nursing facility. Each of these destinations has its own set of requirements and limitations.

Qualifying for Admission to Acute Inpatient Rehabilitation

In order to qualify for an AIR stay, the patient must be able to participate in therapy for at least three hours per day. Patients who are unable to tolerate such a rigorous program can qualify for sub-acute rehabilitation. The purpose of a rehabilitation program is for the patient to participate in therapy and, thus, improve his or her function and activities of daily living. Rehabilitation includes physical therapy, speech therapy, and occupational therapy. These therapies focus on improved nutrition, mobility, and self-care, and therefore support a return to safe independent community-based living. Patients who are unable to gain these skills will likely need to be cared for in a skilled nursing facility rather than at home. The following section will highlight the considerations for a patient with a tracheostomy who is discharged to a rehabilitation facility, and eventually, plan for community-based living.

Tracheostomy in Acute Rehabilitation

Patients with tracheostomy tubes admitted for AIR should be approached with the same systematic and ongoing evaluation as ideally should occur prior to getting there. It should not be assumed that the presence of a tracheostomy at admission is a sign that the tube's continued presence is still warranted. With length of hospital stay being continually challenged, various issues, including the need for a tracheostomy tube, may simply be deferred to the next level of care.

A multitude of injuries and illnesses can result in the placement of a tracheostomy tube. A large percentage of patients admitted for AIR can have their tracheostomy tubes safely progressed and ultimately removed. Regardless of the illness or injury, the same systematic approach to progression and removal should be taken. Generally, all tracheostomy tubes are placed for one or more of the following four indications.[2]

- The need for positive pressure mechanical ventilation
- The need for tracheal suctioning
- The need to relieve upper airway obstruction
- The need for airway protection

The clinician or tracheostomy team should regularly revisit these indications and carefully assess whether they still exist. Clinicians often focus on one indication and fail to consider the others. This bias may be driven by one's area of specialty and familiarity (speech language pathologist, respiratory care practitioner, otolaryngologist, etc.). Common examples might include focusing on the swallowing mechanism (airway protection) but failing to consider airway obstruction. Another example might be focusing on an airway obstruction but failing to consider bronchial hygiene needs. A multidisciplinary approach can help to cover all issues. Additionally, new issues may have evolved since the original reason for the placement of the tracheostomy tube; most notable may be the presence of new airway lesions if the tracheostomy tube has been in place for some time.

In the acute rehabilitation setting, the patient is likely to be more mobile and encounter more health care professionals who may be less familiar with artificial airways. This new environment is likely to present more challenges and potential for problems without the proper precautions.

Clinical Scenario

Patient A John C. is a 23-year-old male admitted to the acute rehabilitation hospital. He had sustained a fracture of the 5th and 6th cervical vertebrae secondary to a diving accident three weeks prior to admission. He required mechanical ventilator support post injury, and at the time of admission to the rehabilitation hospital, he had failed several attempts to discontinue mechanical ventilation support. Neurologically, he was diagnosed as a C6 'incomplete' spinal cord injury.

Progressing the Airway: Taking the First Step

Progressing or removing the artificial airway need not always be a prolonged multi-step process, provided the clinician or tracheostomy team has adequately addressed all issues. Patients should not be subjected to the discomfort and cost of having multiple devices placed if proper evaluation reveals no remaining need for the tracheostomy. The tube might simply be removed, and the stoma allowed to close. The prolonged delay of decannulation with no clear indication remaining can lead to the well-documented sequelae associated with tracheostomy tubes. This could include stenosis, granulation, tracheomalacia, or fistulas.[3] By contrast, certain patients will require a careful, multi-step process to safely advance their airways. It is important for the clinician to know how to individualize plans so the process of advancement can be completed in a timely manner, combining steps when appropriate.

Other patients, however, will require a few or more steps, using varied devices before decannulation can be achieved. It is important for the care team to know the difference.

Clinical Scenario Cont'd.

It was believed by the referring institution that John would need an artificial airway for a prolonged time for mechanical ventilator support and bronchial hygiene needs. Subsequently, before transfer to the acute rehabilitation hospital, his #8 oral endotracheal tube was replaced with a surgically placed #8 Shiley LPC tracheostomy tube.

Choosing the Optimal Tracheostomy Tube

In addition to evaluating the need for an artificial airway, it is important to evaluate the patient for the proper artificial airway. Commonly, patients admitted to the acute rehabilitation setting will have in place whatever device is typically used at the referring acute care hospital, where a standard dual cannula cuffed tracheostomy tube is typical. In an acute care setting, with an immature tracheostomy in place, a tube with an inner cannula can be useful as the tract is not mature enough for the tube to be easily removed or replaced.

This one-size-fits-all approach may suffice for short-term airway management, but it is rarely optimal for someone who is going to need an airway for a longer time.[4,5] A poorly fitting device can lead to a variety of potentially serious problems.[6] In the past several years, the choices available from various manufacturers have become abundant. A multitude of designs and sizes address most patient needs, with only a rare need for customization. Customized tubes can be created with nearly any combination of diameter, length, flange, and cuff style. Custom products, of course, are considerably more costly than standard products, often require laryngoscopy to determine proper size and type, and require additional time to obtain.

Clinical Scenario Cont'd.

On arrival to the rehabilitation hospital, John was alert, oriented, and medically stable, but nonverbal, secondary to an inflated tracheostomy tube cuff. He was receiving Assist Control/Volume Control (AC/VC) ventilation at a rate of 10 breaths/min, tidal volume of 700 ml, and PEEP of 5 cm H_20. No supplemental oxygen was required. Arterial blood gases were acceptable, and the patient had no complaints related to breathing. The patient was easily triggering the mechanical breaths, with a total rate of 12-14 breaths/min. A baseline vital capacity was recorded at 800 ml.

Evaluating the Need for Airway Protection

Protecting the airway is, of course, the concept of attempting to prevent foreign matter from entering the trachea and lungs by sealing off the airway with an inflated cuff (i.e., protection from aspiration). The potential consequences of aspiration are deleterious and well-established. The concept of sealing off the trachea with an inflated cuff to protect the airway is most important during acute care ventilation, when the lung has poor compliance and higher levels of sedation are needed. Controversy exists over when, and for how long, this process should be applied. It is also well-established that attempting to seal off the trachea with a cuffed tracheostomy tube is not a definitive solution to the problem of aspiration.[7] In patients who are eating ad lib, the balloon may actually induce aspiration by compressing the esophagus.[8] In the critical care setting, the serious risks and consequences of aspiration appropriately take priority, and cuff inflation for airway protection remains standard.

Tracheostomy tube cuffs have long been associated with problems.[9,10,11] It is reasonable, therefore, to evaluate the need for a tracheostomy tube with a cuff as a first step when considering progressing the airway in order to minimize potential sequelae.

While cuff inflation for airway protection remains standard in the critical care environment, when the patient has progressed to the acute rehabilitation setting and beyond, other priorities may prevail. Patient disorders that might warrant protection with an inflated cuff include dysphagia as a result of stroke, traumatic brain injury, or other varied pathologies. Cuff inflation may be needed to allow for stable nocturnal ventilation. In addition, a partially inflated cuff may help to reduce alarms in those that are ventilator-dependent. The cuff may be helpful long-term during sleep to reduce episodes of hypoventilation and reduce arousals due to air going through the vocal cords.

When deciding to keep a tracheostomy tube in place for airway protection, the care team must carefully consider the pros and cons. Disadvantages include difficulty or inability to phonate, the potential sequela of a long-term inflated cuff, and the difficulty of maintaining a properly inflated cuff at home or in the extended care setting. The presence of a tracheostomy tube may also limit the discharge destination, as some extended care facilities may not be able to accommodate patients with tracheostomies. Even a return to home may not be an option if there are no caregivers who are willing to be trained on the use and care of the tracheostomy tube.

Evaluating the Need for Suctioning

Clinical Scenario Cont'd.

On day two of admission, the speech language pathologist determined that John was at minimal risk for aspiration and was placed on a regular diet. Plans were made to address phonation as the patient was eager to speak and fully participate in therapy.

Evaluating the need for an artificial airway to facilitate suctioning is primarily a matter of evaluating the effectiveness of the patient's cough. A few simple bedside tests can help with this assessment of an effective cough. Vital capacity (VC) and peak cough expiratory flow rate (PCEF) are the most common. One must fully understand the four factors of an effective cough, as well as what these tests measure to make an informed decision. Shapiro and others,[2] for example, established that patients with spinal cord injuries who had vital capacities equal to or greater than 15ml/kg of ideal body weight should be able to maintain adequate bronchial hygiene without a tracheostomy tube. Bach[12] and Mellies[13] have noted that PCEFs of at least 160 liters/minute appear to be necessary for effective elimination of airway secretions. The clinician must carefully consider, however, that these reduced measurements may only be adequate in conjunction with devices such as the mechanical insufflator-exsufflator (MIE) (**Figures 12.1, 12.2**) or with manual secretion mobilization techniques such as diaphragmatic cough assist or manual inflation hold (**Figure 12.3A-B**).

Figure 12.1 Philips Respironics Cough Assist CA 3000 (shown with circuit)

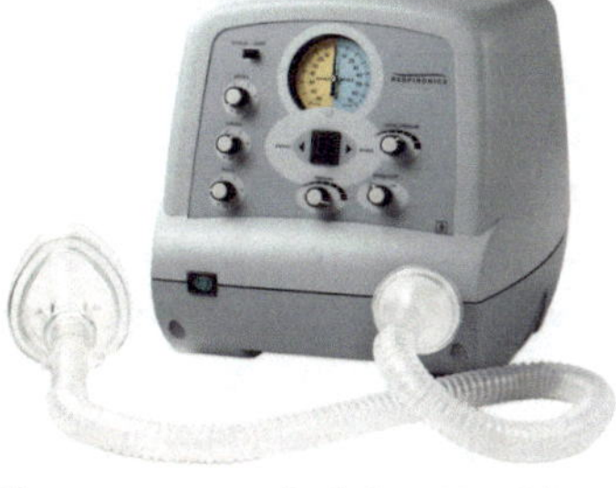

Photo courtesy of Philips Healthcare.

Figure 12.2 Philips Respironics Cough Assist T70 (shown without circuit)

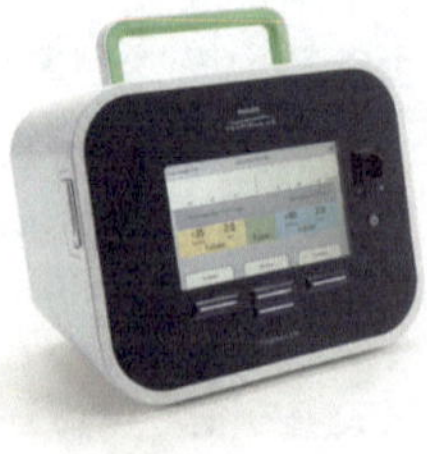

Photo courtesy of Philips Healthcare.

Figure 12.3 Manual ventilation with inflation hold

A) Large breath, inflation hold

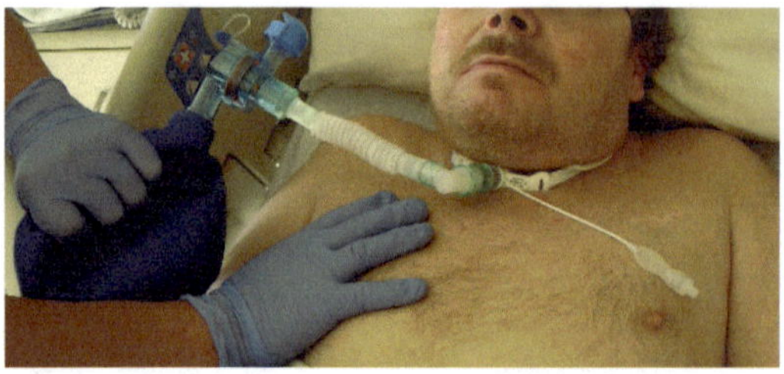

Secretion mobilization using manual ventilation with inflation hold and chest physical therapy techniques. The clinician gives a large manual breath, followed by a short pause (inflation hold), while positioning his or her hand over the patient's chest.

B) Releases grip, exhale, and vibration

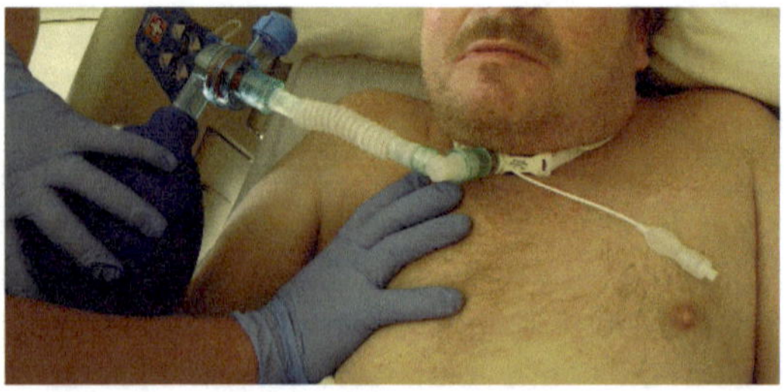

The clinician simultaneously releases his or her grip on the manual resuscitator to allow for exhalation, while vibrating the chest wall to mobilize secretions.

Manual ventilation with inflation-hold requires a cuffed tracheostomy tube for best results. A tracheostomy tube with a low-volume, high-pressure cuff is ideal for patients with chronic but intermittent need for this maneuver. The tube is generally well tolerated for capping purposes, and it has a cuff that may be used for this maneuver or with a mechanical insufflator-exsufflator.

A close look at VC and PCEF provide objective measurements to assess cough. For instance, a measurement of VC looks only at the first step in a cough; that is, the ability to take a large breath. It tells us nothing about the ability to use that breath to forcefully expel air and mobilize secretions. This forceful expelling of air is ultimately what is important, and thus, PCEF is an important supplemental measurement. This measurement reflects the effectiveness of a normal cough. One can easily imagine a patient with an adequate VC, but perhaps a mild upper airway obstruction causing a diminished PCEF; and, thus, a poor cough. Similarly, a patient may have an adequate VC, but poor ability to compress the inspired air due to weak expiratory muscles, or poor glottic closure.

Once more, the result might be a poor cough and inability to maintain adequate bronchial hygiene in spite of an apparently adequate VC.

Importantly, if a patient is to be ultimately discharged to home or to an extended care facility, the resources and skill of the caregivers at that destination must be carefully assessed. A patient whose bronchial hygiene needs are easily managed without a tracheostomy tube in a health care setting might not fare well in the home care setting with less skilled help. All decisions made in the acute rehabilitation setting must be made with the discharge destination and available resources in mind.

Considerable thought should also be given to the predicted course of a patient's condition. For example, a patient with a spinal cord injury and stable ventilatory reserves would be viewed differently from a patient with a progressive neuromuscular disease, where a steady decline might be expected. If there is any doubt about a patient's long-term need for a tracheostomy tube to manage secretions, the stoma can be maintained with a tracheal cannula. Of note, the Olympic stoma button is no longer manufactured. One type of tracheal cannula, a Montgomery cannula, could be placed in the stoma to maintain its patency, and allow for future replacement of a tracheostomy tube, if needed, without requiring a surgical intervention. Tracheostomy cannulas typically require cautious fitting by experienced clinicians. Careful measurement of stoma length and diameter are essential (see Chapter 4 for proper fitting of a tracheal cannula). Proper fitting can prevent closure of the posterior portion of the stoma and airway obstruction resulting from a cannula that protrudes into the tracheal lumen.

Several benefits result from placement of a capped tracheal cannula. Attempting to assess the effectiveness of a patient's cough while a capped tracheostomy tube occupies a large part of the tracheal lumen might be an unfair trial. Secretions often get caught on the tracheostomy tube and cannot be mobilized into the oropharynx. A properly fitted tracheal cannula, however, will eliminate this problem.

If a tracheal cannula cannot be fitted properly, it may be best to maintain a stoma with a cuffless tracheostomy tube of the smallest reasonable outer diameter, thus minimizing obstruction to the mobilization of secretions. If the patient needs frequent suctioning, the inner diameter of the tube must be of adequate size to accommodate an appropriately sized suction catheter.

Bronchial Hygiene Therapy

The indication for an artificial airway usually stated as 'the need for suctioning,' might better be described as the need for bronchial hygiene therapy. Bronchial hygiene therapy encompasses a wide variety of techniques, devices, and pharmacologic agents. The American Association for Respiratory Care (AARC) provides clinical practice guidelines on the effectiveness of both pharmacologic[14] and non-pharmacologic[15] airway clearance therapies in hospitalized patients. It is beyond the scope of this chapter to explore the many options, but a short overview is warranted.

As discussed earlier, the utility of a tracheostomy tube with a cuff can allow the caregiver to deliver a large breath to the patient unable to do so on his or her own. A large breath is the first step of an effective cough, which can be facilitated by using a manual ventilator or MIE. Along with physical therapy techniques such as cough assist, mobilization of secretions is improved. Bach, Saporito, Shah, and Sinquee[16] have reported success in maintaining bronchial hygiene needs using the MIE in patients with severe respiratory muscle insufficiency, which led to subsequent decannulation. Other recent literature, however, has questioned the validity of use of MIE devices in the neuromuscular patient.[17] Our experience, however, has suggested its usefulness in certain patients.

A multitude of devices on the market can be used with tracheostomy patients just as they can in those with an intact airway. Minor adaptations may be needed to integrate these devices with the tracheostomy tube. In addition to the MIE, some of the more commonly used therapies include those summarized in **Table 12.1**.

Table 12.1: Bronchial Hygiene Therapy Techniques

Technique	Use
Mechanical Insufflator/Exsufflator (MIE) **Figures 12.1, 12.2**	Provides positive pressure into the respiratory system during insufflation phase to slowly inflate the lungs. Then, there is an abrupt change to negative pressure, resulting in rapid exhalation, followed by coughing.
Intrapulmonary Percussive Ventilation (IPV)	Intrapulmonary percussive ventilation creates a positive trans-respiratory pressure by injecting short, rapid inspiratory flow pulses into the airway opening, relying on chest wall elastic recoil for passive exhalation.[18]
High-frequency Chest Wall Oscillation	An inflatable vest is used to apply high-frequency, small-volume expiratory pulses to the external chest wall. Negative trans-respiratory pressure is generated by the short, rapid expiratory flow pulses at 2–25 Hz, to loosen, collect, and mobilize airway secretions.[19]
Positive Expiratory Pressure (PEP)	The PEP device consists of a user interface (face mask or mouthpiece) and a one-way valve attached to an expiratory resistor. A manometer may be used to monitor pressures during the maneuver. Tidal breathing, with a slightly active expiration through the expiratory resistor will produce expiratory pressures of 10–20 cm H_2O at mid-expiration to stent airways open or increase intrathoracic pressure distal to retained secretions by increasing functional residual capacity or collateral ventilation.[20]
Meta-Neb **(Figure 12.4)**	Device that combines therapies for lung expansion, secretion clearance, and medication delivery by using CPAP (continuous positive airway pressure), CHFO (continuous high frequency oscillation), and aerosol.

Figure 12.4: Hill-Rom MetaNeb

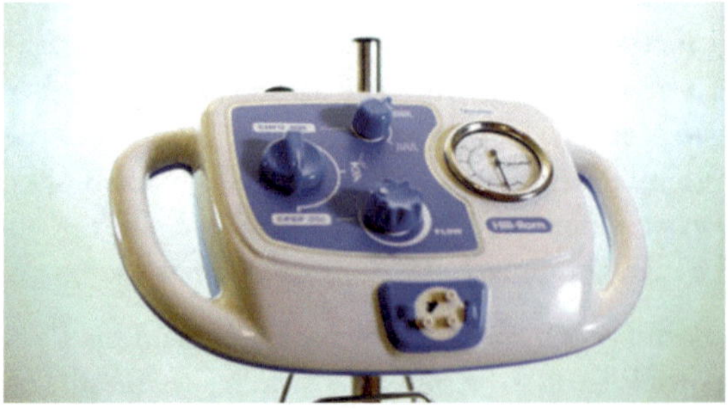

Strong evidence to choose one therapy over another appears to be scant,[21] but numerous resources, as well as experience, can help guide the clinician and patient.[15,18,22,23]

The decision to remove a tracheostomy tube that has been in place for bronchial hygiene needs can be guided by some objective measurements as discussed earlier, but also requires some subjective judgement. Before the tube is removed, one should always review how the patient will fare at the next level of care, whether that is an extended care facility or the home setting. It is also important to assess, at that next level of care, what resources are available, such as personnel or medical devices.

Tracheostomy Tubes and Effective Bronchial Hygiene Therapy

While all tracheostomy tubes may be used for suctioning, not all sizes and styles are optimal for this purpose. The proper choice of tube is essential for maintaining optimal bronchial hygiene therapy, and deciding between a cuffed or a cuffless tracheostomy tube is one important factor. Patients with marginal pulmonary reserves may need a cuff to augment various secretion mobilization devices and techniques such as the MIE and manual ventilation with inflation hold. One must be able to take a large enough breath, or have one manually delivered to the lungs, in order to expel secretions deep in the lungs. The patient who can be capped most of the time, but who requires periodic use of these devices or techniques, is often best served with a tight-to-shaft (TTS) type cuff (**Figure 3.32**). Because these tubes have low profile cuffs, they do not create the resistance of traditional low-pressure cuffs, which may be a good option to facilitate spontaneous breathing around the tube when capped, and mobilize secretions into the upper airway. Thus, the TTS cuffs are very well tolerated for capping, provided the proper size and diameter tube is used. **Figure 12.5** shows the inflation and deflation characteristics of low-pressure, high-volume tubes compared with high-pressure, low-volume tubes.

Figure 12.5 Inflation & Deflation Characteristics

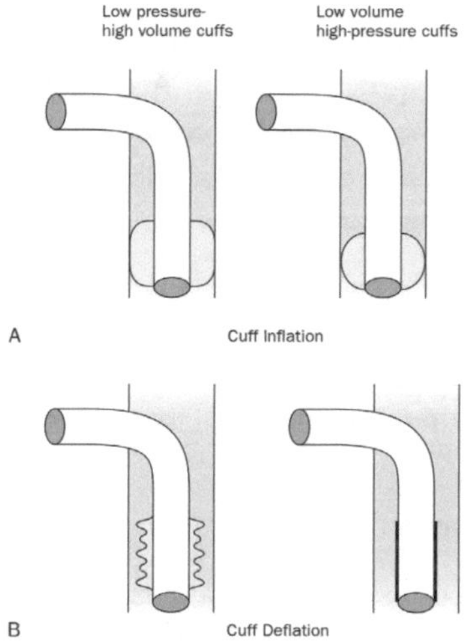

Inflation and deflation characteristics of high-volume, low-pressure cuffs compared to low-volume, high-pressure cuffs.

(A) During cuff inflation, high-volume, low-pressure cuffs distribute pressure over larger surface area. With low-volume, high-pressure cuffs, pressure is concentrated into a very small surface area.

(B) During cuff deflation, the folds of the deflated high-volume, low-pressure cuff occupy a large surface area and create resistance to airflow around the outside of the tracheostomy tube. In contrast, the deflated low-volume, high-pressure cuff lies snugly along the shaft of the tube, creating no resistance to airflow around the outside of the tube.

Strong Cough but Poor Cough Reflex

While it is essential to evaluate the mechanical strength of a cough, it is also important to assess the adequacy of the cough reflex. The neurologically impaired patient (as a result of stroke or traumatic brain injury) may have a strong cough when initiated, but the cough reflex may be delayed or diminished. The clinical picture of rhonchi and congestion must be carefully evaluated when considering removal of the tracheostomy tube. Careful assessment over the course of inpatient rehabilitation can better predict the prolonged need for an airway.

Tracheostomy Tubes and Bronchorrhea

While the need to suction secretions is an indication for having a tracheostomy tube, its presence paradoxically may contribute to secretion problems. The presence of a foreign body (tracheostomy tube), along with the repeated introduction of suction catheters into the airway, may be the cause of irritation and secretion production. Additionally, devices such as heated aerosol tracheostomy collars that add particulate water to the airway may further stimulate excessive secretion production. Tracheostomy tubes develop bacterial biofilms that can precipitate and maintain infection in the airway.[25] Therefore, the tracheostomy tube may be a contribution to, rather than a treatment for, the secretion problem. It is our experience that apparent secretion problems often subside or cease once the tracheostomy tube is progressed and patients are allowed to breathe in a more natural fashion and can cough up secretions rather than be suctioned. This can be especially notable in patients with asthma.

Providing Phonation for Patients Who Require Positive-Pressure Ventilation

The predominance of community-dwelling people who require long-term continuous mechanical ventilation are most commonly treated with a tracheostomy. Those who require nocturnal only ventilator support are often treated with non-invasive ventilation; however, some will be treated with a tracheostomy.[25] The pattern of ventilator support (e.g., continuous versus nocturnal only) influences the choice of tracheostomy tube. Extensive literature exists on assessing patient readiness for weaning and will not be the focus of this discussion.

For the patient who needs continuous mechanical ventilation, choosing the proper tracheostomy tube can greatly influence the success of achieving adequate phonation. Acute medical disorders (e.g., pneumonia, or hemodynamic instability) should be resolved before attempting to achieve phonation. Speech during mechanical ventilation requires adequate cardiopulmonary reserve, so the patient should be hemodynamically stable before attempting phonation.

Traditional mechanical ventilation with an inflated cuff can deliver precise volume ventilation but does not allow for speech since exhaled airflow is diverted away from the vocal cords and through the expiratory limb of the ventilator. The ensuing discussion will assist in choosing the best tracheostomy tube, ventilator adjustments, and strategies to maximize the potential for speech.

Leak Speech with a Deflated Tracheostomy Tube Cuff

It is imperative that clinicians who attempt to facilitate speech by deflating the cuff and manipulating mechanical ventilator settings have a full understanding of the specific ventilator and tracheostomy tube in use. For the patient requiring long-term invasive positive-pressure ventilation, leak speech with a deflated or partially deflated cuff is often the quickest and safest way to achieve phonation. Tube size becomes an important factor when attempting phonation. The tube's outer diameter must allow enough airflow between the tube and the tracheal wall for air to reach the vocal cords and achieve phonation. A tube that is too small, however, may allow too much airflow past the tracheostomy tube and fail to provide adequate ventilation when the cuff is deflated. Furthermore, a small tube may also create undesirably high peak pressures on the ventilator and impede adequate suctioning. Achieving phonation in the chronically ventilated patient through leak speech usually requires a fine balance between achieving adequate phonation and adequate ventilation. One may have to accept a range of clinically acceptable blood gas values since mechanically delivered minute volume may vary. The tracheostomy tube cuff volume usually can be adjusted to achieve this balance if full cuff deflation cannot be tolerated.

In addition to choosing the optimal tube size, cuff inflation volume, and mechanical ventilator settings, it is essential to coach the patient on how their speaking and breathing will be altered when the cuff is deflated. A patient's understanding of the central role of glottic control in balancing breathing and speech is necessary. This can present a challenge to patients, who are likely unfamiliar with upper airway anatomy and may be overwhelmed by their new dependence on a mechanical ventilator. The patient's vocal cords can augment full delivery of the tidal volume when voluntarily adducted, but over time, this may prove tiring for the patient. In the fully adducted position, the vocal cords will be doing what the deflated tracheostomy cuff is no longer doing. Teaching glottic control to variably direct air to the lungs or through the vocal cords for phonation may prove a challenge. Often, patients in the early stages of this process allow too much air to escape through the upper airway, which may lead to shortness of breath, feelings of upper airway dryness, and hypercapnia. The patient's realization that vocal cord adduction can direct more air into the lungs often gives a much-needed feeling of control and lessens the fear of air hunger. Coordination between the speech language pathologist and the respiratory care practitioner is essential in this endeavor.

Careful adjustment of ventilator settings must accompany the leak speech approach. Phonation is limited by the airflow during the inspiratory phase of the ventilator. Speaking during inspiration is, of course, opposite of normal, and, thus, requires learning a new speech mechanism. The key components that ensure adequate and minimally interrupted phonation are experimenting with ventilator rates, longer inspiratory times, and larger delivered tidal volumes. PEEP at varying settings has also been reported to improve speech during mechanical ventilation with cuff deflation.[26] It is important that the clinician not rely too much on a patient's glottic control for delivery of adequate volume. The size of the tracheostomy tube and the degree of cuff inflation, along with the ventilator settings, should be such that acceptable ventilation is achieved regardless of a patient's glottic manipulation. As suggested earlier, the clinician should accept some variation in returned tidal volumes and pCO_2 values with cuff-down ventilation and make adjustments directed by patient comfort within a range of acceptable values.

Mechanical Ventilator Adjustment to Balance Speaking and Breathing

CLINICAL SCENARIO CONT'D.

The speech language pathologist and respiratory care practitioner coordinate their schedules to co-treat the patient. Initially, speech was attempted using simple cuff deflation after clearing the oropharynx of secretions. The patient was coached to speak on the inspiratory phase of the ventilator with minimal success. It was difficult for John to coordinate speaking with the delivery of a positive pressure breath. The patient was instructed to look for visual clues such as chest beginning to rise, as well as sensing the beginning of air flow through the upper airway. Ventilator tidal volume was increased to 900 ml and inspiratory time was increased from one second to two seconds. Some modest improvement in speech was noted with increased number of words per breath and speech volume. Vital signs and arterial blood gases remained stable.

When attempting phonation with simple cuff deflation, phonation is only possible during the inspiratory phase of the ventilator. An examination of different ventilator settings will illustrate how the ability to phonate can vary widely with ventilator settings. For example, a mechanical ventilator set to deliver eight breaths per minute, with an inspiratory time of one second, will only allow for a maximum of eight seconds of potential speaking time per minute, which is typically unsatisfactory. However, if the ventilator is set to deliver 12 breaths per minute, with an inspiratory time of two seconds, the potential time for phonation would increase to 24 seconds, tripling the time available for speech. It is important, however, not to let the desire for adequate speech conflict with other goals and consequences of mechanical ventilation. The long-appreciated effect of mechanical ventilation on venous return and blood pressure, as well as concerns around ventilator induced lung injury (VILI), must be monitored. Higher ventilator rates, which might be preferable for speech, require smaller tidal volumes to maintain a desired pCO_2 level. However, smaller tidal volumes interfere with the prevention of atelectasis. Some authors have advocated the use of the pressure-control ventilation mode to automatically guarantee delivered volumes with leak speech.[27] If small tidal volumes are needed and atelectasis occurs, the addition of aggressive airway clearance is helpful, using the MIE.

Newer ventilators designed for long-term home use have variable options, and intimate knowledge of the particular device being used is important. Some devices have an option to turn off leak compensators, while others do not. Leak compensation may significantly drive up flow and cause CO_2 to plummet. At the extreme, when a fenestration or speaking valve is in place, the drop in CO_2 can be severe. Given these risks, changes should be made in a monitored setting to assure acid-base balance. The resultant metabolic alkalosis can be life-threatening, causing arrhythmia or seizure. The high flow can cause intolerance that limits generation of leak speech. Since leak speak is only a factor in volume-cycled ventilation, switching to pressure-control mode may be helpful.

Leak Speech with Deflated Tracheostomy Tube Cuff and One-Way Valve

Leak speech with the addition of a speaking valve may allow for a more satisfactory speech pattern. This technique essentially prevents the patient's exhaled gas from following the normal pathway through the expiratory limb of the ventilator circuit. Thus, all exhaled gas flow must exit through the patient's upper airway. Optimally, the patient is taught to close his or her glottis during the inspiratory phase of the ventilator, receive the full ventilator breath, and then exhale and speak during the expiratory cycle. Hence, a more normal pattern of speech is approximated. Keeping inspiratory pressure and flow rate modest will help the patient achieve breath-holding during inspiration. In contrast to leak speech without a one-way valve, this method employs shorter inspiratory times and longer expiratory times, since speech occurs primarily during exhalation, and all exhaled gas must be expelled before the next breath is delivered. Ventilator settings (e.g., mode, rate, inspiratory pressure, and flow rate) should be optimized by a methodical trial-and-error approach.

Precautions

Patients unfamiliar with this method initially require instruction, encouragement, and careful monitoring. To assure that neither hypo- nor hyperventilation is occurring, monitoring should include measurement of CO_2 in lieu of exhaled tidal volumes, because exhaled tidal volumes will not be accurate.

- It is vital that the tracheostomy tube cuff never be re-inflated while using the one-way valve, as the patient will not be able to exhale. Ideally, cuffless tubes should be used with speaking valves.
- It is important to select proper tube size and type as well as exclude the presence of any upper airway lesions that may obstruct airflow. This requires the clinician to carefully assess if exhaled gas can flow through the upper airway before the next breath is delivered. Failure to allow complete exhalation may lead to air trapping, with risk of increased intrathoracic pressures, decreased venous return, hypotension, and even pneumothorax.
- Humidification can become problematic with prolonged use of this technique, since an HME attached distally to the one-way valve renders it ineffective.
- A patient with a high secretion burden is not appropriate for the use of a one-way valve because the valve limits the ability to suction, and secretions may occlude the valve, preventing ventilation.

It is a good idea to assess the risks and benefits of the two options (leak speech with and without a valve), and then choose one method. Switching from cuff deflation alone to cuff deflation with a one-way valve can be confusing to the patient and caregiver alike.

Clinical Scenario Cont'd.

On day two of speaking trials with John C., the speech language pathologist requested a trial of leak speech using the Passy Muir speaking valve in an attempt to improve overall speech. He was informed of the different sensation that is experienced with the one-way valve. The patient is instructed to 'hold' the delivered breath and phonate on the expiratory cycle of the ventilator. The same cuff-down settings were used from the previous day, with the inspiratory time decreased to one second, thus allowing more time for exhalation, when the most phonation would occur.

Other Options for Speaking While on a Mechanical Ventilator

Two primary types of tracheostomy tubes address the potential problems encountered when speech is attempted with deflated cuff mechanical ventilation.

Speaking Tracheostomy Tubes

Speaking tracheostomy tubes have long been available but do not appear to have gained widespread acceptance. The design of these tubes is essentially the same as tubes with a subglottic suction port. A feature of these tubes includes a line that can be attached to an external flow of gas. When a thumb port in this line is occluded, the air is diverted above the cuff and through the vocal cords to facilitate speech. One limitation of this design is the possibility of misdirection of airflow if the opening above the cuff is improperly aligned within the tracheal lumen. Without proper alignment, air often exits through the tracheal stoma. Additionally, this small line is prone to clogging with secretions, rendering it useless. The need for an external gas source also creates limitations for the mobile, ventilator-dependent patient. The external gas supply typically comes from portable air or oxygen cylinders or a small air compressor. Patients who are not hypoxemic will not qualify for oxygen in the home environment. Patients who cannot use their hands to occlude the thumb port are dependent on a caregiver for speech. If continuous cuff inflation of the tracheostomy tube is required, however, this tube design may be considered if phonation will be attempted.

Blom Tracheostomy Tube System

The Blom Tracheostomy Tube system offers a different approach to providing speech in the ventilator-dependent patient who requires an inflated cuff. In addition to a fenestrated outer cannula, this tube has a unique inner cannula that allows delivery of the exhaled tidal volume through the vocal cords. This design omits the need for an external gas source. The potential benefit of this system is guaranteed volume delivery, which could not otherwise be achieved with a deflated cuff. The mechanics of the device must be fully appreciated by those using it, and chapter 6 provides more discussion on its use. The redirection of exhaled tidal volume can cause havoc with modern, sophisticated mechanical ventilators and their monitoring systems. An exhaled volume reservoir included in the Blom system attempts to address some of these problems. A detailed understanding of this system, as well as the alarms of the chosen mechanical ventilator, must be clearly identified if this device is to be used successfully.

Characteristics of Tracheostomy Tubes

Size

The size of the tracheostomy tube will have an impact on airflow resistance and cuff-related complications. A small inner diameter may cause excessively high ventilating pressures and increased resistance to spontaneous breathing. A high-volume, low-pressure cuff, if mismatched to the tracheal diameter, may act as a high-pressure cuff.[11]

Ease of Changing

In the patient who is completely dependent on ventilator support, such as the patient with a high-level spinal cord injury, it is critical that the tube be easily reinserted should it become dislodged. A tube with a high-volume, low-pressure cuff can occasionally be difficult to reinsert because, even when deflated, the cuff takes up considerable space, and may not easily pass through a stoma that has closed tightly around the outer cannula. The new Shiley Flexible tracheostomy tube with Taperguard Cuff (**Figure 3.7**) has a thinner, less bulky cuff, which, according to company internal testing, requires 39% less insertion force. The lower insertion force may prove advantageous in difficult tube changes. In contrast to the high-volume, low-pressure cuffs, a low-volume, high-pressure cuff, can typically be inserted with little to no difficulty or trauma. The Bivona TTS tubes, whose cuffs take up virtually no space when deflated, were not designed for continuous cuff inflation. Complications from long-term or improper use of these cuffs have been described previously.

Dual-Versus Single-Cannula

Frequently, the first tracheostomy tube that is placed will have an inner cannula because of the expected volume of secretions. However, the desirable features of some single-cannula tubes may outweigh the advantage of a tube with an inner cannula. One advantage is the increased inner diameter of a single-lumen tube relative to the outer-diameter. Another advantage is the flexibility of many single-cannula tubes that can accommodate variations in anatomy.

With a single-cannula tube, attention should be given to proper humidification and a prescribed tube-change schedule to avoid obstruction and a narrowing of the tube's inner diameter. By comparison, an obstruction of a dual-cannula tube can be easily remedied by changing or cleaning the inner cannula. However, a clogged single-lumen tube may only be remedied by changing the entire device.

CLINICAL SCENARIO CONT'D.

It was suspected that the #8 Shiley LPC tracheostomy tube was too large to allow for complete exhalation between positive pressure breaths when the one-way valve was in place. Without the one-way valve, air-trapping was not a problem since exhaled gas passed through the exhalation valve. However, it appeared that inadequate space around the deflated cuff did not allow enough air flow for acceptable quality speech in the patient. The tracheostomy tube was subsequently downsized to a #6 Shiley LPC.

EVALUATING THE NEED FOR RELIEF OF UPPER AIRWAY OBSTRUCTION

When the clinician decides to progress the tracheostomy tube and allow the patient to breathe through the native airway, it is essential to assess any potential upper airway obstruction. This is especially important in patients who have had artificial airways for a prolonged period, since subtle airway lesions may have developed over time.

At minimum, a simple bedside evaluation should be performed to assess patency of the upper airway; however, a fiberoptic exam may be of value before decannulation.[28] Fully informing patients of these evaluation options is essential to minimize anxiety and fear. Coughing and minor discomfort as well as a sensation of difficulty breathing may be encountered.

The initial step should be clearing secretions above and below the cuff. In a patient with a strong cough, the cuff may be slowly deflated to allow the patient to expel the respiratory secretions. In a patient with a weaker cough, it is helpful to deliver a large breath with a manual resuscitation bag while simultaneously deflating the tube cuff. The large exhaled volume will facilitate blowing the accumulated secretions above the cuff into the oropharynx so they may be expectorated or removed with suction. It may take a few moments for the patient to adjust to the deflated cuff. The clinician should then occlude the tube digitally to assess airflow through the upper airway and look for signs of increased airway resistance:

- Stridor
- Prolonged inspiratory time
- Use of accessory muscles of inspiration
- Intercostal muscle retractions
- Subjective complaints
- Inability to phonate

Any of these signs or symptoms could be attributed to the size of the tracheostomy tube relative to the size of the patient's trachea, resulting in insufficient airflow around the tube and through the upper airway. Typically, this would be a tube with a larger than 10 mm outer diameter, but excessive resistance may be seen in smaller sizes as well. High-volume, low-pressure cuffs, even when completely deflated, can contribute to a significant increase in upper airway resistance.

Eliminate the Tracheostomy Tube as a Source of the Obstruction

In order to exclude the tube as a cause of obstruction, the clinician must remove the tracheostomy tube and reassess airflow. Only clinicians experienced in replacing airways should remove airways. Initial preparation for the procedure includes having immediately available a tube of similar size, a tube one size smaller, and a cuffless tube. The latter two can usually be placed if the original tube proves difficult to reinsert.

When the tube is removed, the clinician should cover the open stoma securely with sterile gauze, apply digital pressure, and assess for upper airway resistance. If no airway resistance is noted, the clinician can reasonably assume that the tracheostomy tube type or size is the problem. If resistance is noted, the airway should be scoped to determine the cause. .

CLINICAL SCENARIO CONT'D.

With the tracheostomy tube downsized in the patient, speech trials were again resumed. Previous cuff-down ventilator settings were resumed: AC/VC with a rate of 10 breaths per minute, tidal volume of 900 ml, PEEP of 5 cm H_2O, and an inspiratory time of two seconds. The smaller tube allowed significantly more air movement around the deflated cuff, with subsequent improvement of phonation. With coaching, John continued to improve coordination of speech with breath delivery. Eventually, the cuff could remain deflated for speech for several hours at a time, while the patient was awake. Periodic arterial blood gas measurements showed somewhat fluctuating arterial pCO_2 levels within an acceptable range. The #6 tube was also deemed to be an appropriate size when the cuff was inflated for nocturnal ventilation. Cuff inflation volume and pressure, as well as ventilating pressures, were all kept within an acceptable range. To avoid confusion, no further attempts with a one-way valve were considered, since a satisfactory result was achieved without it.

Eliminate Soft Tissue as the Source of Upper Airway Obstruction

If increased airway resistance or obstruction remains, one additional maneuver can be performed in select patients, typically in the stroke or traumatic brain injury patient. While one clinician covers the tracheal stoma, another performs a chin lift. If this maneuver eliminates the obstruction, soft tissue is likely the cause. At that point, the tracheostomy tube of choice should be replaced and left uncapped, and a subsequent plan should be devised. Upper airway endoscopy is warranted to verify causes of obstruction. In the patient with mild soft tissue upper airway obstruction, it may be appropriate to cap the tube during periods of supervision, such as during speech therapy sessions. A one-way valve, which bypasses the soft tissue obstruction, might also be trialed.

If soft tissue is clearly the cause of obstruction, it might be helpful to employ CPAP as a way to transition the patient away from an artificial airway. Once daytime capping trials proceed uneventfully, the patient should be screened with the tracheostomy tube capped with overnight oximetry, or type-III limited channel polysomnography. The addition of sleep testing is needed to determine if there is upper airway obstruction that would require the initiation of CPAP therapy.

Conclude the Bedside Clinical Evaluation

If bedside evaluations reveal no upper airway problem, the clinician may proceed to capping trials, with an appropriately chosen tube, as dictated by patient and institution safety measures. If signs of upper airway obstruction persist, the clinician should replace the tracheostomy tube and leave it uncapped. The patient should then be evaluated by an otolaryngologist before the tube is progressed. The incidence of obstructive airway lesions in patients with long-term tracheostomies has been reported as high as 67%.[28] Commonly acquired lesions include tracheal granuloma, tracheomalacia, tracheal stenosis, and vocal cord and laryngeal dysfunction.

Traumatic Brain Injury, Stroke, and Upper Airway Obstruction

Patients impaired by stroke, TBI, or anoxic brain injury often manifest soft tissue upper airway obstruction in the acute rehabilitation setting. In fact, increasing evidence links obstructive sleep apnea (OSA), also known as sleep disordered breathing (SDB) syndrome, as an independent risk factor for stroke,[29,30,31] with sudden cardiac death.[32] Soft tissue upper airway obstruction due to loss of pharyngeal muscle tone may occur during sleep or waking hours. Since an open tracheostomy tube is curative for the obstruction, the clinician must cautiously progress the tracheostomy tube in this patient population. The use of an overnight oximetry with a capped tube will generate an Oxygen Desaturation Index 4% (ODI4%) and indicates the number of events in which desaturation falls below 4% of baseline, and the length of each desaturation event must be at least 10 seconds. An ODI4% between 5-15 events is a reasonable marker for significant mild obstructive sleep apnea. An ODI4% between 15-30 events indicates moderate sleep apnea, and greater than 30 events indicates severe OSA. See Chapter 11, **Figures 11.4, 11.5, and 11.6** for examples of these studies. In many centers, an unattended sleep study can be performed, generating more accurate Respiratory Effort Index (REI), which is now accepted as a technique to diagnose sleep apnea.

Nasal CPAP is the primary supportive mode for patients with soft tissue upper airway obstruction and significant sleep apnea with associated elevated ODI4% or REI. With this therapy, positive pressure throughout the ventilatory cycle acts to stent open the upper airway and relieve soft tissue obstruction. The main limitation to CPAP is the patient's level of alertness and tolerance. It is advisable to attempt nasal CPAP support before decannulation. If the patient does not tolerate the CPAP device, the tracheostomy tube can be left open during sleep. If the patient tolerates nasal CPAP, a tube suitable for capping must be fitted for proper titration of CPAP level. In an adult, a size 6 is usually recommended. Following decannulation of a patient using nasal CPAP, a period of suboptimal CPAP support is expected and should be compensated for while the stoma is closing. Positive airway pressure applied nasally can escape through an open tracheal stoma; therefore, the stoma should be sealed with an occlusive dressing until it closes. Discharge planning should accommodate arrangements for the use of nasal CPAP.

Current devices to treat sleep disordered breathing are numerous, and varied algorithms built into the devices can address a multitude of issues. It is always advisable to consult with a sleep disorder team for diagnosis and optimal treatment.

CONSIDERATION FOR TRANSITIONING TRACHEOSTOMY TUBES

CLINICAL SCENARIO CONT'D.

Serial vital capacity measurements for the patient continued to improve during the stay at the rehabilitation hospital. An admission vital capacity of 800 ml had increased to 1200 ml, and ventilator-free breathing time was gradually increased, until liberation from mechanical ventilation was achieved. John's tracheostomy tube was then changed to a Bivona #6 TTS. This choice allowed for comfortable airflow around the tube when capped, while still having a cuff available for inflation, should bronchial hygiene needs dictate.

The progression of tracheostomy tubes warrants consideration of several important factors, including the presence or absence of a cuff, structure of the tube, and method of downsizing. A description of those factors is provided in the following sections.

Cuffless Tracheostomy Tubes

Cuffless tracheostomy tubes offer an advantage during capping because they offer less airway resistance. However, they will not likely be able to support most attempts at mechanical ventilation, especially nocturnally. They also may be suboptimal for significant bronchial hygiene needs.

TTS Tracheostomy Tubes

The Bivona TTS tracheostomy tube has a low-volume, high-pressure cuff. Consequently, the clinician must pay attention to cuff pressure to avoid tracheal wall damage from long-term exposure to high cuff pressures.

Fenestrated Tracheostomy Tubes

Fenestrated tracheostomy tubes can be used to transition toward decannulation. Their potential advantages during the transitional phase have been introduced elsewhere (see chapters 6 and 11); however, the frequent challenges of properly fitting and positioning these tubes warrant careful observation of the following:

- Fenestrated tubes should be properly fit so the fenestration is located centrally within the tracheal lumen to allow airflow between the upper and lower airways. If it does not fit well, granulation growth and bleeding are frequent complications.
- Proper positioning of the fenestration should be periodically checked by removing the inner cannula or cap and illuminating the opening with a light source. No tissue should compromise the window.

- Changes in patient position, coughing, and too much or too little gauze under the flange are factors that alter the placement of the fenestration within the airway.
- A fenestration in the outer cannula often allows growth into the opening.

One-Way Valves

One-way valves can play a role in the progression of an artificial airway (see chapter 6). They allow inspiration through the tube and direct exhalation through the upper airway. Therefore, an upper airway obstruction should be evaluated prior to the use of a one-way valve. In an attempt to allow patients to phonate, clinicians often use one-way valves with improper tubes, which do not allow easy exhalation. A completely deflated cuff and a tube of appropriate size must be used to allow easy airflow between the tube and the trachea. Many believe that a cuffless tube should be used to promote safety and avoid accidental cuff inflation. Any signs of air-trapping should signal an end to the use of a one-way valve until further assessments of tube size and upper airway patency are carried out. Patients can usually be safely capped instead of using a one-way valve if a cuffless tube of the proper type and size is in place. The advantage of routine capping over the use of one-way valves is the restoration of normal upper airway humidification of inspired air. Prolonged use of one-way valves without supplemental humidification may lead to the formation of thick, inspissated secretions and atelectasis. However, some conditions—such as mild, soft tissue obstruction in the neurologically compromised patient—might benefit from using a one-way valve.

Downsizing Tracheostomy Tubes

Downsizing tracheostomy tubes can play an important role in the progression toward capping and decannulation; thus, the following implications should be considered:

- Increased work of breathing: An increase in airway resistance will occur when the patient breathes through a smaller tube, particularly if the cuff is inflated.
- Adequate removal of secretions: With tube downsizing, the size of the suction catheter will also need to be downsized accordingly. However, it is important to remember that a smaller suction catheter may not be adequate to evacuate thick secretions.
- Appropriate monitoring of cuff pressure: When used to achieve a proper seal, an overinflated high-volume, low-pressure cuff may, in fact, have the effect of a high-pressure cuff. Thus, close attention to cuff pressure is important, particularly when repeated inflation is necessary. Often, over-inflation occurs because clinicians feel that the leak must be 100% eliminated. Learning that leaks can be well tolerated in long-term care patients helps to reduce the urge to over inflate the cuff.

CLINICAL SCENARIO CONT'D.

John C. continued to progress. Vital capacity reached 1600 ml, and cough improved. Secretions were easily mobilized with occasional diaphragmatic cough assist, which family members were taught to perform. To allow for maximal opening of the tracheal lumen for secretion clearance, the patient was fitted with a Montgomery tracheal cannula with plug. Overnight pulse oximetry was performed with no signs of desaturation. With the capped tracheal cannula securely fitted, the decision to decannulate was left for a follow-up visit after discharge.

Discharge to Home

The majority of tracheostomized patients can be decannulated during their acute care stay; however, there are always those who cannot. Cox, Carson, Holmes, Howard, and Carey[33] reviewed a 10-year database of 144,875 patients who required mechanical ventilation in the state of North Carolina. Of 49,872 patients who required intubation for more than four days, nearly 10,000 underwent a tracheostomy. Not only did the rate of tracheostomy increase 200% over the 10-year duration, but also significantly fewer tracheostomized patients were discharged home.

Patients who use oxygen in the hospital must undergo a desaturation trial within three days prior to discharge. In this test, patients are monitored with a pulse oximeter at rest and when the oxygen supplement is removed. If there is no desaturation at rest, the patient is tested during exertion. If the patient desaturates to 88% or less on exertion, he or she qualifies for home oxygen use. Detailed qualifications for the use of long-term oxygen are provided by the Centers for Medicare and Medicaid Services.[34]

Patients who transition to home with tracheostomy tubes warrant careful planning for transition of care. The American Thoracic Society and others have published guidelines that help guide the long-term care of these patients.[35,36,37]

Discharge Planning

In-home Health Care and Provisions

Patients should be given a choice of vendors to provide their tracheostomy supplies and/or support from an in-home medical healthcare provider. In the US, the source of these services is often determined by a patient's insurance. The in-home health provider may be a nurse, respiratory therapist, or home-based physician. Discharge planners should be given a list of the required supplies in order to procure them from appropriate vendors long before the date of discharge. The discharge planner or case manager is usually responsible for investigating the coverage provided by the patient's insurance company, including home care services and supply companies. This process should include the outpatient physician, and if possible, a medical home that should be established for the care of these complex medical patients.[38]

Supplies and Equipment

All equipment should be delivered in the home prior to discharge. It is advisable to have emergency equipment delivered to the patient's bedside for availability during transport. These essential supplies include a manual resuscitation bag for ventilation, a suction machine, suction catheters, and two extra tracheostomy tubes (same size and one size smaller). Insurance will typically cover only one tube every three months.

Caregiver Education

The entire family should be educated to provide routine care and should be aware of the schedule and plan for tracheostomy tube changes and cleaning. Routine care includes suctioning, cleaning the inner cannula and entire tube, cleaning the stoma, and changing the tracheostomy ties or holder.

While doing routine care, patients and family members should be taught to observe color and odor changes in secretions, the presence of fever or bleeding, and an increase in respiratory rate, and then report these signs to their care provider.

Managing Home Emergencies

The family should also be familiar with emergency care. Emergency care includes the management of respiratory distress—most likely a mucous plug. In addition to calling the emergency response system, family members should be taught emergency procedures such as basic life support and the Heimlich maneuver.

When a patient with a tracheostomy is discharged home, a back-up plan should be in place to mobilize prompt and appropriate assistance. Local emergency response personnel should be notified in advance about patients with tracheostomies and their addresses. They should be provided with pertinent medical history and shown how to access the house. This will give paramedics advance notice of what to expect upon arrival, saving precious minutes in an emergency, especially since the patient will likely be unable to speak.

It is also important to make the power company aware that vital emergency equipment—such as suction machines, oxygen extractors, and ventilators—is in the home. In this way, patients and caregivers can be notified in advance of any planned power interruptions. See **Table 12.2** for a home discharge checklist.

Table 12.2: Home Discharge Checklist

Home Discharge Checklist

• Teach patient and family about tracheostomy care and managing emergencies
  o Provide demonstrations, and require return demonstrations and repeated supervised practice to ensure competence prior to discharge
  o Teach caregivers cardiopulmonary resuscitation, especially Heimlich maneuver
• Organize planned discussion among family members regarding shared responsibilities or schedule for care
• Order supplies
• Arrange for home nursing supervision of care
• Complete electrical assessment
• Complete oxygen desaturation test to determine requirement for home oxygen
• Notify power company
• Notify local emergency services

Care for Patients at Home

There are several factors to consider when a patient is discharged home. Is the patient physically able to manage the care of the tracheostomy? Does the patient live alone, or is there someone at home who can assist? When a discharged patient with a tracheostomy is otherwise healthy and strong, he can easily resume a relatively normal life. If the patient is weakened because of disease or disability, destinations other than home should be considered. A ventilator-dependent patient will likely require professional assistance, and consideration should be given for the patient's placement in a specialized facility.

Care for patients at home is a daunting task, but should not overcome a sense of duty, responsibility, or love for a family member. Normal home life is disrupted, and the focus of all activity becomes the care of the patient. There is no reprieve unless arrangements are made for respite care; however, it should be noted that there is no insurance coverage for respite care in the US. Clearly, one person cannot provide round-the-clock care.[39] Continuous professional care at home is a prohibitive out-of-pocket expense for most adults, as it is not covered by adult payors; whereas, in children, these costs are typically covered. For adults, approximately 80% of durable medical equipment cost is covered by Medicare and most insurance companies. Given the high cost of equipment, even the 20% co-pay may be cost- prohibitive.

Tracheostomy Care and Supplies at Home

Care and Cleaning

In contrast to the hospital setting, care of the tracheostomy at home is done with clean rather than sterile technique. **Table 12.3** outlines teaching points for tracheostomy care at home. Patients and caregivers should be taught to clean or change the inner cannula at least twice per day, and more often if necessary. Specific cleaning instructions depend on the type of tube. Inner cannulas made of polyvinyl chloride can typically be cleaned using hydrogen peroxide, which is not recommended for metal or silicone tubes. The manufacturer's recommendations should be consulted regarding specific cleaning procedures. The purpose of cleaning or changing the inner cannula is to keep it free from obstructing secretions. The stoma should also be assessed and cleaned twice per day with cotton-tipped swabs soaked in saline or water. To prevent infection and ensure the integrity of the tube, the entire tracheostomy tube should be changed every month in adults. Typically, pediatric tube changes should be done weekly. In adults who have had multiple episodes of tracheitis or pneumonias, weekly changes should also be considered. Concern for biofilm development leading to ongoing re-infection is concerning in these patients; however, Medicare will only provide new tubes every three months, and families and caregivers will need to be comfortable with cleaning protocols.

Table 12.3 Teaching Points for Tracheostomy Care at Home
• Patients with a tracheostomy have a tendency to develop mucous plugs. Discuss prevention and management strategies in chapter 7. • Use clean technique at home. • Check and clean the inner cannula at least twice per day (refer to the manufacturer's recommendations regarding products to use for cleaning). • Keep stoma clean and dry. Clean the stoma with cotton swabs or gauze. Ensure the stoma is dry before applying a dressing. • Change tracheostomy tube holder (ties) as needed. • Change/clean entire tracheostomy tube at least every month. • Increase fluids as tolerated to keep secretions thin and mobile. • Suction as needed to remove secretions. • Minimize cuff pressure. • Add humidity as needed

Emergency Care at Home

The most common respiratory emergency for the tracheostomy patient at home is mucous plugs causing obstruction within the airway, which is manifested as respiratory distress. In the event of respiratory distress, **Table 12.4** illustrates teaching points for the patient and caretakers in managing a tracheostomy emergency.

Table 12.4: Teaching Points for Managing Tracheostomy Emergencies
• Check the inner cannula for obstruction
• Suction deeply
• Contact emergency services if no relief is noted
• Use the manual resuscitation bag for rescue breathing
• Change the entire tracheostomy tube
• Perform the Heimlich maneuver

The most common cause of cardiac arrest from airway obstruction in the patient with a tracheostomy is mucous plugs. In order to prevent mucous plugs, secretions must remain thin and mobile. The patient must be optimally hydrated and participate in a program of physical mobility. Bedridden patients can perform active or passive range-of-motion exercises. It is essential that secretions are mobilized regularly, and regular airway clearance is indicated for patients whose cough is ineffective. Airway clearance plans could include high-frequency chest wall oscillation therapy, MIE, and/or manual techniques as described above. Routine saline lavage is not recommended as fully discussed in chapter 7.

Patients and their caregivers must ensure the tracheostomy tube is regularly changed. They should be comfortable changing tubes on their own. A standard (non-customized) plastic tracheostomy tube should be changed at least every month. Backman and others[40] demonstrated that polymeric tubes that remained in the trachea for 3–6 months acquired major surface degradation. The tubes in the study were made of polyvinyl chloride, polyurethane, and silicone. Stainless steel and silver tracheostomy tubes can last a lifetime with regular care. Bivona Fome-Cuf™ tubes are made of silicone, but should be changed monthly because of the accumulation of biofilm moisture and debris. The latter can cause infection and hardening of the cuff, making tube removal difficult.

Reimbursement and Medicare Support for Equipment and Supplies

The availability of medical supplies should be periodically checked. A standard Medicare allowance for tracheostomy supplies includes a limited supply of suction catheters, inner cannulas, tracheostomy care kits, and so forth (**Table 12.5**). **Table 12.6** identifies the Medicare coverage for tracheostomy supplies. **Table 12.7** lists the 2019 approximate costs for tracheostomy supplies.

Table 12.5 Tracheostomy Care/Cleaning Supplies
• Gloves • 2 solution basins • Tracheostomy tube brush • Drape • 4×4 gauze sponges • Pipe cleaners • 4×4 nonwoven tracheostomy dressings (precut) • Cotton-tipped applicators • Hydrogen peroxide • Sterile water • Tracheostomy holder or cotton twill tape

Table 12.6: Medicare Allowance for Tracheostomy Supplies (Adult)

Item	**Maximum allowed Frequency**
Suction machine	1
Manual resuscitation bag	1
Yankauer suction catheter	1 monthly
Suction catheter kits	300 per month
Disposable inner cannulas	30 per month
Tracheostomy tube	1 per 3 months
Speaking valve	1 per 6 months
Split gauze (drain sponge)	100 per month
Tracheostomy tube holder (ties)	30 per month
Tracheostomy care/cleaning kits	30 per month
Tracheostomy mask/collar	2 per month
Pulse oximeter	Not covered

Table 12.7: Average Cost of Tracheostomy Supplies (US) (2019)

Item	**Cost**
Plastic tracheostomy tubes	$40-120
Disposable inner cannulas	$3-5
Stainless steel tubes	$80-200
Silver tubes	$300-1,200
Custom tubes	$500-$5,000
Tracheostomy ties	$3-5
Speaking valves	$60-150
Suction catheters	$1
Drain sponges	$0.25
Tracheostomy care/cleaning kits	$2-5

Payment for equipment varies between payors. Durable medical equipment is covered at 80% by Medicare. Aerosol and HMEs are covered by all payors. Medicare and private insurance companies cover manual resuscitation bags. Gloves, peroxide, and normal saline are not covered by

Medicare or private insurance. While Medicaid coverage varies from state to state, most commonly, patients can obtain these items through their pharmacy.

Tracheostomy Care in the Office or Clinic

Unfortunately, insurance regulations do not allow reimbursement for tracheostomy tube changes beyond a certain point in the postoperative period— namely, more than two weeks after the procedure. After that time, a tracheostomy tube change is usually billed through an office visit. For this reason, patients are often given a prescription for the tracheostomy tube and are asked to bring the tube with them for their office visit. Less commonly available for some patients, home care nurses may be able to provide tracheostomy tube changes with a provider's order.

Equipping the Office

Equipment for the well-stocked office should include portable or in-wall suction, with 12-14 French suction catheters, red rubber catheters, and Lukens traps for collecting samples. Exam rooms should be fitted with additional lighting over the exam tables. Positional lighting is preferable because of the challenge of viewing the tracheal area. Available supplies for changing the tracheostomy tube should include sterile gloves, new tracheostomy tubes with obturator, water-based lubricant, split gauze (drain sponges), tracheostomy ties, and a receptacle in which to place the old tracheostomy tube in anticipation of cleaning and processing (See chapter 7 for cleaning instructions).

There should be smaller step-down tubes available in case of emergency. Silver nitrate sticks to treat bleeding granulations should also be available. The room itself should have a disability-friendly environment. Electronic exam tables that can be moved up and down are ideal, so that a patient in a wheelchair can easily transfer, using either a ceiling lift or a transfer board. There should be adequate space for a caregiver, and the office should be equipped with a scale large enough to accept a power chair if needed.

What the Office Staff Needs to Know

The office staff should be aware that, when scheduling a patient with a tracheostomy, they will need to block extra time and have the additional stock items available. If possible, a patient with a tracheostomy tube should be managed in a multidisciplinary clinic for which the underlying need for tracheostomy is appropriate. For example, a patient with muscular dystrophy should be seen in a muscular dystrophy clinic, and a patient with a laryngeal cancer should be see in a head and neck cancer clinic. The office staff should meet the family at every visit to help improve communication in between appointments.

Electronic Medical Record Plan

Standardized flow sheets should be developed within the electronic medical record that include tube size, cuff type, shaft type, specialization or customization, and the durable medical equipment provider. These flowsheets should be exportable into a database for tracking outcomes for research purposes. Each patient should have a comprehensive tracheostomy plan that is reviewed at each visit. **Table 12.8** is an example of a comprehensive tracheostomy plan.

Table 12.8: Comprehensive Tracheostomy Plan

Tracheostomy Plan		Date: ______________________	
Patient Name	**ID Number**	**Birth Date**	**Insurance Carrier**
Home Address	**Phone Number**	**Gender**	**Email Address**
Trach Placement Date	**Last Trach Δ**	**Tube Type**	**Customizations/Specializations**
Tube Size ID, OD, Length	**Cuff type**	**Shaft type**	**Tube material (PVC, silicone, etc.)**
Respiratory Provider	**DME Provider**	**Serial Number(s)**	**Home Nursing Provider**
Airway Clearance Plan (cough assist, therapy vest, Metaneb, Ambu, nebulizers, etc.)			
Trach Change Schedule		**Trach Cleaning Schedule**	
Skin Care Plan		**Communication Plan**	

Review Continued Need for Trach

- ☐ Capping
- ☐ Suction requirements
- ☐ Peak Cough Flow

Trach Progression Plan

- ☐ Oximetry
- ☐ Transcutaneous CO_2
- ☐ Sleep study
- ☐ In-hospital monitoring
- ☐ In-office monitoring

Airway Clearance Plan

As opposed to the initial hospitalization, an outpatient airway clearance plan should try to avoid suctioning as the main technique for clearing secretions because opening the circuit and the tracheostomy tube increases exposure to infection. Frequent introduction of the suction catheter to the trachea can damage the airway and cause bleeding. Alternative devices and treatments to facilitate secretion removal can include the following:

1. ***Mechanical insufflator-exsufflator (MIE).*** The MIE has two jobs in this situation. It can be used to clear secretions, and it can be used for lung volume recruitment, prevention of atelectasis, and active range of motion to the chest wall. Given these goals, the use of an MIE for use in patients with a tracheostomy should always end with an inspiratory maneuver to assure an open lung.
2. ***High-frequency chest wall oscillator.*** These devices provide high vibratory pressure to the chest to loosen and liquify secretions in the small and mid-sized airways, improving ease of cough and opening of the lung. For patients with a tracheostomy tube, often the use of a body wrap is easier than a total vest (**Figure 12.6**), and these wrap devices are often utilized in the ICU and home environments. Therapies that combine positive pressure with vibration have used devices starting in the 1980s, with intrapulmonary percussive ventilation (IPV), to the MetaNeb (**Figure 12.4**) currently on the market. All of these devices can be expensive with limited access in many areas of the world. It is important to remember that a simple manual resuscitation bag can be used on a daily basis with a tracheostomy for lung volume recruitment. No patient should leave the hospital without an airway clearance plan.
3. ***Tracheobronchitis care.*** Regardless of the material, the tracheostomy tube itself is a foreign body, which is at risk for the development of biofilms. Biofilms are sheets of bacteria that change the simple one-celled organism to a more bioactive contaminant in the airway. Over time, these biofilms can re-infect the lung, initially causing infective tracheobronchitis, and ultimately pneumonia. To prevent this process, good oral care, elevation of the head of the bed, and aggressive treatment of reflux is recommended. These practices are helpful, but not sufficient. Often, frequent changes of the tracheostomy tube will be necessary to prevent infection. There is no agreed-upon standard for frequency of tube change, and local practices may vary from once a week, to once every three months. Certainly, all would agree that patients with the highest secretion burden and the most drug-resistant bacteria should have the most frequent tube changes. At each office visit, the care plan should be reviewed, with the development of concordance between patient and physician on the frequency of changes and the technique for cleaning.[41,42]
4. In order to diagnose tracheobronchitis in a patient with a chronic tracheostomy, tracheal aspirates are recommended, as opposed to bronchoalveolar lavage (BAL) that would be needed for a diagnosis of pneumonia. Specifically, the presence of purulence as defined by a tracheal aspirate that contains greater than 25 neutrophils per low-powered field, with less than 10 squamous cells per low-powered field. These patients should be treated with antibiotics, as guided by the results of previous samples and the final culture data from the current sample. There is no agreement on the length of time necessary to treat, and the decision should be made based on the clinical presentation of the patient.[43]

5. ***Skin plans.*** When in the office, the stoma should always be examined. The stoma should be kept clean and dry. Patients who have large secretion burden around the stoma will benefit from foam absorbent dressings to reduce skin irritation. For those who have irritation near the tracheostomy ties, zinc oxide can be protective. If the tracheostomy tube is connected to the ventilator circuit, assure there is no tension, as stretching may cause dilation of the stoma.
6. ***Communication plans.*** During office visits, a communication plan should be reviewed. Patients should have a night-time communication plan so they can easily call for aid, if needed. Voice amplifiers can be helpful to assist with using telephones or baby monitors for this purpose. If a patient is non-verbal, gaze devices can be helpful. For some patients in whom loss of voice is anticipated but has not occurred (such as in ALS or in laryngeal cancers), proactive voice banking can be used to help develop alternative adaptive communication.
7. ***Care coordination with other teams.*** Patients with a tracheostomy tube should become established with a medical home to help coordinate their care. At the heart of a medical home should be an internist or family medicine physician who has been trained in the use and care of a tracheostomy. As medical crises occur, the medical home will need to work with other care teams within the hospital to support this patient, as many teams will be unfamiliar with the needs of a tracheostomy patient. An important consideration is preoperative clearance, where the anesthesia team will need to consider the need for alterative tracheostomy tubes or other airway devices in the perioperative setting.
8. ***Review indications for ongoing tracheostomy.*** At every outpatient visit, the care team should review with the patient the ongoing need for a tracheostomy. A trial of finger capping and measurement of peak cough flow should occur in the office with all routine visits (see chapter 11 for details of downsizing and decannulation).
9. ***Review end of life options.*** In office visits, periods of medical stability are an excellent opportunity to review with patients their health care preferences, advance directives, and assess patients' attitudes toward ongoing aggressive interventions.

Figure 12.6 Hill-Rom Vest Airway Clearance System

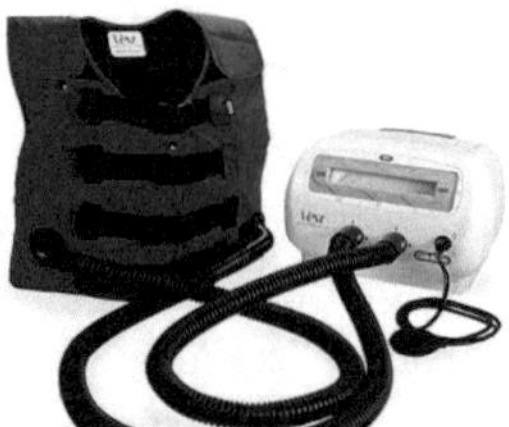

Psychosocial Issues

In addition to physical issues, the patient with a tracheostomy is likely to have numerous psychosocial concerns, including depression, quality of life, body image, and the presence of social support.

Depression

It is common for patients with tracheostomies to become depressed, but it is unknown whether this depression is due to the tracheostomy itself or the underlying conditions. It is well-known that patients with head and neck cancer, especially laryngectomy patients, become depressed.[44] This may manifest itself as poor self-care or avoidance of social activities.[45,46]

Prior to discharge, tracheostomy and laryngectomy patients should be counseled about the likelihood of depression. This is especially true with laryngectomy patients. Not only do these patients have an external reminder of cancer, but they are also grieving the loss of their voice, their natural method of communication, and a personal distinctive feature. Patients need to understand that depression is a natural reaction to what is often a devastating condition. When patients are not given any information about depression, they are often surprised by its onset and need guidance for its management, including medication and psychotherapy. Depression can be worsened by the public reaction of family, friends, and strangers and may amplify the patient's distress at their appearance. At the time of diagnosis, referral to disease-specific support groups for both the patient and the family members can be helpful before depression sets in.

Brook[47] provides an insightful discussion of his experience as a physician who underwent treatment for cancer of the neck. He described how depression and hopelessness were "strangely helpful and calming" as he faced his uncertain future and potentially poor outcome. He described his frustration at his inability to communicate effectively with the health care team and his fear with his inability to summon help when his laryngectomy tube was blocked.

Depression can manifest in the patient as poor self-care. For example, some patients prefer to remove their inner cannula rather than clean it. It is important to reinforce with these patients the purpose of the inner cannula and the fact that secretions will accumulate within the tube and create an obstruction. Guiding these patients to available resources for managing depression will improve long-term tracheostomy care.

Quality of Life

Quality of life data focused on patients with tracheostomies is not prevalent because of the confounding nature of their coexisting disorders.[48] Furthermore, it is difficult to accurately interpret this data, since it is generally known that health care professionals tend to underestimate patients' satisfaction with their lives and overestimate their dissatisfaction.[49]

In the nursing literature, reports of patients with head and neck cancer magnified concerns when they underwent tracheostomy. When vocalization is restored, patients with tracheostomy have an improvement in their quality of life.[50] Restrictions based on the patient's underlying disabilities, and not necessarily the tracheostomy itself, define the patient's psychosocial reactions. Studies of chronic ventilator-dependent patients suggest that the ability to speak plays a large part in quality of life perceptions of patients with tracheostomies. The ability to speak allows a patient to direct their own care, preserves autonomy, and drives improvements in quality of life through independence in all aspects of their lives. One young, ventilator-dependent tetraplegic patient described his quality of life as follows:

> *I feel more normal, less trapped in my body because I can take part— project my personality out of my body with my voice. So, communication is important. It's certainly primary in my life and with my family.*[49]

Babin, Beyneir, LeGall, and Hitier[51] studied quality of life in 150 patients before and after total laryngectomy. They found that there was a significant decrease in smoking, drinking, and dinner outings with friends at home and in restaurants but a significant increase in owning a pet and watching television. The authors concluded that the latter two findings were indicative of feelings of solitude among total laryngectomees and that voice deprivation and the stoma itself are limiting factors in social relationships that push patients into withdrawal.

Caregiver Burden

Ferrario, Zotti, Zaccaria, and Donner[52] studied the burden on those caring for patients with tracheostomies. Their study used interviews with 63 caregivers who completed a family strain questionnaire; 40 of them repeated the questionnaire one year later. The greatest strain was felt by female caregivers. Among the caregivers, 84% reported that their patients experienced emotional distress such as embarrassment, shame, reduction of social contacts, and a feeling of being a burden on their families. A significant number (12 of 63) of these caregivers reported similar feelings themselves. Most caregivers reported restricted social and leisure activities. Very few ever went out to visit friends, to restaurants, or to the cinema. Nearly all caregivers (94.7%) reported they felt better when they were caring for their patients.

Despite the report that caregivers felt better in their role, many reported a sense of intolerance toward their patients. Some patients' wife-caregivers reported disgust with the physical proximity of their partners. Physical intimacy and exchanges of affection were sources of great distress, which also created feelings of guilt.[52]

One study on quality of life in children and their parents found that the quality of life of the caregiver was significantly associated with that of the child. Parents were interviewed with the Pediatric Tracheotomy Health Status Questionnaire. The questionnaire focuses on four domains: physical symptoms of the child, frequency and financial impact of medical visits, quality of life of the child, and quality of life of the caregivers, most of whom were the parents. Most caregivers reported frequent disturbances in their own sleep. Most children woke at night and had at least one nocturnal choking episode per week, and 31% needed help breathing during the night, with 19% needing help every night.[48]

Caring for a child with a tracheostomy has far-reaching effects on the emotional and physical well-being of family members as well as a significant impact on family relationships and the integrity of the family structure. There is a high incidence of divorce among parents of children with a tracheostomy, which places an added burden on the remaining parent. One British study showed that most families received no home nursing care; 73% of the responders did not work outside the home and cared for their child full time, which lowered annual household income. Interestingly, most parents rated the quality of life of their child as better than their own.[48] A plan for respite care is a wise idea for caregivers caring for patients with a tracheostomy. Planned time off can help prevent burnout and nurture relationships between patient and caregiver.

Body Image

The face is considered of high importance in establishing body image perception. Mutilating injuries to the head and neck trigger profound changes that influence self-image, relationships with partners, sexuality, and social isolation. Gilony and others[53] evaluated the effect of tracheostomy and decannulation on body image in noncancer patients. Patients in the study had a tracheostomy for at least three months and were grouped into three categories: those who were waiting for laryngotracheal reconstruction, those who had undergone successful decannulation, and a control group of non-cannulated patients hospitalized for elective surgery with no obvious body defects. They compared long-term and short-term psychological effects. Those patients with tracheostomies in place had been cannulated for a mean of 38.7 months. The investigators found a significant reduction in life satisfaction in patients with tracheostomies in place. After decannulation, there was only mild improvement in life satisfaction and no improvement in body image. Personality tests also revealed that patients became more introverted after prolonged cannulation.[53]

Patients also report embarrassment with the tracheostomy tube. One patient reported that "people's eyes are drawn to the tracheostomy tube."[54] Bowers and Scase[45] reported that one patient avoided social situations because it was "too embarrassing both for other people and me if I had to [give myself] suction." Another patient commented on the ugliness of the tube and its negative impact on her appearance.[55]

Morris, Lupei, and Afifi[56] used a qualitative approach to study body image in 36 patients recruited within one year after discharge from an acute care hospital as well as patients in an online tracheostomy support group. They found that 68% of patients were concerned with others' thoughts about their tracheostomy, but they were not embarrassed or emotionally uncomfortable. In this study, themes revolved around others' reactions during social activities, in which some patients described initial discomfort, but tended to disregard the negative reactions of others over time.

Clinical Follow-Up

Patients with a tracheostomy who live at home should be followed up at regular intervals to ensure they remain otherwise healthy. Frequently, patients are followed up during an office visit; however, patients who are ventilator-dependent and confined to bed may not be able to attend an office visit. In the latter situation, an efficient use of available resources might include ambulance transport for in-hospital care, particularly if there is a suspicion of a co-morbid medical condition such as urinary tract infection or fever. Tracheostomy tube changes can take place during the hospital care. Fortunately, there are now specialized home care nursing services that provide tracheostomy tube changes at home. Some coordination is required by the discharge planner to find an agency, but families are grateful for the convenience and peace of mind.

One of the goals of acute inpatient rehabilitation is to ensure patients who are living at home with a disability have improved access to a full community-based life. This should include training with mobility solutions such as power chairs, etc.

Summary

The purpose of rehabilitation is to optimize the patient's functional level after a long and complicated medical course. It takes patience, methodical planning, continuous assessment, and encouraging support to guide these patients toward optimal function. The debilitation that occurs over the course of a critical illness often takes weeks or months to resolve. As patients become stronger, they become increasingly able to protect their airway and manage secretions. Concurrently, their tracheostomy tube can often be progressed. In the hospital, time to tracheostomy progression and decannulation is often short. By contrast, the process of recovery and tracheostomy tube progression after discharge can take weeks or months. Regardless of discharge destination, patients and their caregivers need information on safe management of the tracheostomy and proper responses to an emergency. Patients and caregivers need to learn good tracheostomy care and the importance of follow-up to prevent major complications. Follow-up visits must be scheduled with providers who are trained in tracheostomy care and will review the continued need for the tracheostomy at each visit.

Finally, caregivers and health professionals must not forget the impact of depression and body image on the recovery process. It is only through teamwork with a group of dedicated professionals that patients can reach their goals.

KEY POINTS

- When progressing tracheostomy tubes, the clinician must always consider the need for mechanical ventilation, suctioning, airway obstruction, and airway protection.
- Patients with a history of stroke, TBI, or sleep apnea have a high frequency of soft tissue upper airway obstruction.
- Patients and their caregivers must be given pre-discharge instructions to become comfortable managing their care at home.
- Patients should be provided with clinical follow-up to manage tracheostomy related issues.
- Close attention to bronchial hygiene needs, skin care, continued need for the tracheostomy, as well as psychosocial concerns, can prevent many complications.

Review Questions

1. A patient will be discharged from the rehabilitation hospital with a tracheostomy in place. His wife wishes to care for the patient at home, despite having had a stroke nine months prior. Which of the following is the next step in the discharge planning process?
    a. Assess the ability and willingness of the family members to provide care
    b. Make a referral to a home care agency
    c. Make a referral to a skilled care facility
    d. Initiate teaching to alternate family members

    ANSWER: A. The best answer is A. If the wife will be the primary caregiver, it is essential to assess her ability to provide care for her husband. If she is not willing or able to provide care, and there is no other caregiver available, then an alternate discharge destination should be sought. Choice B would be correct after the discharge destination is confirmed to the home. Choice C would be correct if no other caregivers are available. Choice D would be correct when the discharge destination is confirmed, and alternate family members live in the home. Generally, it is advisable to teach all family members living in the home, as well as the primary caregiver(s).

2. A patient with a TRACOE uncuffed tube tolerates a speaking valve, but does not tolerate capping. Which of the following is an appropriate next step?
    a. Laryngoscopy to look for cause of airway obstruction
    b. Continue speech therapy with speaking valve
    c. Downsize to smaller TRACOE uncuffed tube
    d. Place a talking tracheostomy tube

    ANSWER: A. The best answer is A. Laryngoscopy will examine the upper airway to determine whether there is an identifiable cause for the inability to tolerate capping (e.g., paralyzed vocal cord(s)). Choice B can be used in the interim if tolerated while a cause for airway obstruction is identified. Choice C might be correct if the tube in situ is large, but does not replace an upper airway laryngoscopy. Choice D is incorrect because a talking tracheostomy tube is a cuffed tube, which is not only a step backward on the decannulation pathway, but would also delay identification of capping intolerance.

3. Which of the following is the best marker for severe sleep apnea?
    a. Nasal CPAP of 15 cm H_2O
    b. ODI4% greater than 30
    c. Daytime sleepiness
    d. Snoring greater than 50 decibels

    ANSWER: B. The answer is B. An Oxygen Desaturation Index 4% indicates the number of events that desaturation falls below 4% of baseline, and each desaturation event must be at least 10 seconds. Greater than 30 episodes during an overnight oximetry test indicates severe OSA.

4. Which of the following is NOT a true statement regarding psychosocial issues of patients with tracheostomies?
    a. Depression can manifest as poor self-care
    b. Caregivers have reported feelings of guilt regarding physical intimacy with their tracheostomized partners
    c. Patients reported embarrassment of their tracheostomy tube that increased over time
    d. There is a high incidence of divorce among parents of children with tracheostomies

    ANSWER: The correct answer is C. Patients have reported embarrassment that decreased over time. The other choices are true.

5. What is the most common cause of cardiac arrest in a patient with a tracheostomy?
    a. Tracheo-innominate fistula
    b. Mucous plugs
    c. Tube dislodgement
    d. Tube decannulation

    ANSWER: B. The incidence of mucous plugs in patients with a tracheostomy is very high; in fact, most patients with tracheostomies will develop mucous plugs at some point. The goal is to keep them small by attending to adequate hydration, humidification, and pulmonary hygiene maneuvers. The other choices are also causes of cardiac arrest in tracheostomy patients, but the incidence is less than that associated with mucous plugs.

REFERENCES

1. Ahmed A, Youssef TA, El-Bergermy MM, Younis HM. Timing of tracheostomy in patients with prolonged intubation: A systematic review. *Eur Arch Oto-Rhino-Laryngol.* 2018; 275(3):679-690.
2. Shapiro BA, Harrison RA, Kacmarek RM, Cane RD. *Clinical Application of Respiratory Care* (3rd ed.). Chicago: Yearbook Medical Publishers, 1985.
3. Fernandez-Bussy S, Mahajan B, Folch E, Caviedes I, Guerrero J, Majid A. Tracheostomy tube placement: Early and late complications. *J Bronchol Intervent Pulmonol.* 2015; 22(4):357-364.
4. Mallick A, Bodenham A, Elliot S, Oram J. An investigation into the length of standard tracheostomy tubes in critical care patinets. *Anaesthesia.* 2008; 63:302-306.
5. Hess DR, Altobelli NP. Tracheostomy tubes. *Respir Care.* 2014; 59(6):956-973.
6. Schmidt U, Hess D, Kwo J, Lagambina S, Gettings E, Khandwala F, Bigatello LM, Stelfox HT. Tracheostomy tube malposition in patients admitted to a respiratory acute care unit following prolonged ventilation. *Chest. 2008;* 134(2):288-294.
7. Dullenkopf A, Gerber A, Weiss M. Fluid leakage past tracheal tube cuffs: Evaluation of the new Microcuff endotracheal tube. *Intensive Care Med.* 2003; 29:1849-1853.
8. Fiorelli A, Ferraro F, Nagar F, Fusco P, Mazzone S, Costa G, DiNatale D, Serra N, Santini M. A new modified Evans blue dye test as screening test for aspiration in tracheostomized patients. *J Cardiothorac Vasc Anesth.* 2017; 31(2):441-445.
9. Grillo HC, Cooper JD, Geffin B, Pontoppidan H. A low-pressure cuff for tracheostomy tubes to minimize tracheal injury. A comparative clinical trial. *Journal of Thoracic Cardiovascular Surgery.* 1971; 62(6):898-907.
10. Kastanos N, Estopa Miro R, Marin Perez A, Xaubet Mir A, Aqusti Vidal A. Laryngotracheal injury due to endotracheal intubation: Incidence, evolution, and predisposing factors. A prospective long-term study. *Crit Care Med.* 1983; 11(5):362-367.
11. Guyton D, Banner M, Kirby R. High-volume, low-pressure cuffs: Are they always low pressure? *Chest.* 1991; 100:1076-1081.
12. Bach JR. Mechanical insufflation-exsufflation comparison of peak expiratory flows with manually assisted and unassisted coughing. *Chest.* 1993; 14:1553-1562.
13. Mellies U, Goebel C. Optimum insufflation capacity and peak cough flow in neuromuscular disorders. *Ann Am Thorac Soc.* 2014; 11(10):1560-1568.
14. Strickland S, Rubin B, Haas C, Volsko T. AARC Clinical Practice Guideline: Effectiveness of pharmacologic airway clearance therapies in hospitalized patients. *Respir Care.* 2015; 60(7):1071-1077.
15. Strickland S, Rubin B, Haas C, Volsko T, Drescher G, O'Mallery C. AARC Clinical Practice Guideline: Effectiveness of nonpharmacologic airway clearance therapies in hospitalized patients. *Respir Care.* 2013;58(12):2187(7).
16. Bach JR, Saporito LR, Shah HR, Sinquee D. Decannulation of subjects with severe respiratory muscle insufficiency: Efficacy of mechanical insufflation-exsufflation. *J Rehabil Med.* 2014; 46(10):1037-1041.
17. Auger C, Hernando V, Galmiche H. Use of mechanical insufflation-exsufflation devices for airway clearance in subjects with neuromuscular disease. *Respir Care.* 2017; 62(2):236-245.
18. Volsko T. Airway clearance therapy: Finding the evidence. *Respir Care*; 2013; 58(10):1669-1678.
19. Chatburn RL. High-frequency assisted airway clearance. *Respir Care.* 2007; 52(9):1224-1235.

20. Myers TR. Positive expiratory pressure and oscillatory positive expiratory pressure therapies. *Respir Care*. 2007; 52(10):1308-1326.
21. Strickland S. Year in Review 2014: Airway clearance. *Respir Care*. 2015; 60(4):603-605.
22. Andrews J, Sathe N, Krishnaswami S, McPheeters M, Nonpharmacologic airway clearance techniques in hospitalized patients: A systematic review. *Respir Care*. 2013; 58(12):2160-2186.
23. McCool FD, Rosen MJ. Nonpharmacologic airway clearance therapies: ACCP evidence-based clinical practice guidelines. *Chest*. 2006; 129(Suppl):2505-2595.
24. Solomon DH, Wobb J, Buttaro BA, Truant A, Soliman AMS. Characterization of bacterial biofilms on tracheostomy tubes. *Laryngoscope*. 2009; 119(8):1633-1638.
25. Rose L, McKim DA, Katz SL, Leasa D, Nonoyama M, Pedersen C, Goldstein RS, Road JD. Home mechanical ventilation in Canada: A national survey. *Respir Care*. 2015; 60(5):695-704.zs
26. Hoit J, Shea S, Banzett R. Speech production during mechanical ventilation in tracheostomized individuals. *J Speech Hear Res*. 1994; 37:53-63.
27. Gilgoff IS, Peng RC, Keens TG. Hypoventilation and apnea in children during mechanically assisted ventilation. *Chest*. 1992; 101(6):1500-1506.
28. Law J, Barnhart K, Rowlett W, de la Rocha O, Lowenberg S. Increased frequency of obstructive airway abnormalities with long-term tracheostomy. *Chest*. 1993; 104:136-138.
29. Martinez-Garcia M, Galiano-Blancart R, Roman-Sanchez P, Soler-Cataluna JJ, CaberoSalt L, Salcedo-Maiques E. Continuous positive airway pressure treatment in sleep apnea prevents new vascular events after ischemic stroke. *Chest*. 2005; 128:2123-2129.
30. Yaggi HK, Concato J, Kernan W, Lichtman JH, Brass LM, Mohsenin V. Obstructive sleep apnea as a risk factor for stroke and death. *NEJM*. 2005; 353:2034-2041.
31. Sico JJ, Taggi HK, Ofner S, Concato J, Austin C, Ferguson J, Qin L, Tobias L, Taylor S, Vaz Fragoso CA, Mclain V, Williams LS, Bravata DM. Development, validation, and assessment of an ischemic stroke or transient ischemic attack-specific prediction tool for obstructive sleep apnea. *Am Heart J*. 2016; 172:135-143.
32. Gami A, Olson E, Shen W, Wright S, Ballman K, Hodge D, Herges R, Howard D, Somers V. Obstructive sleep apnea and the risk of sudden cardiac death: A longitudinal study of 10,710 adults. *J Amer Coll Cardiol.* 2013; 62(7):610-616.
33. Cox CE, Carson SS, Holmes GM, Howard A, Carey TS. Increase in tracheostomy for prolonged mechanical ventilation in North Carolina, 1993-2002. *Crit Care Med*. 2004; 32(11):2219-2226.
34. Centers for Medicare and Medicaid Services (CMS), home oxygen therapy, https://www.cms.gov/Outreach-and-Education/Medicare-Learning-Network-MLN/MLNProducts/MLN-Publications-Items/ICN908804.html. Accessed July 22, 2020.
35. American Thoracic Society. Care of the child with chronic tracheostomy. *Am J Respir Crit Care Med*. 2000; 161:297-308.
36. DeLeyn P, Bedert L, Delcroix M, Depuydt P, Lauwers G, Sokolov Y, Van Meerhaeghe A, Van Schil P. Belgian Association of Pneumology and Belgian Association of Cardiothoracic Surgery. Tracheotomy: Clinical review and guidelines. *Eur J Cardio-Thorac Surg*. 2007; 32:412-421.
37. McKim DA, Road J, Avendano M, Abdool S, Cote F, Duguid N, Fraser J, Maltais F, Morrison DL, O'Connell C, Petrof BJ, Rimmer K, Skomro R. Home mechanical ventilation: A Canadian Thoracic Society clinical practice guideline. *Can Respir J*. 2011; 18(4):197-215.

38. Fonash A. The role of the medical social worker in a pediatric aero-digestive program. *Curr Probl Pediatr Adolesc Health Care*. 2018; 48(4):111-112.
39. Warren ML, Jarrett C, Senegal R, Parker A, Kraus J, Hartgraves D. An interdisciplinary appoach to transitioning ventilator-dependent patients to home. *J Nurs Care Qual*. 2004; 19(1):67-73.
40. Backman S, Bjorling G, Johansson UB, Lysdahl M, Markstrom A, Schedin U, Aune RE, Frostell C, Karlsson S. Material wear of polymeric tracheostomy tubes: A six-month study. *Laryngoscope*. 2009; 119(4):657-664.
41. Mazhar K, Gunawardana M, Webster P, Hochstim C, Koempel JA, Rice DH, Baum M. Bacterial biofilms and increased bacterial counts are associated with airway stenosis. *Otolaryngol Head Neck Surg*. 2013; 149(2 Suppl):P82-P83.
42. Barker JC, Khansa I, Gordillo GM. A formidable foe is sabotaging your results: What you should know about biofilms and wound healing. *Plast Reconstr Surg*. 2017; 139(5):1184e-1194e.
43. Craven D, Hudcova J, Rashid J. Antibiotic therapy for ventilator-associated tracheobronchitis: A standard of care to reduce pneumonia, morbidity and costs? *Curr Opin Pulm Med*. 2015; 21(3):250-259.
44. Murphy BA, Ridner S, Wells N, Dietrich M. Quality of life research in head and neck cancer: A review of the current state of the science. *Crit Rev Oncol Hematol*. 2007; 62:251-267.
45. Bowers B, Scase C. Tracheostomy: Facilitating successful discharge from hospital to home. *Brit J Nurs*. 2007; 16(8):476-479.
46. Mason J, Murty GE, Foster H, Bradley PJ. Tracheostomy self care: The Nottingham system. *J Laryngol Otol*. 1992; 106(8):723-724.
47. Brook, I. A physician's experience as a cancer of the neck patient. *Surg* Oncol. 2010; 19(4):188-192.
48. Hopkins C, Whetstone S, Foster T, Blaney S, Morrison G. The impact of paediatric tracheostomy on both patient and parent. *Int J Ped Otorhinolaryngol*. 2009; 73:15-20.
49. Tippett DC, Vogelman L. Communication, tracheostomy, and ventilator dependency. In D. C. Tippett (Ed.), *Tracheostomy and Ventilator Dependency*. New York: Thieme, 2000.
50. Freeman-Sanderson AL, Togher L, Elkins M, Kenny B. Quality of life improves for tracheostomy patients with return of voice: A mixed methods evaluation of the patient experience across the care continuum. *Intens Crit Care Nurs*. 2018; 46:10-16.
51. Babin E, Beyneir D, LeGall D, Hitier M. Psychosocial quality of life in patients after total laryngectomy. *Revue de Laryngologie Otologie Rhinologie*. 2009; 130(1):29-34.
52. Ferrario SR, Zotti AM, Zaccaria S, Donner CF. Caregiver strain associated with tracheostomy in chronic respiratory failure. *Chest*. 2001; 119(5):1498-1502.
53. Gilony D, Gilboa D, Blumstein T, Murad H, Talmi YP, Kronenberg J, Wolf M. Effects of tracheostomy on well-being and body image perceptions. *Otolaryngol Head Neck* Surg. 2005; 133(3):366-371.
54. Morris LL. (2009). [Outcome evaluation of patients with tracheostomies (short-term), #1429007]. Unpublished data.
55. Sherlock ZV, Wilson JA, Exley C. Tracheostomy in the acute setting: Patient experience and information needs. *J Crit Care*. 2009; 24(4):501-507.
56. Morris LL, Lupei M, Afifi MS. Body image perception after tracheostomy. *ORL Head Neck Nurs*. 2017; 35(4):13-18.

Appendix

APPENDIX A: TRACHEOSTOMY TUBE SIZES (ADULT)

ID=inner diameter
OD=outer diameter
Length of shaft=neck flange to tip
*All measurements are expressed in millimeters.
(Some pediatric sizes are included in adult section.)

Air-Lon Tracheostomy
Low-profile or with 15-mm connector, (called "Inhalation Set")

Size	ID	OD	Length
3	4.0	7.0	70
4	5.0	8.0	76
5	7.0	9.0	83
6	8.0	10.0	89
7	9.0	11.0	95
8	10.0	12.0	102

Angiplast AngelTouch Tracheostomy Tube
*Comes in cuffed and cuffless

Size	ID	OD	Length
14	3.0	4.7	50
16	4.0	5.3	55
18	4.5	6.0	57
20	5.0	6.7	60
22	5.5	7.2	60
24	6.0	8.0	60
26	6.5	8.6	60
28	7.0	9.3	72
28	7.0	9.3	72
30	7.5	10.0	75
32	8.0	10.7	80
34	8.5	11.3	83
36	9.0	12.0	85

Bivona Fome-Cuff

Size	ID	OD	Length
5	5.0	7.3	60
6	6.0	8.7	70
7	7.0	10.0	80
8	8.0	11.0	88
9	9.0	12.3	98
9.5	9.5	13.3	98

Bivona Fome-Cuff With Talk Attachment

Size	ID	OD	Length
5	5.0	7.3	60.0
6	6.0	8.7	70.0
7	7.0	10.0	80.0
8	8.0	11.0	88.0
9	9.0	12.3	98.0
9.5	9.5	13.3	98.0

Bivona Hyperflex–Adjustable Neck (Aire-Cuf, TTS Cuff)

Size	ID	OD	Length
6	6.0	8.7	110
7	7.0	10.0	120
8	8.0	11.0	130
9	9.0	12.3	140

Bivona Hyperflex–Fixed Neck (Aire-Cuf, Cuffless)

Size	ID	OD	Length
6	6.0	8.7	100
7	7.0	10.0	110
8	8.0	11.0	120
9	9.0	12.3	130

Bivona Hyperflex—Fixed Neck TTS Cuff

Size	ID	OD	Length
6	6.0	8.7	70
7	7.0	10.0	80
8	8.0	11.0	88
9	9.0	12.3	98

Bivona Mid-Range Aire-Cuf

Size	ID	OD	Length
5	5.0	7.3	60.0
6	6.0	8.7	70.0
7	7.0	10.0	80.0
8	8.0	11.0	88.0
9	9.0	12.3	98.0
9.5	9.5	13.3	98.0

Bivona Mid-Range Aire-Cuf with Talk Attachment

Size	ID	OD	Length
5	5.0	7.3	60.0
6	6.0	8.7	70.0
7	7.0	10.0	80.0
8	8.0	11.0	88.0
9	9.0	12.3	98.0
9.5	9.5	13.3	98.0

Bivona Uncuffed

Size	ID	OD	Length
5	5.0	7.3	60.0
6	6.0	8.7	70.0
7	7.0	10.0	80.0
8	8.0	11.0	88.0
9	9.0	12.3	98.0
9.5	9.5	13.3	98.0

Bivona TTS Trachs

Size	ID	OD	Length
5	5.0	7.3	60
6	6.0	8.7	70
6.5	6.5	9.4	70
7	7.0	10.0	80
7.5	7.5	10.4	80
8	8.0	11.0	88
8.5	8.5	11.8	88
9	9.0	12.3	98
9.5	9.5	13.3	98

Bivona Sleep Apnea Trachs

Size	ID	OD	Length
6	6.0	9.0	68
6.5	6.5	10.0	73
7.5	7.5	11.0	79

Chiner Silicone

Size	ID	OD	Length
4	7	10	76
5	8	11	76
6	9	12	80
7	10	13	82
8	11	14	82
9	12	15	82

Chiner Polyethylene (inner cannula)

Size	ID	OD	Length
6	8.4 (6.5)	12	77
7	9.4 (7.5)	13	82
8	10.4 (8.5)	14	82
9	11.4 (9.5)	15	82

Cook VersaTube

Size	ID	OD	Length
7	7.0	10	78
8	8.0	11.0	86
9	9.0	12.0	98

Fahl Duracuff

Size	ID	OD Tip-flange	Length
7	7.0	8.8-10.2	65, 75, 100
8	8.0	9.8-11.2	70, 80, 105
9	9.0	11.2-12.4	75, 85, 105
10	10.0	12.2-13.4	85, 95, 110
11	11.0	13.2-14.4	87, 97, 115
12	12.0	14.2-15.4	90, 100, 120

Fahl Duratwix

Size	ID	OD	Length
7	7.0	10.8-11.9	72, 82
8	8.0	11.4-12.5	75, 85
9	9.0	12.5-13.7	78, 88
10	10.0	13.8-15.0	81, 91

Fahl Duravent

Size	ID	OD Tip-flange	Length
3	2.7	3.8-5.2	55
3.5	3.6	4.8-6.2	55
4	4.4	5.8-7.2	55
5	5.4	6.6-8.4	55, 95
6	6.2	7.8-9.4	60, 95
7	7.0	8.8-10.2	65, 100
8	8.0	9.8-11.2	70, 105
9	9.0	11.2-12.4	75, 105
10	10.0	12.2-13.4	85, 110
11	11.0	13.2-14.4	87, 115
12	12.0	14.2-15.4	90, 120
13	13.0	15.2-16.6	90, 125

Fahl Tracheotec

Size	ID	OD	Length
3	3.0	4.7	47.2
3.5	3.5	5.3	50.6
4	4.0	6.0	57.1
4.5	4.5	6.7	57.7
5	5.0	7.3	61.1
5.5	5.5	8.0	63.6
6	6.0	8.7	67.1
6.5	6.5	9.3	73.5
7	7.0	10.0	77.0
7.5	7.5	10.7	81.5
8	8.0	11.3	87.9
8.5	8.5	12.0	90.4
9	9.0	12.7	94.9
10	10.0	14.0	105.3

Fahl Spiraflex

Size	ID	OD	Length
7	7.0	10.4	to 69
8	8.0	11.4	to 96
9	9.0	12.4	to 122
10	10.0	13.4	to 122
11	11.0	14.4	to 123

Moore Tracheostomy Tube

Size	ID	OD	Length
6	6.5	11	109
8	7.5	12	109
10	8.5	13	109

Portex D.I.C. (Cuffed & Uncuffed)

Size	Color	ID	OD	Length
6	Orange	6.0	8.5	64
7	Green	7.0	9.9	70
8	White	8.0	11.3	73
9	Blue	9.0	12.6	79
10	Yellow	10.0	14.0	79

Portex Flex DIC (Cuffed & Uncuffed)

Size	Color	ID	OD	Length
6	Orange	6.0	8.2	64
7	Green	7.0	9.6	70
8	White	8.0	10.9	73
9	Blue	9.0	12.3	79
10	Yellow	10.0	13.7	79

Portex Fenestrated DIC (Cuffed & Uncuffed)

Size	Color	ID	OD	Length
6	Orange	6.0	8.5	64
7	Green	7.0	9.9	70
8	White	8.0	11.3	73
9	Blue	9.0	12.6	79
10	Yellow	10.0	14.0	79

Portex Blue Line (Cuffed & Uncuffed)

Size	ID	OD	Length
6	6.0	8.3	55
7	7.0	9.7	65
8	8.0	11.0	76
9	9.0	12.4	87
10	10.0	13.8	98

Portex Blue Line: Cuffed, Fenestrated

Size	ID	OD	Length
7	7.0	9.7	65
8	8.0	11.0	76
9	9.0	12.4	87

Portex Blue Line, Extra Horizontal Length, Cuffed & Uncuffed

Size	ID	OD	Vert Length	Adj Horiz Length
6	6.0	8.3	23.0	11-31
7	7.0	9.6	26.0	16-36
8	8.0	11.0	35.0	17-37
9	9.0	12.4	38.0	22-42
10	10.0	13.8	41.0	26-46

Portex Per-fit

Size	ID	OD	Length
7	7.0	9.6	82
8	8.0	10.9	86
9	9.0	12.3	93

Portex Blue Line, Trach Talk

Size	ID	OD	Length
7	7.0	9.7	65
8	8.0	11.0	76
9	9.0	12.4	87

Portex Corrugated Inner Cannula for all standard Blue Line Trachs

ID	To fit Tube
5.0	7.0
6.0	8.0
7.0	9.0

Portex Blue Line Ultra, Cuffed & Uncuffed

Size	ID	OD	Length
6	6.0	9.2	64.5
7	7.0	10.5	70.0
8	8.0	11.9	75.5
9	9.0	13.3	81.0
10	10.0	14.0	87.5

Portex Blue Line Ultra Fenestrated, Cuffed & Uncuffed

Size	ID	OD	Length
6	6.0	9.2	64.5
7	7.0	10.5	70.0
8	8.0	11.9	75.5
9	9.0	13.3	81.0
10	10.0	14.0	87.5

Portex Blue Line Ultra, Suctionaid

Size	ID	OD	Length
6	6.0	9.2	64.5
7	7.0	10.5	70.0
7.5	7.5	11.3	73.0
8	8.0	11.9	75.5
8.5	8.5	12.6	78.0
9	9.0	13.3	81.0

Portex Corrugated Inner Cannulas for Blue Line Ultra Trachs

ID	To fit Tube
5.0	6.0
6.0	7.0
7.0	8.0
8.0	9.0

Portex Lo-Profile (Cuffed & Uncuffed; Fenestrated & Non-Fenestrated)

Size	ID	OD	Length
6	6.0	8.5	67
7	7.0	9.9	71
8	8.0	11.3	75
9	9.0	12.6	83
10	10.0	14.0	83

Portex Uniperc

Size	ID With inner cannula	ID Without inner cannula	OD	Length
7	7.0	9.3	11.6	62
8	8.0	10.3	12.6	68
9	9.0	11.3	13.6	74

Rüsch Biesalski

Size	ID	OD	Length
7.0	7.0	8.2	62.8
8.0	8.0	9.3	76
9.0	9.0	10.4	70.6
10.0	10.0	11.4	70.6
11.0	11.0	12.4	78.5
12.0	12.0	13.5	78.5
13.0	13.0	14.6	83.2

Rüsch Crystal Clear Plus

Size	ID	OD	Length
6.5	6.5	8.7	64
7.0	7.0	10.0	70
7.5	7.5	10.7	75.5
8.0	80	11.3	81
8.5	8.5	11.3	81
9.0	9.0	12.7	87
9.5	9.5	12.7	87
10.0	10.0	14.0	95.5

Rüsch Extra Tracheoflex

Size	ID	OD	Length
7.5	7.5	10.3	155
8.5	8.5	11.3	155
9.5	9.5	12.3	155
10.5	10.5	13.3	155

Rüsch SafetyClear

Size	ID	OD	Length
7.0	7.0	10.6	71
8.0	8.0	11.6	86
9.0	9.0	12.7	110
10.0	10.0	13.8	108
11.0	11.0	14.9	105

Rüsch Tracheofix

Size	ID	OD	Length
7.0	7.2	9.0	70
8.5	8.7	10.3	78
10	10.2	12.3	86
11	11.2	13.3	86

Rüsch Tracheoflex

Size	ID	OD	Length
7.0	7.0	10.4	63.0
8.0	8.0	11.4	88
9.0	9.0	12.4	117
10.0	10.0	13.4	117
11.0	11.0	14.4	116
12.0	12.0	15.4	116

Rüsch Trachflex Plus

Size	ID	OD	Length
3.0	3.0	5.3	58
4.0	4.0	6.1	68
5.0	7.6	7.6	72
6.0	6.0	8.6	77
7.0	7.0	10.1	102.5
8.0	8.0	11.1	122.5
9.0	9.0	12.1	152.5
10.0	10.0	13.1	157.2
11.0	11.0	14.2	163.2

Rüsch Ultra Tracheoflex

Size	ID	OD	Length
7.0	7.0	10.4	63
8.0	8.0	11.4	88
9.0	9.0	12.3	117
10.0	10.0	13.4	117
11.0	11.0	14.4	116

Shiley DCT (Cuffed)

Size	ID	OD	Length
4	5.0	9.4	62
6	6.4	10.8	74
8	7.6	12.2	79
10	8.9	13.8	79

Shiley Cuffless Tubes CFS

Size	ID	OD	Length
4	5.0	9.4	65
6	6.4	10.8	76
8	7.6	12.2	81
10	8.9	13.8	81

Shiley Low Pressure Trachs (LPC)

Size	ID	OD	Length
4	5.0	9.4	65
6	6.4	10.8	76
8	7.6	12.2	81
10	8.9	13.8	81

Shiley Disposable Cuffless (DCFS)

Size	ID	OD	Length
4	5.0	9.4	62
6	6.4	10.8	74
8	7.6	12.2	79
10	8.9	13.8	79

Shiley Fenestrated Trachs (Cuffed) FEN

Size	ID	OD	Length
4	5.0	9.4	65
6	6.4	10.8	76
8	7.6	12.2	81
10	8.9	13.8	81

Shiley Disposable Cuffed Fenestrated (DFEN)

Size	ID	OD	Length
4	5.0	9.4	62
6	6.4	10.8	74
8	7.6	12.2	79
10	8.9	13.8	79

Shiley Cuffless Fenestrated Trachs (CFN)

Size	ID	OD	Length
4	5.0	9.4	65
6	6.4	10.8	76
8	7.6	12.2	81
10	8.9	13.8	81

Shiley Disposable Cuffless Fenestrated (DCFN)

Size	ID	OD	Length
4	5.0	9.4	62
6	6.4	10.8	74
8	7.6	12.2	79
10	8.9	13.8	79

Shiley Flexible

Size	ID	OD	Length
4	6.5	9.4	62
5	7.0	10.1	68
6	7.5	10.8	74
7	8.0	11.4	77
8	8.5	12.2	79
9	9.0	12.7	79
10	10.0	13.8	79

Shiley XLT* (Extra Length, Dual cannula)

Size	ID	OD	Length
5	5.0	9.6	90
6	6.0	11.0	95
7	7.0	12.3	100
8	8.0	13.3	105

*Extra length can be either distal or proximal. Comes in cuffed and cuffless.

Shiley Single Cannula Trachs (SCT)

Size	ID	OD	Length
5	5.0	7.0	58
6	6.0	8.3	67
7	7.0	9.6	80
8	8.0	10.9	89
9	9.0	12.1	99
10	10.0	13.3	105

Shiley PERC

Size	ID	OD	Length
6	6.4	10.8	74
8	7.6	12.2	79

Shiley Disposable Inner Cannulas (DIC)

Size	For Use With:				
4	4 DCT	4 DFEN	4 DCFN	4 DCFS	
6	6 DCT	6 DFEN	6 DCFN	6 DCFS	6 PERC
8	8 DCT	8 DFEN	8 DCFN	8 DCFS	8 PERC
10	10 DCT	10 DFEN	10DCFS	10DCFS	

Suru Tracheostomy Tube

Size	ID	OD	Length
2	2.0	2.7	51
2.5	2.5	3.3	51
3	3.0	4.0	53
3.5	3.5	4.7	53
4	4.0	5.3	55
4.5	4.5	6.0	55
5	5.0	6.7	62
5.5	5.5	7.3	65
6	6.0	8.0	70
6.5	6.5	8.9	80
7	7.0	9.5	86
7.5	7.5	10.2	88
8	8.0	10.9	94
8.5	8.5	11.5	100
9	9.0	12.2	102
9.5	9.5	12.9	104
10	10.0	13.5	104
10.5	10.5	14.2	106
11	11.0	14.9	106

TRACOE twist Comes in cuffed, cuffless, with suction line, or with oxygen port

Size	ID	OD	Length
4	4.0	7.2	56
5	5.0	8.6	66
6	6.0	9.2	72
7	7.0	10.4	74
8	8.0	11.4	76
9	9.0	12.5	78
10	10.0	13.8	80

TRACOE Comfort

Size	ID	OD	Length
3	3.5	6.4	46
4	4.0	7.3	55
5	5.0	8.7	57
6	6.0	10.0	60
7	7.0	10.5	65
8	8.0	11.3	70
9	9.0	12.6	75
10	10.0	13.7	85
11	11.0	15.0	87
12	12.0	16.2	90
13	13.0	17.2	100
14	14.0	18.2	105

TRACOE vario

Size	ID	OD	Length
6	6.0	8.2	70
7	7.0	9.7	80
8	8.0	11.2	90
9	9.0	12.3	100
10	10.0	13.7	110
11	11.0	14.8	110

Tracoe Comfort-Extra Long

Size	ID	OD	Length
5	5.0	9.0	92
6	6.0	9.8	95
7	7.0	10.5	100
8	8.0	12.2	105
9	9.0	13.0	110
10	10.0	14.5	115
11	11.0	15.5	120
12	12.0	16.4	125
13	13.0	18.0	130
14	14.0	18.2	135

Metal Tracheostomy Tubes

Chiner Sterling Silver

Size	ID	OD	Length
00	4	5	47
0	5	6	47
1	6	7	52
2	7	8	60
3	8	9	65
4	9	10	68
5	10	11	72
6	11	12	75
7	12	13	80
8	13	14	80
9	14	15	80
10	15	16	80

Fahl Silvervent

Size	ID	OD Tip-flange	Length
0	2.5	4.5-6.1	50
1	3.0	5.0-6.4	50
2	3.7	5.7-6.8	50
3	4.4	6.4-7.5	55
4	5.0	7.0-8.2	55
5	5.7	7.7-9.1	60
6	6.4	8.4-9.8	60
7	7.0	9.0-10.9	65
8	7.7	9.7-11.6	70
9	8.4	10.4-12.3	75
10	9.0	11.0-13.2	80
11	9.7	11.7-13.8	90
12	10.4	12.4-14.6	90
13	11.0	13.0-15.0	90
14	11.7	13.7-15.8	90

Jackson Original (Stainless Steel or Silver) Regular or short length

Size	ID	OD	Length
00	2.4	4.5	33
0	2.8	5.0	36, 38
1	3.0	5.5	44, 51
2	3.4	6.0	48, 58
3	4.3	7.0	48, 58
4	5.3	8.0	52, 62
5	6.2	9.0	56, 68
6	7.2	10.0	56, 69
7	8.3	11.0	56, 69
8	9.2	12.0	56, 69
9	9.9	13.0	56, 69
10	10.6	14.0	56, 69
11	12.3	15.3	56, 69
12	12.7	16.3	56, 69

Jackson Extra Long (Stainless)

Size	ID	OD	Length
5	6.2	9.0	72
6	7.2	10.0	72
7	8.3	11.0	72
8	9.2	12.0	72
9	9.9	13.0	72

Tucker Trachs (Silver)

Size	ID	OD	Length
00	2.4	4.5	31
0	2.9	5.0	36
1	3.0	5.5	48
2	3.3	6.0	50
3	4.4	7.0	53
4	5.3	8.0	55
5	6.1	9.0	60
6	7.1	10.0	60
7	8.1	11.0	60
8	9.1	12.0	60
9	10.1	13.0	60
10	11.2	14.0	60

Luer Tracheostomy

Size	ID	OD	Length
00	2.4	4.5	33
0	2.9	5.0	34
1	3.0	5.5	35
2	3.3	6.0	36
3	4.4	7.0	37
4	5.3	8.0	39
5	6.1	9.0	42
6	7.1	10.0	42
7	8.1	11.0	42
8	9.1	12.0	42
9	10.1	13.0	42
10	11.2	14.0	42

Martin Tracheostomy

Size	ID	OD	Length
6	7.1	10.0	69
7	8.1	11.0	69
8	9.1	12.0	69
8	9.1	12.0	56

Mayo Clinic Tube

Size	ID	OD	Length
3	4.3	7.0	33
4	5.3	8.0	33, 40, 58
5	6.2	9.0	56, 69
6	7.2	10.0	56, 69, 85
7	8.3	11.0	56, 69, 85
8	9.2	12.0	56, 69, 85
9	9.9	13.0	56, 69
10	10.6	14.0	56, 69
12	12.7	16.4	56, 69

Holinger Trachs (Silver)

Size	ID	OD	Length
000	2.1	4.1	26, 27, 30, 33, 40, 46
00	2.4	4.5	24, 25, 26, 27, 30, 33, 40, 46
0	2.9	5.0	25, 27, 30, 33, 40, 46
1	3.0	5.5	33, 40, 46
2	3.3	6.0	33, 40, 46, 50
3	4.4	7.0	33, 40, 50, 55, 60
4	5.3	8.0	40, 50, 55, 60
5	6.4	9.0	50, 63, 68
6	7.4	10.0	63, 68, 73
7	8.3	11.0	68
8	9.2	12.0	78

Talking Tracheostomy Tubes

Portex Blue Line "Trach Talk"

Size	7	8	9
ID	7.0	8.0	9.0
OD	9.7	11.0	12.4
Length	75	82	87

Talk Attachments with Bivona Mid-Range
Aire-Cuf & Bivona Fome-Cuf

Size	ID	OD	Length
5	5.0	7.3	60
6	6.0	8.7	70
7	7.0	10.0	80
8	8.0	11.0	88.0
9	9.0	12.3	98
9.5	9.5	13.3	98

Bivona Fome-Cuff With Talk Attachment

Size	ID	OD	Length
5	5.0	7.3	60.0
6	6.0	8.7	70.0
7	7.0	10.0	80.0
8	8.0	11.0	88.0
9	9.0	12.3	98.0
9.5	9.5	13.3	98.0

Bivona Mid-Range Aire-Cuf with Talk Attachment

Size	ID	OD	Length
5	5.0	7.3	60.0
6	6.0	8.7	70.0
7	7.0	10.0	80.0
8	8.0	11.0	88.0
9	9.0	12.3	98.0
9.5	9.5	13.3	98.0

Blom Tracheostomy Tube System

Size	ID	OD	Length
4	5.0	9.4	62
6	6.4	10.8	74
8	7.6	12.2	79
10	8.9	13.8	79

TRACOE twist with Air Supply Line

Size	ID	OD	Length
4	4.0	7.2	56
5	5.0	8.6	66
6	6.0	9.2	72
7	7.0	10.4	74
8	8.0	11.4	76
9	9.0	12.5	78
10	10.0	13.8	80

APPENDIX B: LARYNGECTOMY TUBE SIZES

ID=inner diameter
Length=neck phalange to tip
OD=outer diameter
*All measurements are expressed in millimeters

Chiner Silicone Laryngectomy Tube

Size	ID	OD	Length
4	7	10	63
5	8	11	63
6	9	12	63
7	10	13	63
8	11	14	63
9	12	15	63

Chiner Silver Laryngectomy (dual-cannula)

Size	ID	OD	Length
00	4	5	42
0	5	6	42
1	6	7	47
2	7	8	55
3	8	9	55
4	9	10	60
5	10	11	60
6	11	12	60
7	12	13	60
8	13	14	60
9	14	15	60
10	15	16	60

Chiner Silver Laryngectomy (single cannula)

Size	ID	OD	Length
5	10	11	63
6	11	12	63
7	12	13	63
8	13	14	63
9	14	15	63

Shiley Laryngectomy Tubes (LGT)

Size	ID	OD	Length
6	6.4	11.1	50
8	7.0	12.6	50
10	8.9	13.7	50

Portex DIC Laryngectomy Tube

Size	8	9	10
Color	White	Blue	Yellow
ID	8.0	9.0	10.0
OD	11.3	12.6	14.0
Length	50	50	50

Size	Color	ID	OD	Length
8	White	8.0	11.3	50
9	Blue	9.0	12.6	50
10	Yellow	10.0	14.0	50

Bivona Laryngectomy Tubes

Size	ID	OD	Length
9.5	9.5	12.0	55
9.5	9.5	12.0	85
11.0	11.0	14.0	55
11.0	11.0	14.0	105
13.0	13.0	16.0	55
13.0	13.0	16.0	85

Fahl Laryngotec

Size	ID	OD	Length
7	7.2	10.2	44, 62, 65
8	8.2	11.2	44, 62, 70
9	9.4	12.4	44, 62, 75
10	10.4	13.4	44, 62, 85
11	11.4	14.4	44, 62, 87
12	12.4	15.4	44, 62, 90

Singer Laryngectomy Tubes SLT

Size	ID	OD	Length
8 x 18	9.5	12.0	18
8x 27	9.5	12.0	27
8 x 36	9.5	12.0	36
8 x 55	9.5	12.0	55
9 x 18	10.5	13.5	18
9 x 27	10.5	13.5	27
9 x 36	10.5	13.5	36
9 x 55	10.5	13.5	55
10 x 18	12.0	15.0	18
10 x 27	12.0	15.0	27
10 x 36	12.0	15.0	36
10 x 55	12.0	15.0	55
11 x 18	13.0	16.0	18
11 x 27	13.0	16.0	27
11 x 36	13.0	16.0	36
11 x 55	13.0	16.0	55
12 x 18	13.5	17.0	18
12 x 27	13.5	17.0	27
12 x 36	13.5	17.0	36
12 x 55	13.5	17.0	55
14 x 18	16.5	20.0	18
14 x 27	16.5	20.0	27
14 x 36	16.5	20.0	36
14 x 55	16.5	20.0	55
16 x 18	20.5	24.0	18
16 x 27	20.5	24.0	27
16 x 36	20.5	24.0	36
16 x 55	20.5	24.0	55

Provox LaryTube (Standard)

Size	ID	OD	Length
8/ 27	9.5	12.0	27
8/ 36	9.5	12.0	36
8/ 55	9.5	12.0	55
9/ 27	10.5	13.5	27
9/ 36	10.5	13.5	36
9/ 55	10.5	13.5	55
10/ 27	12.0	15.0	27
10/ 36	12.0	15.0	36
10/ 55	12.0	15.0	55
12 27	13.5	17.0	27
12/ 36	13.5	17.0	36
12/ 55	13.5	17.0	55

Provox LaryTube Fenestrated

Size	ID	OD	Length
8/ 36	9.5	12.0	36
8/ 55	9.5	12.0	55
9/ 36	10.5	13.5	36
9/ 55	10.5	13.5	55
10/ 36	12.0	15.0	36
10/ 55	12.0	15.0	55
12/ 36	13.5	17.0	36
12/ 55	13.5	17.0	55

Provox LaryTube with Ring

Size	ID	OD	Length
8/ 36	9.5	12.0	36
8/ 55	9.5	12.0	55
9/ 36	10.5	13.5	36
9/ 55	10.5	13.5	55
10/ 36	12.0	15.0	36
10/ 55	12.0	15.0	55
12/ 36	13.5	17.0	36
12/ 55	13.5	17.0	55

TRACOE Twist Laryngecomy Tubes

Size	ID	OD	Length
5	5.0	9.0	47
6	6.0	9.4	50
7	7.0	10.6	52
8	8.0	11.6	55
9	9.0	12.8	57
10	10.0	14.2	60

TRACOE Comfort Laryngectomy Tube

Size	ID	OD	Length
7	7.0	10.5	50
8	8.0	11.3	53
9	9.0	12.6	57
10	10.0	13.7	60
11	11.0	15.0	63
12	12.0	16.2	66

Jackson Laryngectomy Tubes

Size	ID	OD	Length
00	2.4	4.5	33
0	2.8	5.0	38
1	3.0	5.5	44
2	3.4	6.0	51

Air-Lon Laryngectomy Tubes
(also with 15-mm connector, "Inhalation Set")

Size	ID	OD	Length
8	10.0	12.0	63
10	12.0	14.0	63

Martin Laryngectomy Tubes
(regular or with dressing extension)

Size	ID	OD	Length
8	9.0	12.0	42
10	11.0	14.0	42
12	12.7	16.3	42

Holinger Laryngectomy Tube

Size	ID	OD	Length
7	9.0	12.0	50
8	10.0	13.6	50
9	10.6	14.0	50
10	11.2	14.3	50

Appendix C: Tracheostomy Tube Sizes (Neonatal & Pediatric)

ID=inner diameter
Length=neck phalange to tip
OD=outer diameter
*All measurements are expressed in millimeters

Portex FlexTend Plus Neonatal

Size	ID	OD	Shaft Length	FlexTend Length
2.5	2.5	4.0	30	15
3.0	3.0	4.7	32	17
3.5	3.5	5.3	34	20
4.0	4.0	6.0	36	22

Portex FlexTend Plus Standard Pediatric

Size	ID	OD	Shaft Length	FlexTend Length
2.5	2.5	4.0	38	20
3.0	3.0	4.7	39	20
3.5	3.5	5.3	40	25
4.0	4.0	6.0	41	25
4.5	4.5	6.7	42	30
5.0	5.0	7.3	44	30
5.5	5.5	8.0	46	30

Portex FlexTend Plus Pediatric

Size	ID	OD	Shaft Length	FlexTend Length
3.5	3.5	5.3	40	38
4.0	4.0	6.0	44	40
4.5	4.5	6.7	48	43
5.0	5.0	7.3	50	45
5.5	5.5	8.0	52	48

Rüsch Biesalski

Size	ID	OD	Length
4.0	4.0	5.2	47
5.0	5.0	6.2	55
6.0	6.0	7.2	62.8

Rüsch Crystal Clear Plus

Size	ID	OD	Length
3.5	3.5	5.3	47
4.0	4.0	5.9	54
4.5	4.5	6.5	54
5.0	5.0	7.0	57
5.5	5.5	7.5	58
6	6.0	8.7	64

Rüsch Tracheoflex

Size	ID	OD	Length
3.0	3.0	5.0	45
4.0	4.0	6.0	55
5.0	5.0	7.0	59
6.0	6.0	8.4	64.4

Shiley Neonatal NEO

Size	ID	OD	Length
3.0	3.0	4.5	30
3.5	35.	5.2	32
4.0	4.0	5.9	34
4.5	4.5	6.5	36

Shiley Pediatric PED

Size	ID	OD	Length
3.0	3.0	4.5	39
3.5	3.5	5.2	40
4.0	4.0	5.9	41
4.5	4.5	6.5	42
5.0	5.0	7.1	44
5.5	5.5	7.7	46

Shiley Long Pediatric PDL

Size	ID	OD	Length
5.0	5.0	7.1	50
5.5	5.5	7.7	52
6.0	6.0	8.3	54
6.5	6.5	9.0	56

Shiley Cuffed Pediatric PDC

Size	ID	OD	Length
4.0	4.0	5.9	41
4.5	4.5	6.5	42
5.0	5.0	7.1	44
5.5	5.5	7.7	46

Shiley Cuffed Long Pediatric PLC

Size	ID	OD	Length
5.0	5.0	7.1	50
5.5	5.5	7.7	52
6.0	6.0	8.3	54
6.5	6.5	9.0	56

Bivona Uncuffed Neonatal

Size	ID	OD	Length
2.5	2.5	4.0	30
3.0	3.0	4.7	32
3.5	3.5	5.3	34
4.0	4.0	6.0	36

Bivona Uncuffed Pediatric

Size	ID	OD	Length
2.5	2.5	4.0	38
3.0	3.0	4.7	39
3.5	3.5	5.3	40
4.0	4.0	6.0	41
4.5	4.5	6.7	42
5.0	5.0	7.3	44
5.5	5.5	8.0	46

Bivona Uncuffed Neonatal FlexTend Plus

Size	ID	OD	Prox Length	Distal Length
2.5	2.5	4.0	15	39
3.0	3.0	4.7	17	32
3.5	3.5	5.3	20	34
4.0	4.0	6.0	22	36

Bivona Uncuffed Pediatric FlexTend Plus Extra Length

Size	ID	OD	Prox Length	Distal Length
3.5	3.5	5.3	38	40
4.0	4.0	6.0	40	44
4.5	4.5	6.7	43	48
5.0	5.0	7.3	45	50
5.5	5.5	8.0	48	52

Bivona TTS Cuffed Neonatal

Size	ID	OD	Length
2.5	2.5	4.0	30
3.0	3.0	4.7	32
3.5	3.5	5.3	34
4.0	4.0	6.0	36

Bivona TTS Cuffed Pediatric Tubes

Size	ID	OD	Length
2.5	2.5	4.0	38
3.0	3.0	4.7	39
3.5	3.5	5.3	40
4.0	4.0	6.0	41
4.5	4.5	6.7	42
5.0	5.0	7.3	44
5.5	5.5	8.0	46

Bivona Aire-Cuf Neonatal Trachs

Size	ID	OD	Length
2.5	2.5	4.0	30
3.0	3.0	4.7	32
3.5	3.5	5.3	34
4.0	4.0	6.0	36

Bivona Aire-Cuf Pediatric Trachs

Size	ID	OD	Length
2.5	2.5	4.0	38
3.0	3.0	4.7	39
3.5	3.5	5.3	40
4.0	4.0	6.0	41
4.5	4.5	6.7	42
5.0	5.0	7.3	44
5.5	5.5	8.0	46

Bivona Fome-Cuf Neonatal Trachs

Size	ID	OD	Length
2.5	2.5	4.0	30
3.0	3.0	4.7	32
3.5	3.5	5.3	34
4.0	4.0	6.0	36

Bivona Fome-Cuf Pediatric Trachs

Size	ID	OD	Length
2.5	2.5	4.0	38
3.0	3.0	4.7	39
3.5	3.5	5.3	40
4.0	4.0	6.0	41
4.5	4.5	6.7	42
5.0	5.0	7.3	44
5.5	5.5	8.0	46

Bivona Hyperflex, Adjustable-Neck, Uncuffed

Size	ID	OD	Length
2.5	2.5	4.0	55
3.0	3.0	4.7	60
3.5	3.5	5.3	65
4.0	4.0	6.0	70
4.5	4.5	6.7	75
5.0	5.0	7.3	80
5.5	5.5	8.0	85

TRACOE mini (Neonatal)

Size	ID	OD	Length
2.5	2.5	3.6	30
3.0	3.0	4.3	32
3.5	3.5	5.0	34
4.0	4.0	5.6	36

TRACOE mini (Pediatric)

Size	ID	OD	Length
2.5	2.5	3.6	32
3.0	3.0	4.3	36
3.5	3.5	5.0	40
4.0	4.0	5.6	44
4.5	4.5	6.3	48
5.0	5.0	7.0	50
5.5	5.5	7.6	55
6.0	6.0	8.4	62

Index

ID=inner diameter

Made in the USA
Monee, IL
05 November 2026

67806923R00240